Place, Health, and Diversity

Although health equity and diversity-focussed research has begun to gain momentum, there is still a paucity of research from health geographers that explicitly explores how geographic factors, such as place, space, scale, community, and location, inform multiple axes of difference. Such axes can include residential location, age, sex, gender, race/ethnicity, culture, religion, socio-economic status, marital status, sexual orientation, education level, and immigration status. Specifically focussing on Canada's rapidly changing society, which is becoming increasingly pluralized and diverse, this book examines the place-health-diversity intersection in this national context.

Health geographers are well positioned to offer a valuable contribution to diversity-focussed research because place is inextricably linked to differential experiences of health. For example, access to health care and health promoting services and resources is largely influenced by where one is physically and socially situated within the web of diversity. Furthermore, applying geographic concepts like place, in both the physical and social sense, allows researchers to explore multiple axes of difference simultaneously. Such geographic perspectives, as presented in this book, offer new insights into what makes diverse people, in diverse places, with access to diverse resources (un)healthy in different ways in Canada and beyond.

Melissa D. Giesbrecht is a Postdoctoral Fellow in the Centre on Aging at the University of Victoria, Canada.

Valorie A. Crooks is a health geographer and Associate Professor in the Department of Geography at Simon Fraser University, Canada.

Place, Health, and Diversity
Learning from the Canadian Experience

Edited by

Melissa D. Giesbrecht
University of Victoria, Canada

Valorie A. Crooks
Simon Fraser University, Canada

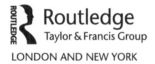

Routledge
Taylor & Francis Group

LONDON AND NEW YORK

First published 2016 by Routledge

2 Park Square, Milton Park, Abingdon, Oxfordshire OX14 4RN

52 Vanderbilt Avenue, New York, NY 10017

Routledge is an imprint of the Taylor & Francis Group, an informa business

First issued in paperback 2020

British Library Cataloguing in Publication Data
A catalogue record for this book is available from the British Library

Library of Congress Cataloguing in Publication Data
Giesbrecht, Melissa D.
Place, health, and diversity: learning from the Canadian experience /
by Melissa D. Giesbrecht and Valorie A. Crooks.
  pages cm. — (Geographies of Health Series)
Includes bibliographical references and index.
ISBN 978-1-4724-4502-5 (hardback: alk. paper) – ISBN 978-1-3156-0059-8 (ebook) –
ISBN 978-1-3170-8055-8 (epub)
1. Medical geography. 2. Medical policy–Canada. 3. Multiculturalism.
4. Health care reform–Canada. I. Crooks, Valorie A., 1976– II. Title.
RA791.G54 2015
614.4′271–dc23   2015018243

ISBN: 978-1-4724-4502-5 (hbk)
ISBN: 978-0-367-66832-7 (pbk)

Typeset in Times New Roman
by Out of House Publishing

Contents

List of Figures   vii
List of Tables   viii
List of Contributors   ix
Acknowledgments   xiv

1   **Place, Health, and Diversity in Canada**   1
    MELISSA D. GIESBRECHT, VALORIE A. CROOKS, AND
    JEFFREY MORGAN

2   **Frameworks, Lenses, and Tools: Approaches to Conducting**
    Diversity-based Health Geography Research   14
    MELISSA D. GIESBRECHT, VALORIE A. CROOKS, AND
    JEFFREY MORGAN

3   **From Embedded in Place to Marginalized Out and Back**
    Again: Indigenous Peoples' Experience of Health in Canada   29
    HEATHER CASTLEDEN, DEBBIE MARTIN, AND DIANA LEWIS

4   **Exploring the Intersections Between Violence, Place, and**
    Mental Health in the Lives of Trans and Gender
    Nonconforming People in Canada   53
    CINDY HOLMES

5   **"I'm a Better Person When I'm Working": Supportive**
    Workplaces, Mental Illness, and Recovery   76
    JOSHUA EVANS AND ROBERT WILTON

6   **Spaces and Places: Engaging a Mixed-methods Approach for**
    Exploring the Multiple Geographies of Pedestrian Injury   96
    JONATHAN CINNAMON AND DANIEL Z. SUI

7   **Countermapping Inner City "Deprivation" in Winnipeg, Canada**   119
    JEFFREY R. MASUDA AND EMILY SKINNER

8 **When Is Helping Hurting? Understanding and Challenging the (Re)production of Dominance in Narratives of Health, Place, and Difference in Hamilton, Ontario** 141
  MADELAINE C. CAHUAS, MANNAT MALIK, AND
  SARAH WAKEFIELD

9 **Constructing the Liberal Health Care Consumer Online: A Content Analysis of Canadian Medical Tourism and Harm Reduction Service Provider Websites** 163
  CRISTINA TEMENOS AND RORY JOHNSTON

10 **Lived Experience in Context: The Diverse Interplay between Women Living with Fibromyalgia and Canada's Health Care System** 183
  VALORIE A. CROOKS

11 **Aging, Gender, and "Triple Jeopardy" Through the Life Course** 200
  RACHEL V. HERRON AND MARK W. ROSENBERG

12 **Does the Compassionate Care Benefit Adequately Support Vietnamese Canadian Family Caregivers? A Diversity Analysis** 220
  IRENE D. LUM AND ALLISON M. WILLIAMS

13 **Conclusion: Ways Ahead in Diversity-based Health Geography Research** 238
  VALORIE A. CROOKS AND MELISSA D. GIESBRECHT

Index 243

Figures

6.1 Pedestrian injury hotspots in Vancouver, 2000–5   103
6.2 Injury hotspot mapping interface   109
6.3 Injury hotspots by type, Cape Town, based on the opinions of emergency medical services personnel   111
6.4 Screenshot of an interactive pedestrian injury story map   113
7.1 Distribution of socioeconomic status in the Winnipeg census metropolitan area   121
7.2 Deprivation map of Winnipeg with Core Area Initiative Boundary   128
8.1 Two professionals featured as experts: Fred Eisenberger and Mark Chamberlain   153
8.2 CT0050, the lowest rated of Hamilton's 130 census tracts, according to Code Red   153

Tables

5.1 Comparison of 2012 welfare income for a single person with disability with after-tax, low income cut-offs (LICO)   79

6.1 Qualitative and quantitative data about injury hotspots in Cape Town   110

7.1 Average values of census valuables by cluster type   129

9.1 The five domains of self-care deficit nursing theory   170

11.1 Demographic and socioeconomic characteristics of older women in Canada, 2008–9   211

11.2 Health, caregiving and care receiving by older women in Canada, 2008–9   213

Contributors

Madelaine C. Cahuas, MA is a doctoral candidate in the Department of Geography and Program in Planning at the University of Toronto, Canada, and was recently awarded a Social Sciences and Humanities Research Council (SSHRC) doctoral fellowship. Her research has examined how complex power relations are navigated when marginalized community members, non-profit organizations and local governments work together to address health inequities. Her doctoral research focuses on the challenges and opportunities that racialized migrant communities face when engaging in environmental health justice activism, both in and beyond the non-profit sector. She is committed to conducting collaborative and community-based research that supports the equity-focused goals of the community groups and organizations with which she is working.

Heather Castleden, PhD is a white settler scholar, health geographer and associate professor jointly appointed to the Departments of Geography and Public Health Sciences at Queen's University, Canada, where she holds a Canada Research Chair in Reconciling Relations for Health, Environments, and Communities. Her scholarship focuses on applying both Indigenous and Western approaches to social, environmental, and health inquiries. She is a recognized leader in community-based participatory Indigenous research, having been awarded the Julian Szeicz Award for significant achievement in 2010, and for her recent guest co-editing (with Monica Mulrennan and Anne Godlewska) of a special issue of *The Canadian Geographer* in 2012 in this area. She has published widely, is regularly sought for peer review, and serves on the advisory board for the Canadian Institutes of Health Research (CIHR) Institute of Aboriginal Peoples' Health.

Jonathan Cinnamon, PhD is a lecturer in human geography at the University of Exeter, UK. His PhD research on geographic injury surveillance and prevention was completed at Simon Fraser University, Canada in 2013. His research interests include injury prevention, health data ethics, health care accessibility, geographic information science, and critical geographic information systems.

Valorie A. Crooks, PhD is a health geographer and associate professor in the Department of Geography, Simon Fraser University, Canada. She is a scholar of the Michael Smith Foundation for Health Research, and holds the Canada Research Chair in Health Service Geographies. Her research examines health services, and currently she is focused on studying emerging global health care mobilities. She has co-edited (with Gavin J. Andrews) a book, *Primary Health Care: People, Practice, Place* (Ashgate, 2008), and recently co-edited (with Sharon-Dale Stone and Michelle K. Owen) a book entitled *Working Bodies: Chronic Illness in the Canadian Workplace* (McGill-Queens University Press, 2014).

Joshua Evans, PhD is an assistant professor in human geography in the Centre for Social Sciences, Athabasca University, Canada. His research interests include inner-city health, housing and homelessness, community care, and social policy. He has published research in peer-reviewed journals such as *Health & Place*, *Social & Cultural Geography*, *Progress in Human Geography*, *Social Science & Medicine*, and *Youth & Society*.

Melissa D. Giesbrecht, PhD is a research associate at Simon Fraser University and a postdoctoral fellow at the University of Victoria, Canada. She recently completed her Social Science and Humanities Research Council (SSHRC)-funded doctoral research in geography at Simon Fraser University. Her research interests include examining diversity within the context of formal and informal palliative caregiving. She has expertise in gender and sex-based analysis, intersectional frameworks, and diversity analysis. She has published in peer-reviewed journals such as *Social Science & Medicine*, *Nursing Inquiry*, and *International Journal for Equity in Health*. She is also co-author (with Olena Hankivsky, Daniel Grace, Gemma Hunting, Olivier Ferlatte, Natalie Clark, Alicia Fridkin, Sarah Rudum and Tarya Laviolette) of *An Intersectionality-based Policy Analysis Framework* (Institute for Intersectionality Research and Policy, 2012).

Rachel V. Herron, PhD is an assistant professor in the Department of Geography, Brandon University, Canada. Her current research examines the continuum of care for people with dementia and their partners in care in rural and small-town settings. Her broader research interests include rural health and aging, care and caregiving, the ethics of doing research with vulnerable populations, and gender and women's health.

Cindy Holmes, PhD is a Michael Smith Foundation for Health Research Postdoctoral Fellow in the Faculty of Health Sciences, Simon Fraser University, Canada, where she coordinates a participatory research project about the connections between safety, well-being, and place in the lives of transgender and gender nonconforming people. She is also a Postdoctoral Fellow with the National Collaborating Centre for Aboriginal Health at the University of Northern British Columbia, Canada. She is an interdisciplinary health scholar examining the intersections between violence, social inequity, health, and place. Her work reflects a commitment to social justice and health equity that is embedded in more than two decades' experience in community health and social work.

Rory Johnston, MA is a PhD candidate in the Department of Geography, Simon Fraser University, Canada. He is a health services researcher whose work focuses on better understanding the international connections between health systems. His work has been published in academic peer-reviewed journals such as *Social Science & Medicine, Globalization and Health*, and *International Journal for Equity in Health.*

Diana Lewis, PhD (ABD) is a Mi'kmaw woman from Nova Scotia and PhD candidate in the Department of Sociology and Social Anthropology, Dalhousie University, Canada. Her research focus uses quantitative, qualitative, and Indigenous methodologies to explore the environmental health of First Nation communities, specifically as these are impacted by resource or industrial development. She helps First Nation communities across Canada understand how resource development impacts their rights.

Irene D. Lum, BASc recently received her undergraduate degree in Honours Arts and Science from McMaster University, Canada. Currently she is continuing her studies at McMaster in the undergraduate medical program.

Mannat Malik, BASc is a Master's of Health Science candidate in the Department of Health, Behavior and Society, Johns Hopkins Bloomberg School of Public Health, USA. She completed an honours BASc degree from McMaster University, Canada. Her undergraduate thesis explored the relationship between the stigmatization of low-income neighborhoods and resident views on community cohesion and sense of place. Her research interests include neighborhood impacts on health, gendered experiences of health marginalization, and community-based health intervention. Her current studies focus broadly on the social determinants of health and illness and health disparities.

Debbie Martin, PhD is a health promotion researcher and assistant professor in the School of Health and Human Performance, Dalhousie University, Canada. Her research focuses on issues related to the health inequities experienced by Indigenous peoples. She is a member of NunatuKavut (southeastern Labrador Inuit). She embraces diverse Indigenous perspectives on health and well-being, and recognizes that much can be learned about social and environmental health inequities when Indigenous knowledge is positioned at the forefront of knowledge generation. She is the principal or co-principal investigator on a number of Indigenous community-based health-related studies, focusing on a range of issues that include oral health, food sovereignty, substance use, and community-based research ethics.

Jeffrey R. Masuda, PhD is an associate professor and Tier II Canada Research Chair in Environmental Health Equity at Queen's University, Canada. His ongoing work includes multi-site investigations of neighborhood-level health inequities in Canadian cities, critical knowledge translation pedagogies in environmental health, and the historical geographies of human rights, health, and place.

Jeffrey Morgan, BA, recently completed his undergraduate degree in geography and gender, sexuality, and women's studies at Simon Fraser University, Canada. His research interests include the intersections between gender and geography, health geography, and urban studies. Currently he is working on his Master's degree in health geography at Simon Fraser University, Canada.

Mark W. Rosenberg, PhD is a professor in the Departments of Geography and Public Health Sciences, Queen's University, Canada. He is also the Tier I Canada Research Chair in Development Studies. He is a past editor-in-chief of the *Canadian Journal on Aging*. He has spent more than 25 years carrying out research on various aspects of the older population of Canada, resulting in numerous publications in refereed journals, book chapters, and reports to all levels of government in Canada.

Emily Skinner, MA is Outreach Coordinator at the First Nations Technical Services Advisory Group in Edmonton, Alberta. She graduated from the geography program at the University of Manitoba, Canada. She partnered with the Graffiti Art Programming Aboriginal Youth Advisory Committee for her thesis project to research neighborhood-level health inequities from youth perspectives, using arts-based methods. She is a former managing director of the Health, Environment, and Communities Research Lab at Dalhousie University.

Daniel Z. Sui, PhD is a professor of geography and Distinguished Professor of Social and Behavioral Sciences at Ohio State University, USA. He also serves as Chair of Geography and Director of the Geographical Analysis Core, Institute of Population Research. His current research interests include geographic information science theory, open or alternative geographic information systems, spatial-temporal synergetics, volunteered geographic information, and crowdsourcing geographic knowledge production.

Cristina Temenos, PhD holds an Urban Studies Foundation Postdoctoral Fellowship at the University of Manchester, UK. She is a geographer interested in the intersection of public health, social policy, and cities, and in the ways that policy mobilities remake urban space. Her work has been published in academic peer-reviewed journals such as *Health and Place*, *Environment and Planning A*, *Geography Compass*, and in *The Routledge Handbook of Mobilities* (edited by Peter Adey, David Bissell, Kevin Hannam, Peter Merriman, and Mimi Sheller, Routledge, 2013).

Sarah Wakefield, PhD is an associate professor in the Department of Geography and Program in Planning, University of Toronto, Canada, where she is also the director of the health studies program. Her research has two main themes: food security policy and practice; and improving neighborhood health through participatory community development and community-based research. These areas are connected by an overarching interest in understanding how individuals and organizations work together to create just, healthy, and sustainable communities. She works closely with community organizations and health policy actors to enhance the relevance of her research.

Allison M. Williams, PhD is a professor in the School of Geography and Earth Sciences, McMaster University, Canada. She leads a research program in various sub-fields of social and health geography including caregiver-employees, quality of life, therapeutic landscapes and sense of place. She currently holds a CIHR research chair in gender, work and health, addressing caregiver-friendly workplaces.

Robert Wilton, PhD is a professor in the School of Geography and Earth Sciences, McMaster University, Canada. He is a social and health geographer with a primary interest in problems of social and spatial exclusion. His research has focused on understanding the experiences of people living with HIV/AIDS, disability, mental ill-health and, most recently, alcoholism and addiction.

Acknowledgments

We would be remiss in not acknowledging some very important contributions to this book. First, we are incredibly thankful to all the chapter authors who agreed to join us in this book project. Second, Jeffrey Morgan and Neville Li have greatly assisted us in formatting the manuscript and coordinating this effort. Finally, financial support for the preparation of this book has come directly and indirectly from Valorie Crooks' scholar award, from the Michael Smith Foundation for Health Research and Canada Research Chair in Health Service Geographies.

1 Place, Health, and Diversity in Canada

Melissa D. Giesbrecht, Valorie A. Crooks, and Jeffrey Morgan

"Diversity is the one true thing we all have in common" (*Anonymous*)

In recent years, use of the word "diversity" has grown tremendously in multiple contexts (Juanita Johnson-Bailey, 2008; Angelini, 2011). This word appears regularly in public media via magazines, advertising slogans, social networking sites, and television, as well as in the scholarly literature. Ideas surrounding the concept of diversity also have become the focus of many public events that aim to increase awareness and celebrate difference, such as pride parades and multicultural fairs. In addition, governmental initiatives and policies have begun embracing the term through various implementations such as the Canadian Multiculturalism Act, 1988, and the vast number of existing employment policies focused on enhancing diversity in the workplace. Despite the popularity of the term, there is no single agreed-upon definition of "diversity." Traditionally, and still today, diversity tends to be associated with culture: more specifically, the languages, values, rules, and beliefs that have been shared, learned, and transmitted throughout generations by specific groups (Hankivsky et al., 2009). In other cases, diversity is used in relation to tolerance and acceptance, eliciting ideas of inclusion or racial and gender differences. Others associate the word with issues of power and inequity, and therefore view it as conjuring affirmative measures designed to insure the representation of minority or marginalized groups. In academia, the term is increasingly ubiquitous.

Although conceptualizations vary widely, for researchers there is a general consensus regarding the significance of acknowledging time, place, and more specifically, context in relation to how diversity is understood, operationalized, and applied. As such, diversity can be seen as a broad lens through which researchers focus on the scale, place, and characteristics that are most relevant and meaningful to the issue, problem, population, or research question at hand. In keeping with this, the conceptualizations of diversity used by authors throughout this collection are diverse, yet collectively focused on the specific context of the research topic being explored; they also all broadly conceptualize diversity as being all the ways in which people and places are both at once unique and different from others (Alberta Health Services, 2011). Therefore, considering that this book is focused on exploring the intersection of diversity, health, and place, we conceptualize diversity as encompassing the multiple, fluid, and relational ways in which differences intersect to influence experiences of health, and the health outcomes of people and population groups in place (James, 2000; Alberta Health Services, 2011).

The Canadian Context

In this book, the focus of diversity is not solely on difference, but also on recognizing and identifying those commonalities shared among particular population groups, places, and contexts. For example, the contributing authors showcase a particular commonality: the contemporary Canadian context. As such, all the diversity-based studies in this collection are anchored geographically, allowing for the examination of those shared, yet unique, aspects of the Canadian landscape that shape diverse health experiences. In other words, the focus of each chapter is situated within this broad yet shared geographic, political, historical, cultural, economic, and social context. This is important to consider, as Canadians experience particular expressions of diversity that are shaped by the country's contexts (Angelini, 2011). It is this situated *place-in-the-world* that directs the way that Canadians live, including their understandings, views, and experiences of health, health care, and health outcomes (Kearns, 1993; Hankivsky and Christoffersen, 2008). At the same time, this situatedness is informed simultaneously by the multiple axes of difference that shape people's social and physical locations, which collectively make up a society's diversity. Thus, although the landscape of Canada shares broad national-level characteristics relative to the global scale, it is also inextricably diverse within its national borders. Today, the Canadian context continues to evolve, and as a result is becoming increasingly pluralized and diverse (Angelini, 2011).

Collectively, Canadians' everyday lived experiences are shaped by the physical geography in which they live. Canada is the world's second largest country, and due to its sheer vastness, it is painted with diverse landscapes and climates ranging from arctic and maritime to prairie and temperate rainforest. From east to west, Canada encompasses ten provinces, three territories, six time zones, and reaches the Atlantic, Pacific and Arctic Ocean coastlines. According to the 2011 census, Canada is becoming increasingly urbanized, with most of the country's 33 million inhabitants living in urban areas (Statistics Canada, 2011). However, more than 6.3 million Canadians live outside cities, throughout rural and remote regions (Statistics Canada, 2011). Together, all Canadians share the reality of living on lands that historically were home to a rich and diverse Indigenous people (as discussed in greater detail in Chapter 3): among them myriad bands and tribes, each with their own rich cultures, spiritual practices, and languages. Despite a direful recent history of colonialism, the Aboriginal population of First Nations, Inuit and Métis peoples remain an active part of Canada today. With the exception of Canada's Indigenous peoples, the remaining population shares a history of immigration at some point in time, and even today Canada continues to boast the highest percentage of foreign-born citizens out of all G8 nations (Evans, 2013). In 2014 alone, Canada welcomed more than 260,000 newcomers to the country, which has created a multicultural society of mixed languages, cultures, and religions (Immigration, Refugees and Citizenship Canada, 2016). Demographically similar to many other countries in the global North, currently the population of Canada is experiencing a rapid overall increase in age whereby, over the next two decades, close to one in four people in Canada will be aged 65 years or over (Statistics Canada, 2014). Importantly, these shared Canadian experiences, among many others not mentioned here, result in very unique and diverse experiences for Canadians at the provincial, regional, neighborhood, community, and individual levels – particularly in regard to experiences and understandings of health, health care needs, and access to such care.

Within Canada, eligibility for, access to, and availability of health care services are not universal; rather, they are largely dependent on where one lives (Williams and Kulig, 2012), a reality that is expanded upon in Chapter 10. This is because of the decentralized nature of the Canadian health care system, and the associated roles and responsibilities of various levels of government in regard to providing such care (Carstairs, 2005). Specifically, it is the individual provincial and territorial governments which have primary responsibility for the delivery of health care services as legislated by the Canada Health Act, 1984, while smaller regional authorities hold responsibility for administering these services. The Canada Health Act sets out the primary objective of Canadian health care policy as it relates to the provision of public services, which is "to protect, promote and restore the physical and mental well-being of residents of Canada and to facilitate reasonable access to health services without financial or other barriers" (Health Canada, 2010, n.p.). Through this Act, the federal government supports the publicly funded health care system through transfer payments to the provinces and territories, health policy creation that falls within its jurisdiction, and some other health care-related activities (Carstairs and MacDonald, 2011). The federal government also has a direct service delivery role for certain populations: First Nations on reserve and Inuit people, military members and veterans, refugee protection claimants, and inmates of federal penitentiaries (Carstairs and MacDonald, 2011). The federal government can provide leadership to the provinces through the creation of policy directives, and also administer health-related programs. Although the federal government plays a major role in the funding of health care in Canada, it is the provincial and territorial governments that are responsible for providing local leadership and setting the overall direction for the health systems that fall under their jurisdiction. For example, in the province of British Columbia, this involves the provincial government undertaking actions such as policy creation and enactment, legislative changes, and allocating funds to organizations and individuals who provide services. As such, the provincial government is responsible for legislative changes that are necessary to improve services that fall within the scope of the public health care system (British Columbia Ministry of Health, 2006).

In the remainder of this chapter we provide a broad overview of the concepts of health, place, and diversity from a Canadian perspective. We also review key developments in existing research focused on diversity and health, and discuss how health geographers are well positioned to address this knowledge gap regarding the interconnections of health, place, and diversity. We conclude by providing an overview of the book. Ultimately, this chapter emphasizes that in order to gain a more nuanced understanding of how health and/or health care is experienced in Canada and beyond, place must be considered in relation to the diverse social conditions and unique socioeconomic, political, cultural, and historical axes that shape people's lived realities.

Diversity and Health

From the international reach of the World Health Organization (WHO) to the micro-realm of local municipal governance, the consideration of diversity in prevailing institutional constructions of health transcends geographic scale, and represents a significant paradigm shift that is continuously evolving. Differing from the previous positivist and biomedical conceptions, health today is commonly understood as being much more than the mere absence of disease; instead, it is thought of as a complete state of social, physical, and mental well-being (World Health Organization, 2014). This framing increases the complexity of what it means to be healthy, or experience good or bad health outcomes, by emphasizing the social construction and subjective nature of health. As such, a diverse range of understandings of what constitutes health – from scales of the individual to particular population groups, regions, and beyond – have emerged in recent decades (Kearns and Collins, 2010).

In Canada, a social understanding of health was first advocated for in a national report written by Lalonde (1974), "A New Perspective on the Health of Canadians." In this report, Lalonde stated that:

> [T]he traditional view of equating the level of health in Canada with the availability of physicians and hospitals is inadequate ... there is little doubt that future improvements in the level of health of Canadians lie mainly in improving the environment, moderating self-imposed risks and adding to our knowledge of human biology. (1974, p. 18)

Here, Lalonde emphasized the critical role that physical and social environments (or determinants) play in shaping the health of Canadians, effectively calling for a diversity perspective to be employed (Coburn et al., 2003). Since this time, Canadian conceptions of health have continued to evolve, resulting in the development of frameworks that encompass diversity, particularly those social determinants that have been found to directly or indirectly shape health and health-related opportunities, choices, decisions, and outcomes (Public Health Agency of Canada, 2011). Such frameworks have since been adopted within Canada through, for example, the Public Health Agency of Canada's listing of the social determinants of health facing Canadians (discussed further in Chapter 2), as well as international health agencies such as the WHO.

Despite the common recognition that social and environmental factors play a critical role in shaping health, and acknowledging the role that diversity plays in health, no universal framework has been developed to encompass these diverse determinants. Instead, health agencies at various levels tend to prioritize differing social determinants, again emphasizing the critical role of context and the need to adapt such perspectives to the issues, questions, or population groups at hand. As the WHO states, "action on the social determinants of health should be adapted to the national and sub-national contexts of individual countries and regions to take into account different social, cultural and economic systems" (World Health Organization, 2011b, p. 2). Determinants of health frameworks can be focused and adapted even further to a specific target population group, community, or neighborhood, such as a specific immigrant group or residents in an isolated area (for example, see Dysart-Gale, 2010; Tindale et al., 2011; Greenwood and Leeuw, 2012). As such, developing a universal social determinant of health framework is not desirable, as such an approach would fail to take into consideration the inevitable nuances of any population-specific or place-specific health profile, thereby not reflecting a diversity approach to health.

Since its inception as an international health agency, the WHO has been a leader in acknowledging the diverse social impacts on health. In fact, in its 1948 charter there is a call for "collaboration with sectors such as agriculture, education, housing, and social welfare to achieve health gains" (World Health Organization, 2010, p. 10). The recognition that health is determined by such diverse and far-reaching factors gained further prominence with the WHO's Declaration of Alma-Ata on primary health care (World Health Organization, 1978), which asserted the significance of primary health care and health equity for ensuring the health of populations, and laid the foundations for the social determinants of health framework that would be adopted later. Finally, in 2005 the Commission on Social Determinants of Health was launched and its resulting report, "Closing the Gap in a Generation: Health Equity through Action on the Social Determinants of Health", was published (Commission on Social Determinants of Health, 2008). The WHO has effectively advocated for a diversity approach to health at the global level for the last several decades.

Collectively, key WHO reports emphasize that social factors, including education, employment status, income level, gender, and ethnicity have a marked influence on the health of every person. Furthermore, they stress that in all nations, including high, middle, and low-income, great disparities exist in the health statuses of different social groups. For example, the lower an individual's socioeconomic position, the higher their risk of poor health, regardless of their country's development status (World Health Organization, 2011a). It is in effect the unequal distribution of power and resources that are responsible for such health disparities or inequities, which are defined as "those systematic differences in the health status of different population groups" (World Health Organization, 2011a, n.p.). As such, addressing health inequities while acknowledging diversity is highly complex and seen as a shared responsibility, requiring the engagement of all sectors of government and society (World Health Organization, 2011b).

In the Canadian context, a particular population that faces disproportional health inequities are Aboriginal groups. Monette et al. (2011) examined differences in the determinants of health-related and housing-related characteristics between groups of Aboriginal and Caucasian adults living with HIV/AIDS in the Canadian province of Ontario. Using a quantitative approach, the authors found that compared to Caucasian participants, Aboriginal participants living with HIV/AIDS were more likely to be younger, female or transgender women, less educated, unemployed, and homeless or unstably housed (Monette et al., 2011). In addition, they were more likely to have low incomes and to have experienced housing-related discrimination (Monette et al., 2011). Richmond and Ross (2009) emphasize the significant link between environmental dispossession and adverse health effects for Aboriginal populations. Expanding beyond the proposed institutionalized social determinants of health put forward by the Public Health Agency of Canada (see Chapter 2), Richmond and Ross suggest the need to include six additional Aboriginal-specific social determinants of health:

1) balance;
2) life control;
3) education;
4) material resources;
5) social resources; and
6) environmental and cultural connections (Richmond and Ross, 2009).

They argue that because of the deep and profound connections between place, land, and Indigenous culture, a health geography perspective is particularly apt in addressing these place-based health profiles (Richmond and Ross, 2009). Although Aboriginal health is of concern to Canadian health policymakers, the inequities faced by this group are not unique to Canada and reflect the global marginalization of Indigenous populations (World Health Organization, 2007). To help restore Indigenous peoples' control over their lives and destinies, it is argued that reversing the colonization process (globally through locally) through self-determination is necessary (World Health Organization, 2007). Similarly, Canada's National Collaborating Center for Aboriginal Health identifies self-determination as the most important determinant of health among Aboriginal peoples (Reading and Wien, 2009). Such research demonstrates the importance of recognizing diversity and adapting social determinants of health to particular times, contexts, and peoples in order to illuminate the unique histories, experiences, and realities of particular population groups, such as the Aboriginal populations of Canada (and beyond).

Overall, the recognition that various axes of difference – such as residential location, age, sex, gender, "race" and ethnicity, culture, religion, socioeconomic status, marital status, sexual orientation, education level, and immigration status – simultaneously shape all health-related opportunities, experiences, and outcomes has become widely accepted, including by health geographers. However, although health equity and diversity-focused research has begun to gain momentum, there is still a paucity of research from health geographers that *explicitly* explores how geographic factors such as place, space, scale, community, and location inform the multiple axes of difference referred to above (see also Chapter 2). This very argument has been raised by Dunn et al. (2007) in the context of income inequality and population health, who state that despite a clear association between place, scale, and the social determinants of health, there is a peculiar dearth of geography in this academic literature. They contend that the absence of geographic research and approaches may be a product of epistemological tension between nomothetic and idiographic research approaches (Dunn et al., 2007). Undoubtedly, this tension also emerges beyond the domain of geographic research, but does present the common challenge of considering relational, subjective, and fluid diversity while still generating useful knowledge that can be meaningfully applied in health policy and practice.

Diversity, Health, and Place: A Health Geography Perspective

Fittingly, the discipline of health geography is broad, interdisciplinary, and inherently diverse (Luginaah, 2009; Kearns and Collins, 2010). This is the result of a continued evolution in both the epistemological underpinnings and philosophical understandings of what constitutes "health" and "place" – two cornerstone concepts upon which health geography is built. Contemporary health geography is rooted within the field of medical geography, which emerged in the early 1970s and held an explicit focus and interest in positivist pathologies and sites, and systems of care (Andrews, 2003). In 1993, a highly influential paper by Kearns titled "Place and health: Towards a reformed medical geography" called for the reformation of the discipline of medical geography to a more qualitative *health* geography that would include a greater emphasis on subjective experiences of place and a greater integration of social theory (Kearns, 1993). This publication resulted in a flurry of arguments, debates, and explanations; however, the end result has been a qualitative, cultural, and postmodern shift within the field and a renaming of the discipline to the current, more encompassing *health geography*, which emphasizes the multidimensional, constructed, fluid, dynamic and diverse experiential aspects of place, space, health, and well-being (Kearns and Collins, 2010).

Contemporary geographies of health consider place as central to the study of health, and increasingly draw from disciplinary fields from outside geography such as medical health sciences, epidemiology, and various social sciences such as sociology and anthropology, which emphasize the application of cultural theory as well as more critical perspectives. Today, health geographers commonly perceive place as an "operational and living construct which matters, as opposed to being a passive container in which things are simply recorded" (Kearns and Collins, 2010, p. 17). Thus, place must be understood as dynamic, fluid, multidimensional, contestable, and importantly, as holding *different meanings* to *different individuals and social groups* (Andrews, 2003). This description signifies that place is doubly constructed: built physically but socially interpreted, narrated, perceived, felt, understood, and imagined (Easthope, 2004). Building upon this definition, place in the physical sense also can be understood as a material artefact, a literal location, and a setting for social relations; while the social dimensions of place include the meanings that people attribute to places, the ways that they engage in place-making activities or place-specific behaviors, how they understand their place in the social hierarchies, how they develop a sense of place, and how they create emotional attachments to places (Castleden et al., 2010). Although places hold significant meanings for people, a person's history and experiences will influence his/her perceptions and experience of places, while at the same time places will affect that same person's opportunities and activities (Easthope, 2004). Therefore, places are linked together complexly in unequal ways through social relations of power (Easthope, 2004). Places are shaped also by context, as is diversity.

Reflecting the spectrum of health geographic inquiry, research in the discipline is broad and methodologically diverse (Kearns and Collins, 2010). Especially within Canada, the field of health geography encompasses diverse scholars who, arguably, have been at the cutting edge of exploring and documenting place and its complex relationship to health (Luginaah, 2009; Williams and Kulig, 2012; Giesbrecht et al., 2013). Considering this, health geographers are well positioned to offer a valuable contribution to diversity-focused health research, particularly because of their firm disciplinary base in understanding place and its link to differential experiences of health (Kearns, 1993; Moss, 1997; Dolan and Thien, 2008).

A core area of exploration for health geographers is access to health care and health-promoting services and resources, which are largely influenced by where one is physically and socially situated within the web of diversity (French et al., 2006; Hwang et al., 2010; Maddison et al., 2011). Some individuals and/or population groups are subjected to systematic discrimination based on axes such as "race," religion, ethnicity, or language, which renders service provision as inequitable (Hankivsky et al., 2011). By applying geographic concepts such as place in both the physical and social sense, researchers are able to explore multiple axes of difference and oppression simultaneously, which can inform policymaking and practice that account for issues of diversity while acknowledging inequity. Such geographic perspectives have the potential to offer new insights into what makes diverse people, in diverse places, with access to diverse resources healthy or unhealthy in different ways (Abelson and Giacomini, 2003).

Overview of this Volume

Although place, health, and diversity have been explored in numerous ways by various researchers, a paucity of research still exists by health geographers who *simultaneously* acknowledge and investigate these complex concepts in differing Canadian contexts. As such, this volume offers a unique glimpse of the ways in which place, health, and diversity are inextricably linked within the Canadian landscape. At the same time, its chapters provide readers with examples of the various approaches and methods that can be used by others wishing to explore similar themes in their own research domains. By focusing on the place–health–diversity intersection in the Canadian context, this book provides a uniquely Canadian perspective on diversity and health that is transferable to other contexts. Also, as Canadian scholars are leaders in the field of health geography, a geographic focus on Canada is fitting in order to learn of geographers' unique perspectives when exploring place–health–diversity intersections.

In Chapter 2, an introduction to some commonly employed methods and frameworks used by health researchers to conduct diversity-based analyses is provided. The following ten chapters provide examples of such analyses from various contemporary Canadian health geographers. In each chapter, the authors examine no fewer than two intersecting axes of difference relevant to their specific area of health geography inquiry, while explicitly situating their discussion in the relevant Canadian context. Collectively, these ten chapters offer multiple perspectives on diversity within a variety of contemporary health geography research domains.

In Chapter 3, Castleden, Martin, and Lewis look to Canada's Aboriginal population, which is often thought of as a single homogenous group, and explore why acknowledging diversity is critical to making sense of the health disparities that can be found across and within Indigenous populations in Canada today. Also looking at health disparities, in Chapter 4, Holmes examines the links between mental health, violence, and place in the lives of transgender and gender nonconforming people. In this chapter, Holmes emphasizes the need to acknowledge gender diversity, while also highlighting the diverse lived experiences of Canada's transgender, gender nonconforming, and Two-Spirit populations. Continuing this focus on mental health, in Chapter 5, Evans and Wilton explore the relationship between poverty and mental illness and examine the role of employment in the recovery process. More specifically, they examine issues of social class, employment status, and psychiatric disability within the diverse context of Canadian workplaces.

Chapters 6, 7, and 8 collectively emphasize the benefits of employing mixed- and multi-methods approaches in diversity-based health geography research. In Chapter 6, Cinnamon and Sui state that it is by combining spatial analysis and qualitative data that specific locations and population groups disproportionately at risk of pedestrian injury in Canada and elsewhere can be identified and targeted for prevention purposes. In Chapter 7, Masuda and Skinner examine deprivation mapping and find that when this technique is applied in a traditional way, it can undermine its equity-based goals unless qualitative participatory methods are employed simultaneously in order to provide contextual narratives. Building on the limits of deprivation mapping, in Chapter 8 Cahuas, Malik, and Wakefield contend that in fact, efforts to document geographic disparities in health can work to further marginalize and stigmatize particular people and places. Here, the authors conduct a content analysis of media reporting and qualitative interviews to provide a case study on how underlying, often unconscious, narratives of dominance are reproduced in the Canadian media and reports on health inequities.

Chapters 9, 10, 11, and 12 examine various issues regarding health care and services, and their implications for health in Canada. In Chapter 9, Temenos and Johnston seek to understand better the ways in which Canadian private service providers of medical tourism and harm reduction – two very different health practices with two very different patient groups – each mobilize liberal concepts in online promotional materials in an effort to present themselves as relevant and legitimate options to their potential users. In Chapter 10, Crooks qualitatively explores how the structure and organization of Canada's health care system shapes the experiences of chronically-ill women managing fibromyalgia syndrome. More specifically, she shows how factors as diverse as access to care, social location, and the body shape, mediate and guide their experiences and decisions regarding health care. In Chapter 11, Herron and Rosenberg explore the differences that affect Canada's oldest women, particularly in relation to the provision and receipt of care. Here, they conduct a descriptive statistical analysis of the Canadian Community Health Survey and in so doing, emphasize the value of pursuing intersectionality from a quantitative perspective. Finally, in Chapter 12, Lum and Williams examine informal family caregiving within the Vietnamese Canadian community, and investigate the specific axes of diversity that exist among this population which shape diverse caregiving experiences.

Collectively, the contributed chapters (3 to 12) provide multiple examples of how various methods and frameworks can be employed to explore diversity within various health geography domains. We believe that they provide important lessons for conducting diversity-focused health geography research within Canada and beyond. In Chapter 13 we conclude the book by tying together the various ways that diversity has been understood and operationalized within the ten contributed chapters, emphasizing what was gained by employing a diversity-based analysis in each of these contexts. We also discuss the lessons learned from these chapters by specifically examining the Canadian experience and context. Lastly, we identify areas for future research, so that other health geographers can pick up where this book leaves off.

References

Abelson, J. and Giacomini, M., 2003. Appendix: What is health policy analysis? CHEPA working paper. Hamilton, ON: McMaster University.

Alberta Health Services, 2011. Towards an understanding of health equity: Annotated bibliography. Available online at www.albertahealthservices.ca/poph/hi-poph-surv-shsa-tpgwg-annotated-glossary.pdf (accessed January 28, 2016).

Andrews, G.J., 2003. Locating a geography of nursing: Space, place and the progress of geographical thought. *Nursing Philosophy*, 4(3), pp. 231–48.

Angelini, P. ed., 2011. *Our society: Human diversity in Canada*. Toronto: Nelson Education Ltd.

British Columbia Ministry of Health, 2006. *A provincial framework for end-of-life-care*. Victoria: Ministry of Health.

British Columbia Ministry of Health, 2013. *BC Palliative Care Benefits Program: Information for prescribed*. Available online at www2.gov.bc.ca/gov/content/health/practitioner-professional-resources/pharmacare/prescribers/plan-p-bc-palliative-care-benefits-program (accessed January 28, 2016).

Carstairs, S., 2005. *Still not there. Quality end-of-life care: A progress report*. Available online at http://www.chpca.net/media/7883/Still_Not_There_June_2005.pdf (accessed January 28, 2016).

Carstairs, S. and Macdonald, M.L., 2011. The PRISMA Symposium 2: Lessons from beyond Europe. Reflections on the evolution of palliative care research and policy in Canada. *Journal of Pain and Symptom Management*, 42(4), pp. 501–4.

Castleden, H., Crooks, V.A., Schuurman, N. and Hanlon, N., 2010. "It's not necessarily the distance on the map...": Using place as an analytic tool to elucidate geographic issues central to rural palliative care. *Health & Place*, 16(2), pp. 284–90.

Coburn, D., Denny, K., Mykhalovskiy, E., Mcdonough, P., Robertson, A. and Love, R., 2003. Population health in Canada: A brief critique. *American Journal of Public Health*, 93(3), pp. 392–6.

Commission on Social Determinants of Health, 2008. *Closing the gap in a generation: Health equity through action on the social determinants of health*. Geneva: World Health Organization.

Dolan, H. and Thien, D., 2008. Relations of care: A framework for placing women and health in rural communities. *Canadian Journal of Public Health–Revue Canadienne de Sante Publique*, 99(supp. 2), pp. S38–42.

Dunn, J.R., Schaub, P. and Ross, N.A., 2007. Unpacking income inequality and population health. *Canadian Journal of Public Health–Revue Canadienne de Sante Publique*, 98(supp. 1), pp. S10–17.

Dysart-Gale, D., 2010. Social justice and social determinants of health: Lesbian, gay, bisexual, transgendered, intersexed, and queer youth in Canada. *Journal of Child and Adolescent Psychiatric Nursing*, 23(1), pp. 23–8.

Easthope, H., 2004. A place called home. *Housing, Theory and Society*, 21(3), pp. 128–38.

Evans, L., 2013. *Diversity in Canada: An overview.* Available online at http://canadian immigrant.ca/guides/moving-to-canada/diversity-in-canada-an-overview (accessed February 17, 2015).

French, J., McGahan, C., Duncan, G. Lengoc, S. Soo, J. and Cannon, J. 2006. How gender, age, and geography influence the utilization of radiation therapy in the management of malignant melanoma. *International Journal of Radiation Oncology*, 66(4), pp. 1056–63.

Giesbrecht, M., Cinnamon, J., Fritz, C. and Johnston, R., 2013. Themes in geographies of health and health care research: Reflections from the 2012 Canadian Association of Geographers annual meeting. *The Canadian Geographer*, 58(2), pp. 160–7.

Greenwood, M.L. and Leeuw, S.N.D., 2012. Social determinants of health and the future well-being of Aboriginal children in Canada. *Les déterminants sociaux de la santé et le futur bien-être des enfants autochtones au Canada*, 17(7), pp. 381–4.

Hankivsky, O. and Christoffersen, A. 2008. Intersectionality and the determinants of health: A Canadian perspective. *Critical Public Health*, 18(3), pp. 271–83.

Hankivsky, O., Cormier, R. and De Merich, D., 2009. *Intersectionality: Moving women's health research and policy forward.* Vancouver: Women's Health Research Network.

Hankivsky, O., De Leeuw, S., Lee, J.A., Vissandjée, B. and Khanlou, N. eds., 2011. *Health inequities in Canada: Intersectional frameworks and practices,* Vancouver: UBC Press.

Health Canada, 2010. *Canada Health Act.* Available online at www.hc-sc.gc.ca/hcs-sss/medi-assur/cha-lcs/index-eng.php (accessed February 25, 2015).

Hwang, S.W., Ueng. J.M. and Chiu, S. 2010. Universal health insurance and health care acess for homeless persons. *American Journal of Public Health*, 100, pp. 1454–61.

Immigration, Refugees, and Citizenship Canada, 2016. Facts and figures – Immigration overview: Permanent residents. Available online at: www.cic.gc.ca/english/resources/statistics/facts2014/permanent/index.asp (accessed January 28, 2016).

James, C.E., 2000. *Experiencing difference.* Halifax: Fernwood Publishing.

Juanita Johnson-Bailey, N.M.R., 2008. Diversity issues. In: L. Given, ed. *The SAGE encyclopedia of qualitative research methods.* Thousand Oaks, CA: Sage Publications, pp. 226–30.

Kearns, R.A., 1993. Place and health: Towards a reformed medical geography. *Professional Geographer*, 45(2), pp. 139–47.

Kearns, R. and Collins, D., 2010. Health geography. In: T. Brown, S. Mclafferty and G. Moon, eds. *A companion to health and medical geography.* Chichester: Blackwell. pp. 13–32.

Lalonde, M., 1974. *A new perspective on the health of Canadians: A working document.* Ottawa: Government of Canada.

Luginaah, I., 2009. Health geography in Canada: Where are we headed? *The Canadian Geographer*, 53(1), pp. 91–9.

Maddison, A.R., Asada, Y. and Urquhart, R., 2011. Inequity in access to cancer care: A review of the Canadian literature. *Cancer Causes & Control*, 22(3), pp. 359–66.

Monette, L.E., Rourke, S.B., Gibson, K., Tsegaye, M.B., Ruthann, T., Greene, S., Sobota, M., Koornstra, J., Byers, S., Amrita, A., Dunn, J.R., Guenter, D., Hambly, K. and Bhuiyan, S., 2011. Inequalities in determinants of health among Aboriginal and Caucasian persons living with HIV/AIDS in Ontario: Results from the Positive

Spaces, Healthy Places study. *Canadian Journal of Public Health–Revue Canadienne De Sante Publique*, 102(3), pp. 215–19.

Moss, P., 1997. Negotiating spaces in home environments: Older women living with arthritis. *Social Science & Medicine*, 45(1), pp. 23–33.

Public Health Agency of Canada, 2011. *What determines health?* Available online at www.phac-aspc.gc.ca/ph-sp/determinants/index-eng.php (accessed June 9, 2014).

Reading, C.L. and Wien, F., 2009. *Health inequalities and social determinants of Aboriginal peoples' health.* Prince George: National Collaborating Centre for Aboriginal Health.

Richmond, C.A. and Ross, N.A., 2009. The determinants of First Nation and Inuit health: A critical population health approach. *Health Place*, 15(2), pp. 403–11.

Statistics Canada, 2011. *Population, urban and rural, by province and territory.* Available online at www.statcan.gc.ca/tables-tableaux/sum-som/l01/cst01/demo62a-eng.htm (accessed February 25, 2015).

Statistics Canada, 2014. *Population projections: Canada, the provinces and territories, 2013 to 2063.* Available online at www.statcan.gc.ca/daily-quotidien/140917/dq140917a-eng.htm (accessed February 25, 2015).

Tindale, J., Denton, M., Ploeg, J., Lillie, J., Hutchison, B., Brazil, K., Akhtar-Danesh, N. and Plenderleith, J., 2011. Social determinants of older adults' awareness of community support services in Hamilton, Ontario. *Health & Social Care in the Community*, 19(6), pp. 661–72.

Williams, A. and Kulig, J.C., 2012. Health and place in rural Canada. In: J.C. Kulig and A. Williams, eds. *Health in rural Canada.* Vancouver: UBC Press, pp. 1–22.

World Health Organization, 1978. *Declaration of Alma-Ata.* Geneva: World Health Organization.

World Health Organization, 2007. *Social determinants and Indigenous health: The international experience and its policy implications.* Geneva: World Health Organization.

World Health Organization, 2010. *A conceptual framework for action on the social determinants of health,* Social determinants of health discussion paper 2. Geneva: World Health Organization.

World Health Organization, 2011a. *10 facts on health inequities and their causes.* Available online at www.who.int/features/factfiles/health_inequities/en/ (accessed June 21, 2011).

World Health Organization, 2011b. *Rio political declaration on social determinants of health.* Geneva: World Health Organization.

World Health Organization. 2014. *Social determinants of health.* Available online at www.who.int/social_determinants/en/ (accessed June 9, 2014).

2 Frameworks, Lenses, and Tools

Approaches to Conducting Diversity-based Health Geography Research

Melissa D. Giesbrecht, Valorie A. Crooks, and Jeffrey Morgan

The traditional emphasis for social science research to focus on a single category of identity, or a small number of dominant expressions of identity, has been the subject of growing scrutiny among experts (Hankivsky and Christoffersen, 2008; Juanita Johnson-Bailey, 2008). While often it is simpler for researchers to categorize people into single or separate population groups, according to Wilkinson, "[i]t has become increasingly apparent ... that this way of doing research is rather limited in its ability to accurately represent the complexity of social life" (2003, p. 27). In terms of policy and practice, government services that target only one category of identity cannot be considered inclusive (Hankivsky and Cormier, 2010). For example, even though gender is important, if it is the only axis of difference considered then the full scope of the social, political, and economic determinants of health that shape people's lives will not be fully captured; neither will adequate solutions to existing health disparities be found. In this chapter we will present an overview of some existing frameworks, lenses, and tools that can be (and sometimes already have been) employed by health geographers to acknowledge diversity among target population groups in their research. More specifically, we provide overviews of gender and sex-based analysis, social determinants of health and health equity impact assessment approaches, as well as intersectionality – all of which are commonly employed diversity frameworks in health research. We begin with a brief introduction to diversity-based health research.

Diversity-based Research

Health geography is inherently interdisciplinary in nature. It is this very characteristic that places health geographers in an excellent position to apply frameworks, lenses, approaches, and methods that are conducive to understanding the spatial aspects of everyday lives and experiences of diverse population groups in relation to health. The most general approach to exploring differentials within health research falls under the broad umbrella of what can be called "diversity-based analyses." This approach to analysis is not tied to particular theoretical paradigms or methods, but aims simply to explore and uncover differences between or within population groups. Here, diversity is used as a term to define all the ways in which people are unique and different from others (Alberta Health Services, 2011). Such analyses can take place at various scales, from examining individual narratives in order to explore in-depth how diverse social locations influence a particular person's experiences, to investigating how diverse processes and structures of power influence the health experiences and outcomes of particular population groups. Generally, many of these analyses aim to uncover differentials among or within particular population groups who self-identify their membership based on a collective experience: such as those who belong to a particular socioeconomic status, culture, gender, or groups identified by sexual orientation (Women in Employment Committee, 2003).

Broadly speaking, diversity-based analyses not only provide an understanding of how social (and spatial) patterns interact and have an impact on an individual's health, but also often emphasize (directly or indirectly) issues of inequity by generating critical knowledge about how differences continually affect people's opportunities, choices, decisions, and health outcomes. In other words, diversity-based analyses aim to probe deeply into issues in order to understand better the complex relationships and outcomes shaped by differing experiences of socioeconomic, cultural, sex, gender, historical, racial, and geographic lived positions, among others (Women in Employment Committee, 2003). This differs greatly from more traditional approaches to social science research, which tend to focus on and prioritize singular categories of difference such as gender, which assume that all population groups are homogenous. This traditional approach has become increasingly criticized in recent years: for example, black, Indigenous, and Chicana feminists all have highlighted that women differ from men greatly in their experiences of oppression, "race," and cultural realities (Crenshaw, 1994; Hankivsky, 2005; Juanita Johnson-Bailey, 2008). Diversity-based research, which considers multiple categories of difference simultaneously, has emerged over the last ten years as a promising step forward in capturing the complexity of lived realities and experiences (Juanita Johnson-Bailey, 2008). It has been argued that diversity-based research approaches can lead to findings that ultimately help to inform more effective health and health-related care, support, programs, and policies.

Regardless of the type of research, whether qualitative, quantitative, or spatial, researchers are guided by their own beliefs about what constitutes knowledge within a particular subject area. This epistemological stance informs the work of all researchers – particularly the theoretical perspective taken in generating research questions, developing research design, and the approaches taken to conduct such research. For example, qualitative diversity-based researchers often employ a variety of theoretical perspectives such as critical, feminist, postcolonial feminist, and postmodern, which commonly emphasize relativity and the shifting and changing nature of reality and identities (Juanita Johnson-Bailey, 2008). Quantitative researchers using diversity-based approaches may or may not apply such theoretical perspectives, but generally will employ population-level spatial and/or determinants of health perspectives in their work that enable them to examine differences, as well as address power and social justice (Hankivsky and Christoffersen, 2008). Some argue that in order for diversity to be truly captured in research, mixed-method approaches are required. This is because such approaches can integrate simultaneously the macro-scale quantitative and/or spatial data with that of more micro-scale contextual and grounded qualitative data (Hankivsky et al., 2011). Clearly, the knowledge garnered from diversity-based research will become only further enriched by the diversity of perspectives and epistemological approaches taken by interdisciplinary researchers.

One common thread uniting the range of approaches and theoretical positions undertaken by qualitative and quantitative researchers using diversity-based approaches is the understanding that diverse lived experiences, or social and physical locations, have multiple impacts on one's health and health outcomes (Hankivsky, 2012). There is also the common belief that knowledge generated from diversity-based analyses has the potential to inform more effective health and health service programs and initiatives. With differential experiences being revealed, findings also will be more conducive to achieving equity through policy, programs, and support. Currently, many health-related policies and programs in Canada and elsewhere are characterized by a "one-size-fits-all" approach, which attempts to achieve equality by treating a greatly heterogeneous population as all the same (Women in Employment Committee, 2003; Hankivsky and Cormier, 2010). Those who advocate for diversity-based approaches to research contend that if decision-makers continue to ignore the lived complexity of people's lives, the evidence base that is generated will only reify inequities (Hankivsky and Cormier, 2010). It is through recognizing and acknowledging diversity via research-based evidence that health care, social support, programs, and policies can be responsive to the *real needs* of citizens – which, ultimately, can lead to more equitable health and health outcomes.

In the following sections we examine three broad examples of approaches to undertaking diversity-based analysis, specifically: gender and sex-based analysis, social determinants of health and health equity impact assessments, and intersectionality. These are examples of approaches available to health geographers to unpack the complex roles that diversity plays in mediating the health–place relationship.

Gender and Sex-based Analysis

Gender and sex-based analysis (GSBA) is one of the first diversity-based approaches that emerged: it is considered to be at the heart of feminist health research (Grant, 2008; Greaves, 2012; DAWN-RAFH, 2014). This method of analysis can be thought of as a systematic approach to health research and policy formation that inquires about biological (sex-based) and sociocultural (gender-based) differences between women and men, and boys and girls (Health Canada, 2003; Hankivsky et al., 2009; Johnson et al., 2009; Greaves, 2012). It challenges the assumption that women and men are affected in the same way by research, policies, programs, and/or the causes and effects of health issues and health care delivery (Health Canada, 2003). Sex refers to the biological characteristics such as anatomy (for example, body size and shape) and physiology (for example, hormonal activity or functioning of organs), that distinguish males and females (Health Canada, 2003). Gender refers to the array of socially constructed roles, attitudes, personality traits, behaviors, values, and relative power and influence that society ascribes to two sexes on a differential basis (Health Canada, 2003). By considering both sex and gender, GSBA acts as a tool for understanding and accounting for biological and social processes of health, allowing for responses that embrace more equitable options (Disabled Women's Network Ontario, 2014).

Various forms of gender-based, sex-based, or gender and sex-based analysis have become the most common approach for identifying and responding to health-based diversity in Canada (Hankivsky et al., 2009). This approach has gained much currency in recent years among researchers, as well as within government and policy circles, becoming the most widely recognized and applied approach used today by both quantitative and qualitative health researchers to uncover "difference" (Hankivsky et al., 2009; Disabled Women's Network Ontario, 2014). For example, Status of Women Canada, a federal government organization, reinforces the government's commitment to strengthen the use of gender-based analysis as a key tool for developing public policy and informing decision-making (Status of Women Canada, 2014a). Furthermore, the Canadian Institutes of Health Research (CIHR), Canada's main health research funding agency, now requires all grant applicants to submit a statement outlining how they will account for gender and sex in their research, when appropriate (Canadian Institutes of Health Research, 2014). The widespread recognition of differences in health experiences and outcomes between men and women that has been brought about by the popularity of GSBA is a promising step forward in recognizing diversity in health research.

Recently, traditional applications of GSBA have received much criticism from an increasing number of experts, as such research still tends to assume that all men and women belong to one of these two sex-gender groupings – thereby reinforcing this binary and focusing on equality rather that moving the agenda forward to a focus on equity (Johnson et al., 2009; Greaves, 2012; Hankivsky et al., 2012; Status of Women Canada, 2014a). Moreover, GSBA research approaches have been strongly focused on the needs and experiences of women, particularly white women, which is another emerging critique. Further, it is believed that understandings of "sex" or "gender" differences within GSBA-based research ultimately call for stratification and disaggregation, which leads simply to comparing men and women or males and females (Johnson et al., 2009; Greaves, 2012). Consequently, GSBA approaches are not designed to insure that the differences between different groups of women and men are examined, or that different types of population groups are interrogated (Crenshaw, 1994; Juanita Johnson-Bailey, 2008; Waldegrave, 2009; Hankivsky et al., 2012).

Recent applications of GSBA stress using critical thinking to avoid the limitations of such approaches: for example, by considering sex and gender as *relational* issues that are context-specific and evolve across space and time (Greaves, 2012). However, this recognition certainly adds complexity to the research process, as our understanding of the concepts "sex" and "gender" continuously evolve. Today, sex and gender are recognized as concepts that are "tightly interrelated, exist on a continua, and simultaneously interact iteratively with each other" (Greaves, 2012, p. 4). In addition, recent applications of GSBA emphasize that such approaches always should be undertaken in the context of *diversity*, whereby it is recognized that the differences between men and women are influenced by a variety of factors, including class, socioeconomic status, age, sexual orientation, gender identity, "race," ethnicity, geographic location, education, and physical and mental ability (Health Canada, 2003). Clow et al. (2009) explain that:

> From its roots as a white, middle-class urban women's movement, based largely in North America and Europe, sex and gender-based analysis has become more inclusive and expansive, embracing both the analysis of diversity and an understanding of global perspectives on the health and well-being of women and girls as well as for men and boys. (p. 158)

By embracing diversity, GSBA recently has undergone a renaming and is now known in some circles as "GSBA(+)," the plus sign highlighting that the approach goes beyond gender to include an examination of a range of other intersecting identity factors (Status of Women Canada, 2014b). A common example of this approach has been applied in anti-smoking campaigns, where GSBA+ encourages consideration of gender differences, whereby young women and men cite different reasons for smoking – for example, girls cite curiosity, making friends, and fitting in, while boys cite pleasure, looking tough, and being independent – in addition to other aspects of smokers' social locations, such as levels of education, that combine to inform smoking behavior (Status of Women Canada, 2014b). Therefore, it is the combination of these and other factors, along with gender, that are important for designing and implementing anti-smoking campaigns (Status of Women Canada, 2014b), which is in keeping with a GSBA(+) approach.

Health geographers have much to offer through using GSBA(+) approaches, because some existing place-based health research has been found to emphasize this complex link between sex, gender and diversity. For example, it is now well-known that cardiovascular disease tends to appear about ten years later in women than in men due to biological, sex-based differences, including the protective effect of women's higher levels of estrogen before menopause

(Health Canada, 2003). However, when non-biological factors are considered, it becomes apparent that there are social differences in gender-related risk factors, such as smoking, depression, low income, obesity and lack of physical activity (Health Canada, 2003), which carry spatial implications for implementing targeted public health initiatives. Setia et al. (2011) applied GBA+ to illuminate sex and gender differences, among various other social factors, in the healthy immigrant effect – another prominently geographic process. Setia et al. (2011) found that country of origin played a role in the ethnic differential between women and men's self-rated health statuses and had independent negative effects, particularly among women. As such, women from "less developed" countries appear to be at greater risk of poor self-rated health, which holds great implications for public health programs aimed at assisting new immigrants in Canada (Setia et al., 2011).

Wiles (2002) considered the gendered implications of health care reform in New Zealand, emphasizing a fluid conceptualization of women's health whereby emphasis is placed on the gendered social context of women's lives. More specifically, Wiles (2002) recognizes that individual women have different, even contradictory, health care issues and needs that will vary according to their differing roles, identities, contexts, and access to resources. This conception of gender is applied to explore situated ideas about place and identity in relation to access to health care services in New Zealand's restructured health care system (Wiles, 2002). Clearly, there is great potential for health geographers to contribute further to GSBA(+) research, particularly by applying their specialized knowledge of space and place, and how such dimensions shape the health experiences and outcomes of diverse men and women, and boys and girls.

Social Determinants of Health Frameworks and Health Equity Impact Assessments

As mentioned in the previous section, understandings of gender and sex in regard to health have evolved considerably in recent years, notably in response to the social determinants of health (SDOH) approach (Greaves, 2012). SDOH approaches differ from GSBA and GSBA+ as primacy is not given to one category of identity – notably, sex and/or gender – in the research or policymaking process. Rather, SDOH approaches encourage the examination of multiple factors which potentially can result in differentials in health and health outcomes among diverse population groups.

The World Health Organization (WHO) defines SDOH as the diverse "conditions in which people are born, grow, live, work and age" that shape one's health and health outcomes (World Health Organization, 2014). The SDOH perspective recognizes that these determinants are dynamic, fluid, interrelated, and continuously evolving across space and time (Pederson et al., 2007; Hankivsky and Christoffersen, 2008). Since the emergence of this approach, which is said to have been sparked by a Canadian governmental report published in 1974 (see Lalonde, 1974) and the WHO's Alma-Ata Declaration (1978), several determinants of health models have been developed at the national and international levels to guide health policy creation and evaluation (see for example, Raphael, 2006; Native Women's Association of Canada, 2007; Commission on Social Determinants of Health, 2008; Public Health Agency of Canada, 2011). For example, the Public Health Agency of Canada has identified 12 determinants of health that represent the myriad social, cultural, environmental, genetic, and biological factors that shape the health of Canadians (Public Health Agency of Canada, 2011):

1) income and social status;
2) social support networks;
3) education and literacy;
4) employment and working conditions;
5) social environments;
6) physical environments;
7) personal health practices and coping skills;
8) healthy child development;
9) biology and genetic endowment;
10) health services;
11) gender; and
12) culture.

While the SDOH models developed in different countries have some commonalities, they do differ with regard to which socio-biocultural factors are included or excluded, and in the ways in which these factors are interrelated.

Rather than seeing health as simply an outcome of individual-level susceptibilities, choices, and behaviors, the SDOH approach emphasizes that health is shaped largely by broader processes that occur at various scales, from the global to the local levels (Pauly et al., 2013; World Health Organization, 2014). From this perspective, one can see that differences in health are influenced largely by unequal distributions of money, power, and resources (World Health Organization, 2014). As such, SDOH frameworks have become increasingly popular for use in health research aiming to understand and address health inequities, which are the disparities in health outcomes that are avoidable, unfair, and systemically related to social inequality and marginalization (Braverman and Gruskin, 2003; Pederson et al., 2007; Commission on Social Determinants of Health, 2008; Ontario Ministry of Health and Long-term Care, 2012; World Health Organization, 2014). Not only are these differences in health an important social justice issue, but acknowledgment of their importance has led to a growing understanding of the sensitivity of health to the social and physical environments in which we live our everyday lives (Pauly et al., 2013) – something quite pertinent to the discipline of health geography.

Importantly, attentiveness to health inequity via the SDOH approach has drawn attention to identifying *"opportunities for health"* (Greaves, 2012, p. 8;

emphasis in original) as being the key measure for addressing diversities and disparities in health status. Grounded in the SDOH framework, health impact assessments and health equity impact assessments (HIA and HEIA) have become invaluable tools for identifying such opportunities while underscoring the variety of factors that influence and shape health, and at the same time promoting equity, sustainability, and healthy public policy (Hankivsky et al., 2012). The main difference between GSBA(+) (described previously as giving primacy to gender and/or sex), the SDOH approach, and HIAs/HEIAs is that the latter are focused on issues of power and equity more broadly. That is, while still being anchored within SDOH frameworks (which recognize a plethora of structural and social factors that affect health), HIAs and HEIAs must consider both power and inequity when identifying opportunities for health, which is not true of GSBA(+) and SDOH approaches alone (Hankivsky et al., 2012).

The WHO defines HEIA/HIAs as "a combination of procedures, methods and tools by which a policy, program or project may be judged as to its potential effects on the health of a population" (World Health Organization, 1999, n.p.). Although these assessments have a variety of interpretations and applications, their general aim is to determine the potential negative or positive effects of policy in terms of increasing or reducing health inequities across different population groups, in a move to create healthier societies (Simpson et al., 2005; Hankivsky et al., 2012). Such an approach holds great potential for generating research and findings which can improve the quality of decision-making, promote social and environmental justice, encourage public participation in public policy, prioritize both qualitative and quantitative evidence, and bring attention to how policy, in all sectors, affects health (Scott-Samuel and O'Keefe, 2007).

Although the SDOH that produce health inequities are complex – with many falling outside the reach of the health care system itself – through employing this framework or undertaking HIA/HEIAs, research and analysis of the broader determinants of health have the potential to clarify important pathways to health outcomes, suggesting solutions that may lead towards addressing health disparities (Pauly et al., 2013). As the importance of the social environment becomes clearer in determining health, research into various ways that such approaches can be applied is increasing (Pauly et al., 2013). For example, Canada's National Collaborating Center for Aboriginal Health has created its own framework and categorizes, in a very scalar way, the social determinants of Aboriginal health as being: distal (e.g. historic, political, social, and economic contexts); intermediate (e.g. community infrastructure, resources, systems, and capacities); and proximal (e.g. health behaviors, physical and social environment) (Reading and Wien, 2009). Another example is offered by Benoit and Shumka (2008), who build on previous SDOH models to propose a dynamic framework that differentiates among various macro, meso, and micro-scale determinants for shaping health outcomes. Here, the macro determinants refer "to the primary importance of some determinants for shaping health outcomes" (2008, p. 18). These include sex, gender, social class, "race," ethnicity, immigrant status, geographic location, and age. Meso-level determinants refer primarily to access to key resources such as employment, education, childcare, safe neighborhoods, and health services. Micro-level determinants refer to behaviors such as smoking, diet, and exercise. In their SDOH framework, macro-level and meso-level variables are thought to interact in shaping individual behavior, ultimately determining health outcomes (Benoit and Shumka, 2008).

Health geographers have begun to contribute valuable research to the literature on SDOH, yet still have much more to offer in regard to understanding health and the impacts that social and physical determinants have in shaping our experiences and health outcomes. For example, Dunn et al. (2007) argue that there has been an absence of geography in studies on the relationship between income inequality and population health. In their study, Dunn et al. (2007) use methods of spatial pattern visualization, outlier analysis, and comparative case study analysis to investigate the role of geography in understanding the relationship between income inequality and health in Canada and the USA. Their findings demonstrate that by applying a spatial approach, otherwise obscure patterns emerge, which opens the door for new questions regarding how unequal places may be less healthy than more egalitarian ones (Dunn et al., 2007).

Other scalar and place-based inquiries into the relationship between health and socioeconomic status have been put forward by health geographers. For example, Wilson et al. (2009) deploy a highly geographic approach to SDOH research, and review the relative importance of the determinants for different health outcomes among those living in four neighborhoods in Hamilton, Ontario. Using a neighborhood-level inquiry and applying both qualitative and quantitative methods, their study reveals how varying health determinants impact neighborhoods with disparate socioeconomic status (e.g. income, education, housing tenure) and demographic diversity (e.g. percent married, visible minorities, etc.) (Wilson et al., 2009). With an explicit focus on the social and environmental factors that determine health, there is great potential for geographers to employ SDOH or HIA/HEIA approaches further in their research.

Intersectionality

Health researchers, policymakers, and practitioners in many countries, including Canada, have growing concerns about issues of diversity and how best to acknowledge the importance of the SDOH, such as gender, "race"/ethnicity, class, income, education, ability, age, sexual orientation, immigration status, and geography (Health Canada, 2003; Bates et al., 2009; Greaves, 2012; Hankivsky, 2012; Hankivsky et al., 2012; Status of Women Canada, 2014a). However, as raised by health geographers Richmond and Ross (2009), there has been much debate regarding how best to conceptualize, research, and respond to these issues of diversity (Young, 1994; Benoit and Shumka, 2008; Bowleg, 2012; Bauer, 2014). The newly-emerging framework of intersectionality has much to offer in this domain, particularly in providing a more precise identification of inequities, developing equitable health intervention strategies, and ensuring that research results are relevant within specific communities (Hankivsky, 2012; Bauer, 2014). Intersectionality has been identified as an important framework because it incorporates the SDOH (Hankivsky and Christoffersen, 2008), and thus can be meaningfully applied in population health (Bauer, 2014), public health (Bowleg, 2012) as well as sex, gender, and health research (Hankivsky, 2012; Bauer, 2014). Furthermore, it has been cited as holding great potential for advancing feminist geography (Valentine, 2007), as well as for improving researchers' collective ability to document inequities within diverse population groups more precisely, and study the potential individual-level and group-level causes of observed inequities (Bauer, 2014).

Broadly, intersectionality is concerned with building on and moving beyond existing GSBA, GSBA+, SDOH, and HEIA frameworks in order to bring about a conceptual shift in how we understand diverse determinants, social locations, their relationships, and interactions (Hankivsky et al., 2012). More specifically, it requires consideration of all the complex relationships between mutually constituting factors of social location and structural disadvantage in order to map more accurately the determinants of equity and inequity both within and beyond health (Hancock, 2007; Valentine, 2007; Grace, 2010). This approach is rooted in the history of black feminist writing, Indigenous feminism, Third World feminism, and queer and postcolonial theory (Crenshaw, 1994; Collins, 2000; Hankivsky et al., 2011). The central tenets of intersectionality assert that human lives cannot be reduced to single categories; neither can the complexity of lived human experiences be understood by prioritizing one single factor (e.g. gender), or a constellation of factors purposely selected in an additive manner (Bauer, 2014). Rather, intersectionality emphasizes that categories of differentiation are fluid and dynamic and, in essence, inseparable: they are shaped by interacting and mutually constituting social processes and structures which, in turn, are shaped by power and influenced by both time and place (Hankivsky et al., 2012). Also, differing from SDOH approaches but somewhat similar to HEIA, social justice and equity are central aims of intersectional approaches (Grace, 2010). Therefore, intersectional approaches enable the exploration of simultaneous impacts of oppressions on health, such as classism, sexism, ableism, and heterosexism (Hankivsky et al., 2009).

Although public health researchers and professionals hold a strong commitment to social justice, intersectional approaches have been rarely applied by these groups (Boleg, 2008). Understandably, one of the most salient challenges faced by those wishing to apply intersectionality in their research and practice is to come to grips with how to manage the complexity of such an analysis (McCall, 2005; Hankivsky, 2012; Bauer, 2014). Since its emergence, discussions of how to actually apply intersectionality in health research and practice remain quite limited (McCall, 2005). Furthermore, intersectionality has been criticized as being overly relativistic and simply too difficult to operationalize (McCall, 2005). Nevertheless, this approach is praised continuously as having much unrealized potential in diversity research, as it opens up new intellectual spaces for knowledge and research production, which can lead to theoretical and methodological innovation (Valentine, 2007; Bowleg, 2012; Bauer, 2014).

Intersectionality approaches can and have been used in quantitative, qualitative, and mixed-methods health research. For example, in an attempt to address how intersectionality can be incorporated into a quantitative analysis, Wilkinson (2003) suggests that categories that are highly correlated – for example, immigrant status and visible minority status – should be combined into a single variable. This then allows for examination of the difference between immigrants that are not visible minorities in relation to the variable of interest: in this case, educational outcome (Wilkinson, 2003). The strength of qualitative methods such as ethnography, neighborhood studies, participatory action research, historical analyses, and interviews, among others, lies in their ability to generate in-depth data on individuals' personal unique social locations and experiences with power and privilege (McCall, 2005; Hankivsky, 2012). As such, there is a natural alignment between the use of qualitative methods and the tenets of an intersectional approach.

Despite the challenges that researchers and policy experts face in actually applying intersectional approaches, there are a number of intersectional analyses beginning to emerge in the health geography literature. For example, Valentine (2007) applied intersectionality using a case study narrative technique in order to gain a better understanding of the ways that gender, sexuality, class, motherhood, disability, and the cultural and linguistic identity of D/deaf interact with specific spatial contexts and biographical moments. D/deaf is a term that includes those who are Deaf (sign language users), and deaf (who are hard of hearing, but who have English as their first language and may lipread and/or use hearing aids). Her findings emphasize the spatial components and fluidity of identity in relation to the constant process of becoming (Valentine, 2007). Another example comes from Cairns (2013), who used an ethnographic approach to conduct an intersectional analysis of rural imaginaries. The analysis focused on white, working-class, rural youth and demonstrated how young people construct their own rural identities through racialized representations of urban and global "others" (Cairns, 2013). Using interview data, Boleg et al. (2013) used an intersectional approach to explore the experiences of black heterosexual men, and how their interlocked multiple identities of "race," gender, and socioeconomic status held implications for HIV prevention research and interventions for this particular population group. Using a quantitative approach, Veenstra (2011) applied an intersectional lens to Canadian Community Health Survey data in order to investigate the interconnections between "race," gender, class, and sexuality and self-reported hypertension. Using binary logistic regression modeling on fair or poor self-rated health, Veenstra (2011) found that the poorest self-rated health outcomes were reported by respondents claiming Aboriginal, Asian, South-Asian, or bisexual identities, and also who were lower class. Furthermore, each axis interacted significantly with at least one other resulting in compounding effects pertaining to, most prominently, poor homosexuals and South-Asian women who were at unexpectedly high risk.

Looking Forward: Health Geographers and Diversity Research

Considering the inherent nature and diversity of the discipline, health geographers hold the potential to offer valuable contributions to diversity-based research through applications of various approaches, such as GSBA(+), SDOH, HIA/HEIAs, and intersectionality. Building on contemporary understandings that health is experienced *in place*, a key project for health geographers is to assess the place-based dimensions of the various categories of difference that people occupy, in order to gain a better understanding of how such complex social locations relate to, intersect with, and co-constitute place. Understanding place from a relational perspective is a promising approach for health geographers who wish to examine diversity, because the social conditions that shape our health are unbounded, dynamic processes that are constructed and shaped by various relational processes stretching across multiple scales, times, and spaces (Dolan and Thien, 2008; Hankivsky et al., 2011). Taking a step further, and echoing Kearns' (1993) call for understanding place in light of one's "place-in-the-world," there is a need for health geographers to expand their scope. This would be to consider how place is experienced in relation to the social conditions that so greatly shape health and health inequities, in order to truly tackle issues of diversity in their research (Valentine, 2007; Dolan and Thien, 2008). Thus, in order to gain a more nuanced understanding of how health and/or health care is experienced by diverse people in diverse locations, place must be considered in relation to social conditions and the socioeconomic, political, cultural, and historical axes that shape people's lived realities (Moss, 1997; Dolan and Thien, 2008). In the final chapter, we put forth a fuller discussion about the ways ahead for health geographers engaging in diversity research.

References

Alberta Health Services, 2011. Towards an understanding of health equity: Annotated bibliography. Available online at www.albertahealthservices.ca/poph/hi-poph-surv-shsa-tpgwg-annotated-glossary.pdf (accessed January 28, 2016).

Bates, L.M., Hankivsky, O. and Springer, K.W., 2009. Gender and health inequities: A comment on the Final Report of the WHO Commission on the Social Determinants of Health. *Social Science & Medicine*, 69(7), pp. 1002–4.

Bauer, G.R., 2014. Incorporating intersectionality theory into population health research methodology: Challenges and the potential to advance health equity. *Social Science & Medicine*, 110, pp. 10–17.

Benoit, C. and Shumka, L., 2008. *Why gender matters: Extending the ehealth determinants framework to better understand girls' and women's health.* Vancouver: Women's Health Research Network.

Boleg, L., 2008. When black + lesbian + woman ≠ black lesbian woman: The methodological challenges of qualitative and quantitative intersectionality research. *Sex Roles*, 59(5–6), pp. 312–25.

Boleg, L., Teti, M., Malebranche, D.J. and Tschann, J.M., 2013. "It's an uphill battle everyday": Intersectionality, low-income black heterosexual men, and implications for HIV prevention research and interventions. *Psychology of Men & Masculinity*, 14(1), pp. 25–34.

Bowleg, L., 2012. The problem with the phrase "women and minorities": Intersectionality – an important theoretical framework for public health. *American Journal of Public Health*, 102(7), pp. 1267–73.

Braverman, P. and Gruskin, S., 2003. Poverty, equity, human rights and health. *Bulletin of the World Health Organization*, 81(7), pp. 539–45.

Cairns, K., 2013. Youth, dirt, and the spatialization of subjectivity: An intersectional approach to white rural imaginaries. *Canadian Journal of Sociology*, 38(4), pp. 623–46.

Canadian Institutes of Health Research, 2014. *CIHR grants and awards guide: Section 1-A2 – gender, sex, and health research.* Available online at www.cihr-irsc.gc.ca/e/22630.html#1-A2 (accessed June 8, 2014).

Clow, B., Pederson, A., Haworth-Brockman, M. and Bernier, J., 2009. *Rising to the challenge: Sex- and gender-based analysis for health planning, policy and research in Canada.* Halifax: Atlantic Centre of Excellence for Women's Health.

Collins, P.H., 2000. *Black feminist thought: Knowledge, consciousness, and the politics of empowerment.* New York: Unwin Hyman.

Commission on Social Determinants of Health, 2008. *Closing the gap in a generation: Health equity through action on the social determinants of health.* Geneva: World Health Organization.

Crenshaw, K.W., 1994. Mapping the margins: Intersectionality, identity politics, and violence against women of color. In: M.A. Fineman and R. Mykitiuk, eds. *The public nature of private violence.* New York: Routledge, pp. 93–120.

DAWN-RAFH Canada, 2014. Inclusive Practices Toolkit, 2014. Available online at http://www.dawncanada.net/?attachment_id=1208 (accessed January 28, 2016).

Dolan, H. and Thien, D., 2008. Relations of care: A framework for placing women and health in rural communities. *Canadian Journal of Public Health–Revue Canadienne de Sante Publique*, 99(Supp. 2), pp. S38–42.

Dunn, J.R., Schaub, P. and Ross, N.A., 2007. Unpacking income inequality and population health. *Canadian Journal of Public Health–Revue Canadienne de Sante Publique*, 98(supp. 1), pp. S10–17.

Grace, D. 2010. When oppressions and privileges collide: A review of research in health, gender, and intersectionality in late (post)modernity. *Canadian Journal of Humanities and Social Sciences*, 1(1), pp. 19–23.

Grant, L., 2008. *Gender issues. In: L. Given, ed. The SAGE Encyclopedia of Qualitative Research Methods.* Thousand Oaks, CA: Sage Publications, pp. 365–70.

Greaves, L., 2012. Why put gender and sex into health research? In: J.L. Oliffe and L. Greaves, eds. *Designing and conducting gender, sex, and health research.* Thousand Oaks, CA: Sage Publications, pp. 3–14.

Hancock, A.-M., 2007. Intersectionality as a normative and empirical paradigm. *Politics & Gender*, 3(2), pp. 248–54.

Hankivsky, O., 2005. Gender vs. diversity mainstreaming: A preliminary examination of the role and transformative potential of feminist theory. *Canadian Journal of Political Science*, 38(4), pp. 977–1001.

Hankivsky, O., 2012. Women's health, men's health, and gender and health: Implications of intersectionality. *Social Science & Medicine*, 74(11), pp. 1712–20.

Hankivsky, O. and Christoffersen, A., 2008. Intersectionality and the determinants of health: a Canadian perspective. *Critical Public Health*, 18(3), pp. 271–83.

Hankivsky, O. and Cormier, R., 2010. Intersectionality and public policy: Some lessons from existing models. *Political Research Quarterly*, 64(1), pp. 217–29.

Hankivsky, O., Cormier, R. and De Merich, D., 2009. *Intersectionality: Moving women's health research and policy forward*. Vancouver: Women's Health Research Network.

Hankivsky, O., De Leeuw, S., Lee, J.A., Vissandjée, B. and Khanlou, N. eds., 2011. *Health inequities in Canada: Intersectional frameworks and practices,* Vancouver: UBC Press.

Hankivsky, O., Grace, D., Hunting, G., Ferlatte, O., Clark, N., Fridkin, A., Giesbrecht, M., Rudrum, S. and Laviolette, T., 2012. An intersectionality-based policy analysis framework. In: O. Hankivsky, ed. *An intersectionality-based policy analysis framework*. Vancouver: Institute for Intersectionality Research and Policy, Simon Fraser University.

Health Canada, 2003. *Healthy living*. Available online at www.hc-sc.gc.ca/hl-vs/pubs/women-femmes/gender-sexes-eng.php (accessed June 8, 2014).

Johnson, J.L., Greaves, L. and Repta, R., 2009. Better science with sex and gender: Facilitating the use of a sex and gender-based analysis in health research. *International Journal for Equity in Health*, 8(14), pp. 1–11.

Juanita Johnson-Bailey, N.M.R., 2008. Diversity issues. In: L. Given, ed. *The SAGE Encyclopedia of Qualitative Research Methods*. Thousand Oaks, CA: Sage Publications, pp. 226–30.

Kearns, R.A., 1993. Place and health: Towards a reformed medical geography. *Professional Geographer*, 45(2), pp. 139–47.

Lalonde, M., 1974. *A new perspective on the health of Canadians: A working document*. Ottawa: Government of Canada.

McCall, L., 2005. The complexity of intersectionality. *Signs*, 30(3), pp. 1771–1800.

Moss, P., 1997. Negotiating spaces in home environments: Older women living with arthritis. *Social Science & Medicine*, 45(1), pp. 23–33.

Native Women's Association of Canada, 2007. *Social determinants of health and Canada's Aboriginal women,* Submission to the World Health Organization's Commission on the Social Determinants of Health. Ottawa: Native Women's Association of Canada.

Ontario Ministry of Health and Long-term Care, 2012. *Health equity impact assessment workbook*. Toronto: Ontario Ministry of Health and Long-term Care.

Pauly, B., Macdonald, M., Hancock, T., Martin, W. and Perkin, K., 2013. Reducing health inequities: The contribution of core public health services in BC. *BMC Public Health*, 13(1), pp. 1–11.

Pederson, S., Barr, V., Wortman, J. and Rootman, I., 2007. *Evidence review: Equity lens*. Victoria: British Columbia Ministry of Health.

Public Health Agency of Canada, 2011. *What determines health?* Available online at www.phac-aspc.gc.ca/ph-sp/determinants/index-eng.php (accessed June 9, 2014).

Raphael, D., 2006. Social determinants of health: Present status, unanswered questions, and future directions. *International Journal of Health Services*, 36(4), pp. 651–77.

Reading, C.L. and Wien, F., 2009. *Health inequalities and social determinants of Aboriginal peoples' health*. Prince George: National Collaborating Centre for Aboriginal Health.

Richmond, C.A. and Ross, N.A., 2009. The determinants of First Nation and Inuit health: A critical population health approach. *Health & Place*, 15(2), pp. 403–11.

Scott-Samuel, A. and O'Keefe, E., 2007. Health impact assessment, human rights and global public policy: A critical appraisal. Special theme – health and foreign policy. *Bulletin of the World Health Organization*, 85, pp. 212–17.

Setia, M.S., Lynch, J., Abrahamowicz, M., Tousignant, P. and Wuesnel-Vallee, A., 2011. Self-rated health in Canadian immigrants: Analysis of the Longitudinal Survey of Immigrants to Canada. *Health & Place*, 17(2), pp. 658–70.

Simpson, S., Mahoney, M., Harris, E., Aldrich, R. and Williams, S., 2005. Equity-focused health impact assessment: A tool to assist policy makers in addressing health inequalities. *Environmental Impact Assessment Review*, 25(7–8), pp. 772–82.

Status of Women Canada, 2014a. *Introduction to gender-based analysis plus framework*. Available online at http://www.swc-cfc.gc.ca/gba-acs/course-cours/eng/mod00/mod00_01_01.html (accessed January 28, 2016).

Status of Women Canada, 2014b. *What is GBA+?* Available online at http://www.swc-cfc.gc.ca/gba-acs/intro-en.html (accessed January 28, 2016).

Valentine, G., 2007. Theorizing and researching intersectionality: A challenge for feminist geography. *Professional Geographer*, 59(1), pp. 10–21.

Veenstra, G., 2011. Race, gender, class, and sexual orientation: Intersecting axes of inequality and self-rated health in Canada. *International Journal for Equity in Health*, 10(1), pp. 1–11.

Waldegrave, C., 2009. Cultural, gender, and socioeconomic contexts in therapeutic and social policy work. *Family Process*, 48(1), pp. 85–101.

Wiles, J., 2002. Helath care reform in New Zealand: The diversity of gender experience. *Health & Place*, 8(2), pp. 119–28.

Wilkinson, L., 2003. Advancing a perspective on the intersections of diversity: Challenges for research and social policy. *Canadian Ethnic Studies Journal*, 35(3), pp. 3–23.

Wilson, K., Eyles, J., Elliot, S. and Keller-Olaman, S., 2009. Health in Hamilton neighbourhoods: Exploring the determinants of health at the local level. *Health & Place*, 15(1), pp. 374–82.

Women in Employment Committee, 2003. Gender and diversity analysis: Discussion paper and lens, August 8. Women in Employment Committee of the Canadian Association of Administrators of Labour Legislation.

World Health Organization, 1978. *Declaration of Alma-Ata*. Geneva: World Health Organization.

World Health Organization, 1999. Health impact assessment: Main concepts and suggested approach, Gothenburg consensus paper. Brussels: European Centre for Health Policy, World Health Organization.

World Health Organization, 2014. *Social determinants of health*. Available online at www.who.int/social_determinants/en/ (accessed June 9, 2014).

Young, I.M., 1994. Gender as seriality: Thinking about women as a social collective. *Signs*, 19(3), pp. 713–38.

3 From Embedded in Place to Marginalized Out and Back Again

Indigenous Peoples' Experience of Health in Canada

Heather Castleden, Debbie Martin, and Diana Lewis

If you are reading this chapter somewhere in Canada, then the chances are you are in the traditional territory of an Indigenous nation that has occupied this land since time immemorial. The land you are on may be ceded – that is, surrendered by treaty or other form of compensation – or it may not; but either way, this has a bearing on how Indigenous peoples experience health in place. There is a strong probability that you do not know whose territory you are on, as most non-Indigenous Canadians are ill-informed about this aspect of the Canadian "story" (Godlewska et al., 2010). So, before you read this chapter, we invite you to do a Google search to figure out whose territory you are on, and whether or not it has been ceded through a historic or modern-day treaty (comprehensive land claim). By the end of this chapter, we hope you will have an appreciation for why territoriality, self-determination, and place-in-the-world matter for Indigenous health and well-being in Canada. We also hope you will appreciate the diversity of Indigenous health-related opportunities, experiences, and outcomes, and why an equity framework that recognizes Indigenous and treaty rights, as well as the United Nations International Declaration on the Rights of Indigenous Peoples, is needed to address the grievous health incongruities that exist between Indigenous and non-Indigenous peoples in Canada.

While many parallels exist across Indigenous cultures in Canada, the world-views, values, norms, and experiences found within and between these populations are diverse. Similarly, their colonial encounters with European settlers over the past 500 years have some commonalities as well as contrasts. Despite this centuries-old connection between Indigenous peoples and European settlers, which has shaped the social, political, economic, and health landscape of Canada, Canadians in general have a superficial understanding of Indigenous peoples' social and physical place within the fabric of Canadian society, as well as the ways in which the Indigenous–settler relationship has had a significant bearing on Indigenous peoples' health and well-being across the nation.

This chapter explores why understanding diversity is critical to making sense of the health disparities across and within Indigenous populations in Canada today. It begins with an overview of Indigenous health in Canada, from pre-contact to contemporary times, providing critical historical context and tracing how Indigenous peoples, once were – and in many ways still are – embedded in place, and have been marginalized out through multiple pathways, but are now finding ways to recover a healthy (social and physical) place in Canada.

Indigenous Health in Canada

Pre-contact

Indigenous peoples throughout Canada have their own origin stories, and rely on oral histories to trace their roots to the landscape (Atleo, 2007). The archaeological record reveals evidence of human presence here for tens of thousands of years (Deloria, 1995). Complex social and cultural institutions and customary laws helped govern the ways in which Indigenous peoples stayed healthy. Moreover, generally low population density and relatively small groupings of people, as well as mobility and intimate knowledge of the local environment and climate conditions, promoted good health (Waldram et al., 2006). Although there is limited knowledge about infant mortality rates, it is known that life expectancy worldwide was generally much shorter (around 40 years) than it is today, and that mortality tended to be related to accidental deaths, aging, and periods of scarcity.

Prior to contact, Indigenous peoples lived largely off what the local lands, water, and air provided them. At times it was feast, at other times famine (Waldram et al., 2006). Trade for goods and services between groups took place, as well as warfare (causing injury and death). There is no significant documentation of infectious or chronic diseases (except arthritis), in the literature or oral histories (First Nations Health Authority, 2014). Instead, Indigenous peoples led relatively healthy and active lifestyles. Their health could be characterized as generally strong, especially when foods were abundant; however, starvation did occur periodically (First Nations Health Authority, 2014). Injuries and accidental death sustained from land-based and water-based activities were a health consequence of their way of life, but a depth of knowledge of the local environment often protected them from mishaps. When individuals were sick or injured, or experienced mental, emotional, or spiritual ills, they would turn to respected traditional herbalists, healers, and spiritual guides for help (First Nations Health Authority, 2014).

Early Contact

Upon contact, North American Indigenous peoples began to experience dramatic health impacts. Early European explorers and settlers brought infectious and chronic diseases to which Indigenous people had had no previous exposure and limited immunity. Many populations were decimated – some as much as by 90 percent – with people of all ages succumbing to epidemics such as the common flu, smallpox, tuberculosis, measles, whooping cough, and venereal diseases (Waldram et al., 2006). Worse, the historical record suggests that the transmission of some of these diseases was not accidental; rather, some Europeans were intentionally infecting trade goods and gifts to destabilize populations and shift power dynamics from local, Indigenous health, healing, and spiritual providers to Western care providers who had already been exposed to these diseases for longer periods and had developed effective antidotes, which they shared or withheld at their discretion (Heagerty, 1928 and Stearn and Stearn, 1945 cited in Houston and Houston, 2000).

Late Contact

As Indigenous populations collapsed from an onslaught of multiple epidemics, an ever-increasing stream of European settlers was arriving in the New World. As the population scales tipped in favor of the settlers, colonial governmental authorities and various religious sects sought to civilize, colonize, Christianize, and control Indigenous peoples in an attempt to dominate them, and to make the extraction and export of natural resources conflict-free (Cardinal, 2011). In so doing, colonial policies and practices were established, setting in motion mechanisms that served to undermine and delegitimize a number of Indigenous methods of healing, as well as midwifery and child-rearing, use of traditional and herbal medicines, and spiritual ceremonies (First Nations Health Authority, 2014).

A series of key colonial policies during this later period of contact help to contextualize the dramatic shift for Indigenous peoples, from being generally healthy and having health-protecting characteristics, to being disparate from the settler population across virtually every health measure (Adelson, 2005): the Indian Act, the reserve system, residential schools, forced relocations, and intentional neglect. The Indian Act, 1876 controlled virtually every aspect of the lives of registered Indians, from their identity as Indigenous peoples to their movements (e.g. when registered Indian women married non-Indigenous men, they lost their right to be registered as Indians; and federally appointed Indian agents issued passes allowing or denying people the right to leave their reserve). The creation of Indian reserves (small parcels of generally unproductive or game-poor land set aside for registered Indians) served to displace them from, and dispossess them of, their traditional territories. Indian residential schools (discussed later in this chapter) were the federal government's strategic attempt to, as Canadian Prime Minister Sir John MacDonald put it, "do away with the tribal system and assimilate the Indian people in all respects with the inhabitants of the Dominion, as speedily as they are fit for change" (Royal Commission on Aboriginal Peoples, 1996, p. 165).

In 1920 the process was still in motion, as noted by Duncan Campbell Scott, Superintendent of the federal Department of Indian Affairs, who informed a parliamentary committee that "Our objective is to continue until there is not a single Indian in Canada that has not been absorbed into the body politic" (in Miller, 1991, p. 191). The early processes of European colonization in Canada were, for the most part, an organized attack on all Indigenous social, economic, political, cultural, educational, and health institutions vis-à-vis residential schools, out-of-culture adoptions, forced relocations, imposed starvation, intentional neglect, destruction of sacred objects and sites, and other externally imposed influences. The continued effects of this attack are evident in Indigenous peoples' health status today (Bombay et al., 2009).

Contemporary Times

Indigenous health in Canada today is the epitome of inequity: no population is in a more disadvantaged health position (Adelson, 2005). Indigenous people have substantially lower life expectancies, significantly higher rates of suicide, mental illness, chronic illness and disease (e.g. obesity, diabetes, tuberculosis, asthma), violent injury, substance abuse, poverty, and infant mortality (to name but a few examples) compared to non-Indigenous people in this country. They also experience segregation, exploitation, and persecution in exponentially greater proportions than other members of Canadian society (Battiste and Youngblood Henderson, 2000). Colonial and racist approaches to health research, policy, and practice continue to have strong links to current health inequalities relative to Canada's national averages (these effects are expanded on below).

How Are Indigenous Peoples Embedded in Place?

Attachment to Land

Origin stories place people physically in relation to the contours and rhythms of their local natural environment, as well as socially in relation to other human lineages and non-human species. As a means to offer answers to fundamental questions about human beings and their relationship to the rest of the world, origin stories offer guiding principles for how to live upon the earth in ways that respect local ecosystems, such that they continue to provide for future generations. These guiding principles translate into values and beliefs about how one should interact with the local natural environment: for example, which plants and animals should be eaten and when, and how one should express gratitude and respect for the bounties of one's surroundings (Castleden et al., 2009). In short, the local natural environment provides the context in which culture is created. Thus, it may be said that the multitude of cultures that characterize the Indigenous peoples of Canada are as diverse as the Canadian landscape itself.

However, while Indigenous peoples have a deep and intimate connection to their local natural environment, it does not follow that *being* Indigenous bestows an innate ability to live off the land. Rather, the guiding principles, values, and beliefs that have given rise to diverse Indigenous cultures are the hard-won results of trial and circumstance, and traumatic experiences of drought, extreme cold, famine, and disease (Kalland, 2003; Radkau, 2008). The intimate knowledge referred to as traditional or Indigenous knowledge (which encompasses physical, mental, emotional, relational, and spiritual knowledge) that Indigenous peoples have with respect to place must be passed on in order to survive – and in order for it to be passed on, deep and lasting relationships to the local natural environment must persist.

Wholistic Health

For many Indigenous peoples in Canada, the concept of health extends well beyond mainstream definitions that focus mainly on physical and mental health and the absence of illness and disease. Even the World Health Organization's (WHO) definition, "a state of complete physical, mental and social well-being and not merely the absence of disease or infirmity" (World Health Organization, 2012, para. 1), fails to truly encompass what *wholistic* (not holistic) health means from an Indigenous perspective. Many, but certainly not all, Indigenous peoples view health as a balance of physical, mental, emotional, and spiritual well-being. The Medicine Wheel, a familiar concept in many Indigenous contexts, is used to represent this balance. Embodying multiple representations of health and healing, the Medicine Wheel is a way of teaching about and broadly applying *whole-ism*, from aspects of life (as noted above) and stages of life (birth, youth, adult, elder) to seasons of the year (spring, summer, fall, winter) and directions (east, south, west, north); and elements of nature (fire, air, water, earth) and ceremonial medicines (tobacco, sage, sweet grass, cedar) to peoples of the world (Indigenous, black, Asian, Caucasian) and spiritual entities (Grandfather Sun, Grandmother Moon, Father Sky, and Mother Earth) (adapted from a teaching given by Maliseet knowledge-keeper, Ken Paul, personal communication).

Those who embrace this wholistic approach to health are also embracing traditional or Indigenous knowledge, which values alternative medicine practices (e.g. traditional medicines and ceremony) as well as Western medicine, and recognizes the interconnectedness of people to the food they eat, the water they drink, the air they breathe, and the land on which they live. While this might make a lot of intuitive sense, our Western health care system in Canada is not designed to support such an approach. However, we are seeing some advances: for example, one of the 13 institutes of the federally funded Canadian Institutes of Health Research (CIHR) focuses on Indigenous peoples' health from a wholistic perspective.

Healthy Lands, Healthy People

For Indigenous peoples, the relationship between healthy lands and healthy people is interdependent (Simpson, 2004; McGregor, 2005; Atleo, 2007;

Wilson, 2008; Cajete and Pueblo, 2010; Prosper et al. 2011; Tobias and Richmond, 2014). A brief example from Nuu-chah-nulth territory helps to illustrate this ontology and epistemology. The Nuu-chah-nulth people, on the west coast of Canada, have had a symbiotic relationship with cedar and salmon since time immemorial (Castleden et al., 2009). When one is not healthy, the others are negatively impacted. The Nuu-chah-nulth worldview stands on its own, but it has also been corroborated with Western science. Scientists have found that when a cedar grove is subjected to an extensive clear cut to the edge of salmon-spawning streams, the riverbeds are compromised in their ability to incubate salmon eggs, thus negatively affecting the salmon population (Helfield and Naiman, 2006). The Nuu-chah-nulth population is similarly affected: economic opportunities (commercial fishing) and healthy food sources (fish for sustenance and social and ceremonial purposes) are reduced, thereby compromising Nuu-chah-nulth identity, relationships, health, and spirituality (Castleden et al., 2009).

Why Have Indigenous Peoples Been Marginalized Out of Place?

Land Dispossession and Residential Schools

While literature on culture, place, and health is well-established (for a seminal text, see Gesler and Kearns, 2002) the literature connecting Indigenous peoples' health to place, and how place matters, is only beginning to emerge (see for example, Wilson, 2003; Castleden et al., 2009; Richmond and Ross, 2009; Harper et al., 2012). For many Indigenous peoples in Canada, health and well-being is closely linked to their connection to the land, as strength of culture grows from that connection (Greenwood and de Leeuw, 2007). Indigenous scholar and educator Gregory Cajete (2000) coins this relationship "ensoulment" – a metaphysical attachment at the deepest level of psychological involvement with the land. Any disassembly of this essential component of being has implications for the health and wellness of Indigenous people (Walters et al., 2011).

Colonial policies, such as the protracted effects of land dispossession, have had (and continue to have) direct effects on Indigenous health. New research also is emerging about the health impacts on Indigenous populations of anthropogenic climate change and nonpoint-source pollution creeping into Indigenous lands, water, and air. Cunsolo Willox and colleagues (2013) discuss the mental health effects of place-based distress known as "solastalgia" (see Albrecht, 2005; see also Chapters 4 and 5 of this volume for other perspectives on mental health and well-being), in the eastern Arctic. Cunsolo Willox and colleagues found that for the Inuit, anthropogenic climate change was compromising the local weather and land and ice conditions in the Arctic. Being unable to use the land to hunt, fish, trap, and simply *be there* in the way that they had been for generations was eliciting anxiety, sadness, depression, fear, and anger, and was impacting their cultural continuity, sense of self-worth, and overall health and well-being.

Since as early as the 1820s, residential schools have been a way for the colonial state to disconnect people from their families and communities, cultures, languages, and spirituality, and most of all, their lands (Waziyatawin, 2009). More than 130 federally funded residential schools across Canada were operated by mainstream churches (Catholic, Anglican, Presbyterian, and United), and although many believe that all the schools closed in the 1960s and 1970s, the last one did not close until 1996. Some 150,000 or more Indigenous children were removed from families and communities: they were forced to attend residential schools and were often verbally and/or physically punished for speaking their own languages (Truth and Reconciliation Commission, 2015). Although it was done ostensibly to educate children in the ways of the dominant society, clearly government policies were aiming for assimilation (Harrison, 2009; Spears, 2014). Worse still, in addition to physical punishment, many children were subjected to nutritional deprivation, unhygienic conditions, and sexual abuse (Truth and Reconciliation Commission, 2015). In 2008, Canadian prime minister Stephen Harper issued a formal apology for this national disgrace, and a year later the Truth and Reconciliation Commission was established with a mandate to inform all Canadians about what happened at the residential schools.

Multigenerational Trauma

As a result of these travesties, multigenerational trauma has been found in many Indigenous communities across Canada – both urban and rural. It can be defined as trauma that is transmitted across generations through oral history and social modeling (Jones, 2008; Czyzewski, 2011). The historical events of the past, which disrupted cultural practices, continue to resonate in the present (Wesley-Esquimaux, 2007). Symptoms of social disorders are caused not only by immediate trauma but by the memories of past trauma, disrupting adaptive social and cultural patterns of behavior, diminishing social skills, and normalizing social disorder (Castellano and Archibald, 2007; Wesley-Esquimaux, 2007). These memories and images become so powerful in subsequent generations that they constitute memories in their own right (Bombay et al., 2009). Resignation and shame are the primary intergenerational effects of historical trauma, joined with a sense of fatalism, inevitability, and permanence, culminating in a poverty of spirit or wound of the collective soul (Wesley-Esquimaux, 2007; Bombay et al., 2009; Spears, 2014).

Although intergenerational trauma is the result of multiple stressors (mistreatment and oppression, racism, forcible expulsion from lands), residential schools are considered the major perpetrator. Many residential school survivors lived their formative years in an environment where parental practices were modeled on abuse and neglect, resulting in persistent negative learned behaviors (Bombay et al., 2009; Harrison, 2009). Poor social modeling received as children is then passed on to the next generation of children, and on it goes (Rice and Snyder, 2008). While some would suggest that residential school survivors (those who actually attended, as well as their descendants) should "get over" the trauma of those experiences, this sentiment reveals a fundamental misunderstanding of the human condition, and the difficulty in coping with trauma (Harrison, 2009).

Racism

Racism is a known stressor that contributes to disparities throughout Indigenous people's lives, and negatively impacts their physical, social, emotional, and spiritual health and well-being (Frohlich et al., 2006; Reading and Wien, 2009; (James et al., 2010 chart the experiences of racism in Canada). Indigenous people continue to report encounters of individual and institutional racism in the health care system, despite various attempts to create culturally safe spaces and cross-cultural competencies among health care professionals (Guilfoyle et al., 2008; Castleden et al., 2010). Experiences of discrimination, prejudice, and racism are so widespread, and so much a part of many Indigenous people's collective memory (Cannon and Sunseri, 2011), that many individuals suppress their Indigenous identity in mainstream health care spaces (Browne and Fiske, 2001) or avoid treatment (Patterson et al., 2011). It is not surprising that fear of discrimination – a form of racism – keeps Indigenous people from accessing public services, including the health care system (Guilfoyle et al., 2008). Besides individual encounters with racism, systemic barriers impact Indigenous people's ability to access timely and effective health services; these barriers exist at proximal, intermediate, and distal scales in relation to the social determinants of health (as discussed in Chapter 2), and operate throughout the life cycle within physical, social, emotional, and spiritual realms (Reading and Wien, 2009).

Although the lived experience of Indigenous people often points to the existence of racism within the health care system, the pathways through which racism transcends to negatively influence Indigenous health in Canada are seldom addressed (Brondolo et al., 2009a, 2009b). We do know that chronic and acute stress (from racism, poverty, etc.) triggers neuro-endocrine responses (e.g. release of cortisol), which may be adaptive in the immediate situation, but over time can damage organs such as the heart and brain (Paradies, 2006a; Jackson et al., 2010; McEwen and Gianaros, 2010). There are other relevant pathways: the history of racism and colonialism has created mistrust and suspicion, which may lead some Indigenous people to avoid seeking health care or to avoid taking medication, thereby exacerbating their health conditions (for an example with respect to non-attendance at diabetes clinics, see Patterson et al., 2011).

Moreover, experiences of racism can lead to awkward interactions and poor communication with health care providers, whose decisions and behavior also may be affected by stereotypes (Tang and Browne, 2008). In addition, how pain is expressed differs across cultures, leading to misdiagnosis and/or inadequate treatment (Latimer et al., 2012). General reviews of racial discrimination and health seem to find that the most significant impacts are on mental health and health behaviors (e.g. smoking, substance abuse), but evidence also suggests that there are effects on physical health and self-rated health (e.g. Krieger, 2000; Paradies, 2006b). While this is only an emerging body of literature, what is firmly established is that Indigenous health is not only influenced by genetic factors, but also sociopolitical, economic, historical, legal, and environmental ones (Reading and Wien, 2009; Richmond and Ross, 2009). Although these hold true for the entire human population, within the Canadian population's settler ideology, there tends to be a failure to understand or accept these factors when it comes to marginalized populations (Guilfoyle et al., 2008). Thus, Indigenous people often are blamed for their health issues (lifestyle) or viewed as having genetic faults; these have obvious links to racism (Smith, 1999). While other marginalized populations (e.g. African Canadians, see James et al., 2010) also experience racism and disproportionate health burdens, Indigenous peoples' experiences are distinct because of their specific colonial experiences with the influx of the settler population to their traditional territory (Czyzewski, 2011). Consequently, Indigenous people's health, as well as their ability to access equitable health care, is impacted by a "double-edged burden" of colonialism and racism (Awofeso, 2011).

Recognising Diversity: Limits to Umbrella Labels

First Nations, Inuit, and Métis

In the vast and diverse physical landscape of Canada we can find everything from mountains to grasslands, arctic tundra to rainforests, marshy wetlands to desert, and much in-between. As mentioned earlier, Indigenous peoples consider themselves of the land: their languages, ceremonies, beliefs, and practices have all emerged from their interaction with local natural environments. For example, Inuit who live primarily in Canada's Arctic are known to have extensive knowledge of, and language to describe, the local climate; they are attuned to weather patterns, the seasonal migrations of animals, and the cyclical abundance that characterizes local wildlife. Indigenous peoples within other parts of Canada are similarly knowledgeable about their own respective territories and landscapes – e.g. Cree, Anishinaabe, Nuu-chah-nulth, Dene, Mi'kmaq, Métis – and their languages reflect that cultural diversity. Yet in spite of this tremendous diversity of cultures, languages, and ceremonies, there continues to be a tendency to describe the Indigenous peoples of Canada as being homogeneous, or to use a *pan-Indigenous* approach to examine and understand Indigenous peoples. This is problematic, because it fails to account for the rich, ever-changing diversity that exists between and among Indigenous populations in Canada.

This ever-changing element of Indigenous cultures and identities is important to highlight. There is often an unwritten or unspoken assumption that to be Indigenous is to be required somehow to strictly adhere to conventional stereotypes about how an Indigenous person should act or appear. For example, if an Indigenous person dresses in a suit, talks on a cell phone, or eats fast food, then that is somehow equated with a desire to relinquish his/her Indigenous identity (King, 2012). Embracing modernity is considered – by some, nay many – as evidence of the inevitable demise of Indigenous identity. Such logic fails to recognize that the very survival of all cultures, not just those that are Indigenous, depends to a large extent on the ability of people within it to adapt to changing circumstances and to absorb elements of other cultures in ways that support, and even enhance, the existence of one's own culture. In fact, many would argue that Indigenous cultures, by their very nature, are characterized by their acceptance of diverse perspectives and new ideas (Battiste, 2000; Loppie, 2007).

Rural and Urban Diversity

When conceptualizing the diversity of Indigenous peoples within Canada, it is important to consider the starkly different lived experiences and health differences of Indigenous peoples living in rural and urban environments, although limitations in data collection and reporting make it difficult to pinpoint the extent and nature of such differences (see Browne et al., 2009; Place, 2012). For example, some data suggest that, generally speaking, the health of Indigenous people living in urban areas is better than that of those living on-reserve and in rural areas (Place, 2012). However, this may not hold true for all health conditions: for example, HIV/AIDS prevalence is particularly high among urban Indigenous peoples, although this should not be constructed as only an "inner-city problem" (Browne et al., 2009). Moreover, not all studies agree with this assessment. A study by Tjepkema (2002) found that on-reserve and off-reserve populations had very similar rates of smoking, drinking, inactivity, and obesity. Clearly, this points to the need for greater insight into the health differences between those living in rural and urban areas.

Any discussion of this issue must consider the extent to which Indigenous people (particularly First Nation peoples and Métis) have moved into urban centers over the past 60 years. In the 1950s, for example, fewer than 10 percent of all Indigenous people in Canada lived in urban areas. As of 2006, more than 50 percent of the Indigenous population within Canada live in urban centers, and most of these (nearly 95 percent) are First Nation peoples and Métis (Browne et al., 2009), whereas most Inuit continue to live in sparsely populated rural and/or remote communities across Canada's north (it is worth noting that more than 80 percent of non-Indigenous people are urban-based).

So, why the exodus out of rural areas? For many, the reasons are similar to those explaining the out-migration of young people in virtually all rural

Canadian communities. There is a desire to move closer to urban areas to access what are perceived to be better health and social services and amenities, as well as a desire to pursue greater educational or employment opportunities. Historically, Indigenous peoples settled or gathered at the confluences of major waterways for transportation, trade, and abundant wild food sources; it was the reserve system that situated communities on lands intentionally away from the waterways, where cities such as Winnipeg or Halifax eventually developed. However, cities are also places where Indigenous people experience marginalization, racism, and other forms of social exclusion that may negatively impact their health (Peters, 2004; Browne et al., 2009), including having difficulty finding the housing, employment, and social safety nets they were seeking. This may result in homelessness, gang activity, prostitution, substance abuse, violence, and regular trips back to the reserve. As shown in Chapter 7, these forms of marginalization manifest themselves in areas of Winnipeg, Canada. In response, Native Friendship Centres, which can be found in more than 115 communities across Canada, offer a safe haven and support services (health, social, spiritual) for more than 700,000 urban Indigenous people, regardless of whether they are First Nations, Inuit, or Métis.

Gender Diversity

Gender roles provide another prominent example of the diversity within and between Indigenous peoples across Canada. Traditionally, Indigenous men and women held distinct gendered roles in their communities. For example, men were largely responsible for hunting, trapping, fishing, protecting the community, and making tools, while women were largely responsible for hunting smaller game, gathering berries, roots, and other herbal foods and medicines, as well as child-rearing, caring for the elderly, and making and mending clothing for the family. In many societies, women were also the water keepers. While clearly the position of men and women was divided along gendered lines, it was not one of unequal power and authority, but rather one of recognized interdependence (Gunn Allen, 1986). For example, warm clothing and medicines (the purview of women) enabled hunting (largely the purview of men). Should either a man or a woman be rendered incapable of completing their tasks, the results could mean starvation or hunger for a family or community.

The term "Two-Spirit" – a relatively new term in the English language and used in many Indigenous contexts – has begun to emerge in recent years to recognize the fluid nature of gender and sexual identity, and the interconnectedness between these identities with spirituality and traditional worldviews (Wylie, 2012). It is often used to indicate those who hold both feminine and masculine identities within one body; but beyond this, sometimes it is also used as a politicized term that recognizes the role that colonization has played in undermining and ignoring the fluidity and diversity of gendered identities within traditional First Nations, Inuit, and Métis cultures. Although the term "Two-Spirit" may be newly coined, there is evidence that prior to contact, First Nations, Inuit, and Métis peoples not only recognized Two-Spirit individuals within their communities, but also placed these individuals in positions of high esteem. They were counselors, healers, or visionaries, as they were thought to have a special connection with the Creator by carrying not just one gendered spirit, but two (Wylie, 2012). It is thought that a great deal of the stigma and discrimination faced by Two-Spirited individuals today can be traced to the influence of colonial perspectives on sexuality and gender identity, which often hold a much more rigid, binary conception of sexuality that requires individuals to identify as either male or female. (Chapter 4 offers a closer look at the health issues among gender nonconforming people, including those who identify as Indigenous.)

Aside from acknowledging the particular role of Two-Spirited individuals within many First Nations, Inuit, and Métis societies, there are other reasons why gender diversity is an important consideration with respect to Indigenous peoples' health in Canada. Statistical analyses of gender reveal differences in life expectancy between men and women: specifically, that despite similar social, cultural, political, and economic circumstances, outcomes are very different. For example, among the Mi'kmaq people of Nova Scotia, changing economic circumstances on reserve have differentially influenced men and women, with women surpassing men in terms of educational achievement and employment outcomes (e.g. unemployment rates of 25 percent for women and 41 percent for men) (Union of Nova Scotia Indians, 2013). At the same time, only 38 percent of youth in the sample report that they live with their biological father (down from 46 percent in 2002–3); and the proportion of single-parent families on reserve is more than double the provincial average (Union of Nova Scotia Indians, 2013). These, and many other *upstream* determinants, are known to have different (gendered) impacts on individual health and well-being (and they fall within the GSBA framework introduced in Chapter 2).

Socioeconomic Diversity

Another upstream determinant of health is socioeconomic status. There is a general perception that regardless of where they live, all Indigenous people are living on huge handouts from the government. The reality is that Canada is failing with respect to social justice and basic human rights: for example, 50 percent of First Nations children live in poverty, and if Indigenous poverty were taken into account in the Human Development Index, Canada would drop in rank from fourth to 78 (Palmater, 2011). Conversely, to assume that all Indigenous people are impoverished neglects the socioeconomic diversity of this population and the associated links to health. What is important to note is that poverty increases the risk of infectious and chronic illnesses due to factors such as poor nutrition, overcrowding, and lack of access to safe drinking water. In turn, poor health increases poverty because of the costs associated with treatment (e.g. lost wages, medicine costs, transportation and accommodation fees, etc). It is well established that wealthier people are generally healthier and live longer (which leads to different health issues and associated long-term care costs). Although these issues can be applied across the board to Indigenous and non-Indigenous peoples, the complex issues associated with isolation and exclusion compound the health impacts experienced by Indigenous people (Reading and Wien, 2009).

While socioeconomic indicators measure quality of life, life satisfaction, income, education, employment, housing, working conditions, and access to health services, these indicators do not tell the whole story. Indigenous health inequalities arise from general socioeconomic factors in combination with cultural and historical factors (Adelson, 2005; King et al., 2009; Richmond and Ross, 2009). The inequities produced by social norms, policies, and practices – inequities that tolerate or produce unequal access to power, wealth, or other social resources – manifest in high rates of unemployment, scarce community resources and economic opportunity, poor housing, violence, and low literacy and educational attainment. Until the link between inequality and poor health is addressed, reducing health disparities in Indigenous communities will remain extremely difficult to realize (Adelson, 2005; Reading and Wien, 2009; Czyzewski, 2011).

Although Indigenous peoples continue to work towards socioeconomic parity with the rest of Canada, and although there have been remarkable successes, the limited autonomy they have to make their own health decisions, or to effect change in health policies and practices, continues to impact how such decisions are being made. We have only to look at Jordan's Principle to illustrate the jurisdictional nightmares in which many communities find themselves embroiled, and that continue to affect the delivery of health and social services, despite the jurisdictional certainty and clarity provided by the courts.

Jordan's Principle was a "child first" Bill unanimously passed in the House of Commons in 2007 after Jordan River Anderson, a Cree child, died at the age of five, having lived his entire life in a hospital while the federal and provincial governments disputed who had jurisdiction to pay for his complex health care needs. In short, the federal government must act in good faith for the good of all Canadians, and not in its own best interests – especially regarding its fiduciary responsibility to Indigenous peoples – in order for effective change to take place for *all* communities. We turn next to that responsibility in the context of applying an equity framework that recognizes Aboriginal and treaty rights.

Applying an Equity Framework: Indigenous Autonomy and Self-determination

Aboriginal Rights

In seeking an understanding of how we might achieve Indigenous health equity in Canada, first it is critical to have a functional understanding of

Aboriginal and treaty rights. Aboriginal rights are those collective rights that flow from the use and occupation of land prior to contact, and include the right to continue practicing one's customs and traditions, including practices of healing and medicine. Treaty rights (rights specified in a treaty) may include rights to hunt, fish, and sustain a moderate livelihood, and in the modern land claim agreements, the right to self-determination. Aboriginal and treaty rights are recognized under Section 35(1) of the Canadian Constitution Act, 1982, which states that "existing aboriginal and treaty rights of the aboriginal peoples of Canada are hereby recognized and affirmed" (Government of Canada, 2015a, para. 1).

Violation of the rights of Indigenous peoples is at the root of current health inequities: any disruption of the right to pursue cultural practices, customs, or traditions can impact on positive self-image and a healthy identity (King et al., 2009). Briefly, some political determinants, including the inability to exercise Aboriginal rights, have profoundly negative effects on Indigenous health (Reading and Wien, 2009). Conversely, research shows that the ability to carry on activities such as traditional harvesting leads to an enhanced sense of self-reliance and overall health (Long, 2014).

Returning to the rural exodus, Senese and Wilson (2013) remind us that colonial policies have linked Indigeneity with rural settings (i.e. on reserve), effectively making urban spaces fundamentally incompatible with Indigenous identity. This has significant implications with respect to the assertion of Aboriginal rights in urban settings, and consequently for urban Indigenous health. The federal government claims jurisdictional responsibility to those living *on-reserve*; those Indigenous people living in urban areas are claimed to be under the jurisdiction of the provinces, like all other citizens, leading to jurisdictional gaps in services when it comes to rights or benefits. Thus, in terms of rights and benefits, where one lives is implicated in increasing health inequities among urban Indigenous people.

Historic and Modern Treaties

Indigenous peoples' treaty rights in Canada are based on historic treaties (i.e. the peace and friendship treaties and numbered treaties) between the British Crown and various Indigenous nations; or on modern-day treaties (also known as "comprehensive land claims") between the federal and provincial or territorial governments and First Nations and Inuit (none exist with Métis at this time). Generally, historic treaties were understood as nation-to-nation pacts for peace or access to resources, and often came with provisions (if the peace is kept, then land, resources, medicine, etc. will be provided in return). It is important to note – but often not understood – that treaties remain intact until such time as they are broken, or a new treaty has been negotiated. While both types of treaties cover much of the Canadian landscape, a substantial area still exists that remains unceded by the original inhabitants of the land (e.g. much of British Columbia, and all of the Atlantic provinces).

Historic treaties also often included a "medicine chest" clause, which has been interpreted literally by the federal government as providing medicine, and interpreted metaphorically by Indigenous peoples as providing comprehensive health care in perpetuity (Boyer, 2003). The spirit and intent of the historic treaties have been widely debated by scholars, policy analysts, and governments, and they remain contested to this day. An enormous amount of time and financial and human resources are dedicated to fighting over the modern interpretations; this is deeply problematic, because the federal government is in a constant conflict of interest. On the one hand, it has to uphold its fiduciary responsibility to Indigenous peoples (as outlined in the Indian Act, 1876); but on the other hand, it continues to resist honoring the various promises laid out in the treaties. Modern treaties often spell out in far greater detail what the signatories' responsibilities are to each other. Having said that, it is important to recognize that both types have been entered into under at least some degree of duress. Regardless, the great challenges that Indigenous peoples face today in operationalizing their treaty rights play out in the form of health impacts, ranging from environmental health to economic health, and from political health to spiritual health, and everything in-between.

United Nations Declaration on the Rights of Indigenous Peoples

A working group of the United Nations (UN) began developing a Declaration on the Rights of Indigenous Peoples in 1982: it took more than 25 years for the UN to vote in favor of the draft. No other declaration has taken so long. Particularly noteworthy is the fact that when it came time to vote, four countries voted against it: Australia, Canada, New Zealand, and the USA. Perhaps it is no surprise that these four countries did not support even a non-binding UN declaration on the matter of Indigenous rights: they are all former colonies of the British Empire and share similar colonial histories. Moreover, they have the most to lose – or put differently, give back – in recognizing such rights. For example, with respect to health, the Declaration states in Article 24, paras 1 and 2:

1. Indigenous peoples have the right to their traditional medicines and to maintain their health practices, including the conservation of their vital medicinal plants, animals and minerals. Indigenous individuals also have the right to access, without any discrimination, all social and health services.
2. Indigenous individuals have an equal right to the enjoyment of the highest attainable standard of physical and mental health. States shall take the necessary steps with a view to achieving progressively the full realization of this right. (United Nations, 2007, p. 9)

Clearly, to honour the essence of what is laid out in this Article would require a substantially different and more robust engagement between the state and

Indigenous peoples in Canada. An equity framework with Indigenous peoples leading the way is the logical path forward; however, the political will is lacking.

Conclusion: Indigenous Pathways to Health

A Young and Growing Population

Today, approximately 1.5 million people in Canada (approximately 5 percent of the Canadian population) identify as Indigenous. This figure is approximately 20 percent higher than what was reported in the 2006 census, indicating that Indigenous populations are the youngest and fastest growing demographic in the country. (Note that this rapid increase in population also reflects legislative changes, such as Bill C-31, An Act to Amend the Indian Act, 1985, which reinstated individuals who lost their status when they married "out" or were enfranchised, as well as an increase in numbers of people self-identifying as Indigenous; Peters, 2004.) This contrasts sharply with the national demographic trend toward a steadily aging population. With a young and growing Indigenous population, opportunities to increase health equity will present themselves through education and capacity building, but particular health issues associated with child, youth, and maternal health also will need to be the focus of Indigenous health leaders' attention. We conclude our chapter with a look at ways in which Indigenous peoples are recovering their health and well-being.

Better Health Research, More Health Education and Capacity

When it comes to Indigenous health, it is important to acknowledge the legacy of unethical research that has taken place over the past several decades, ranging from a lack of informed consent to misappropriated and misunderstood uses of Indigenous knowledge – all of which cause harm in various forms to individuals and communities. A number of different responses to this legacy have occurred, many in the last ten to 15 years. Decolonizing approaches to research (Smith, 1999) and Indigenous research methodologies (Kovach, 2010) have been important contributions to mainstream academic discourse. Policy on ethical research has been transformed, first with the federal 1998 Tri-Council Policy Statement on Research Ethics involving Human Subjects (Canadian Institutes of Health Research and National Sciences and Engineering Research Council of Canada, 1998), which included brief mention of particular considerations for academic research involving Indigenous peoples; and later a revised Policy Statement in 2010 (Canadian Institutes of Health Research (CIHR), National Sciences and Engineering Research Council of Canada, and Social Sciences and Humanities Research Council of Canada, 2010), which included an entire chapter devoted to such ethical considerations.

Perhaps most important has been the work done by Indigenous organizations and communities themselves to protect against the consequences of unethical research. For example, the National Aboriginal Health Organization (2014) developed a policy referred to as OCAP™ (Ownership, Control, Access, and Possession of Data involving Indigenous Peoples in Canada) to insure the proper handling of data and allow decision-making authority to reside in the place where the data were generated. In addition, a number of community, tribal, and nation-based ethics boards have been established (e.g. Mi'kmaw Ethics Watch and NunatuKavut Research Ethics Committee) to provide additional ethical supervision for research in Indigenous communities and throughout their traditional territories. Often, the focus of such boards has been relational ethics, not simply procedural ethics, the latter of which has been (and largely continues to be) the focus of institutions.

As noted earlier, the federally funded CIHR Institute of Aboriginal Peoples' Health (IAPH) is dedicated specifically to Indigenous health research and capacity-building, and has supported the development of a cadre of Indigenous and non-Indigenous health researchers through a supportive network of research environments. A key goal is to bring Indigenous health in Canada onto a level playing field with the health of all Canadians: to do this requires an approach framed around health equity (Reading, 2003). Since its inception, IAPH has supported more than 650 graduate students across Canada through the Network Environments for Aboriginal Health Research (NEAHRs) (Richmond et al., 2013). At the same time, these NEAHRs have supported opportunities for Indigenous communities and organizations to identify and address their own health research objectives and priorities, working in collaboration with Indigenous health researchers (Reading, 2003), and promoting the rapid uptake of new health knowledge generated through research (Richmond et al., 2013). We are seeing a surge in community-based Indigenous health research, management, and service capacity, as well as more educated Indigenous people taking up health-focused careers.

An important caveat to this is that the signs *were* positive in terms of more education and more capacity. However, at the time of writing, CIHR is taking steps towards dismantling the progress that has been made, the NEAHRs have had their funding cut, IAPH has had its budget cut in half (along with that of all the other 12 CIHR institutes), and there is a movement away from context-specific research to scaled-up models of health research that suggest a "one-size-fits-all" approach – an approach that has failed already in most contexts, not just Indigenous ones.

Idle No More: A Groundswell of Political Action

Along with a growing Indigenous population, a rise in its educational attainment, and the overall growing capacity to address health issues in ways that are culturally relevant, we are seeing also a groundswell of Indigenous political consciousness and action to address the ongoing legacy of health inequities.

This groundswell has roots in the creation of the National Indian Brotherhood (later morphing into the Assembly of First Nations) by Indigenous leaders across Canada, who recognized the need to band together and fight the proposed federal White Paper on Indian Policy in 1969. Subsequently, the Berger Inquiry (Berger, 1977) was a response to the Mackenzie Valley Pipeline proposal in the 1970s, which threatened the on-the-land livelihoods, health, and well-being of Indigenous peoples. The Oka Crisis in 1990 prompted a much-needed Royal Commission on Aboriginal Peoples (Government of Canada, 1996), resulting in a 4,000-page report outlining more than 400 recommendations and a 20-year plan to improve relations between Indigenous peoples and the state. In addition, in the 1993 "War in the Woods," hundreds of Indigenous and non-Indigenous environmentalists and protestors peacefully protested in Clayoquot Sound to prevent clear-cutting of an old-growth rainforest; it was one of the largest acts of civil disobedience in Canada, with more than 800 arrests (D'Auria et al., 2013).

These and many other Indigenous-led protests against extractive resource industries that impact environmental and human health are going on across the country today. The grassroots "Idle No More" movement began reacting against federal legislative abuses of Indigenous rights two years ago through teach-ins, flash mob "round dances" (contemporary "friendship dances" welcoming all to hold hands and dance), and road or rail blockades, and continues today. Moreover, we are hearing calls for inquests about Indigenous health and racism (e.g. into the tragic but preventable emergency room death of Brian Sinclair in Winnipeg, ignored for 34 hours seemingly because he was Indigenous and staff assumed he was drunk and seeking shelter; Provincial Court of Manitoba, 2014); for national inquiries into Indigenous health and violence against women (e.g. into the hundreds of missing and murdered Indigenous women in this country; Government of Canada, 2015b); and for human rights tribunals about health inequalities between Indigenous and non-Indigenous Canadians (e.g. over the federal government's chronic underfunding of First Nations child welfare programs; CBC News, 2016). We have seen court battles over constitutionally protected rights to use traditional medicines in place of Western medicine (for example, *Hamilton Health Sciences Corp.* v. *D.H.* (2015 ONCJ 229, CanLII); Mehta, 2014), and most recently, open letters from the Indigenous health research community critiquing the CIHR's inequities in funding for Indigenous health research (Aboriginal Health Research Steering Committee, 2014).

Our final message is this: nowhere in Canada has a uniquely situated place-in-the-world been more shaped by external forces than in the case of Indigenous peoples. As Indigenous peoples continue to gather strength through physical, cultural, political, economic, emotional, and spiritual healing, embodied health inequities cannot be overlooked any longer. Recognizing Indigenous spaces and creating culturally safe places is a step in the right direction. Cultural safety includes an understanding of colonial forces and its impacts; an understanding of the relationships between residential school experiences and negative intergenerational health outcomes; knowledge of historical and current policies and practices towards Indigenous peoples that have perpetuated health inequities; a commitment to relationship-building based on respect and collaboration, with Indigenous peoples setting priorities and leading the way; and recognition of Indigenous knowledge systems and practices regarding health and well-being rooted in the land.

References

Aboriginal Affairs and Northern Development Canada, 2011. *Aboriginal demographics from the 2011 National Household Survey*, Planning, Research and Statistics Branch. Ottawa: Planning, Research and Statistics Branch.

Aboriginal Health Research Steering Committee, 2014. *What is Kahwa:tsire? A response to the emerging crisis between CIHR and the Aboriginal health research community*. Available online at http://kahwatsire.com (accessed January 30, 2016).

Adelson, N., 2005. The embodiment of inequity: Health disparities in Aboriginal Canada. *Canadian Journal of Public Health*, 96(2), pp. S45–61.

Albrecht, G.A., 2005. Solastalgia: A new concept in human health and identity. *PAN: Philosophy Activism Nature*, 3, pp. 41–55.

Atleo, E.R., 2007. *Tsawalk: A Nuu-chah-nulth worldview*. Vancouver: UBC Press.

Awofeso, N., 2011. Racism: A major impediment to optimal Indigenous health and health care in Australia. *Australian Indigenous Health Bulletin*, 11(3), pp. 1–14.

Battiste, M., 2000. *Reclaiming indigenous voice and vision*. Vancouver: UBC Press.

Battiste, M.A. and Youngblood Henderson, J.Y., 2000. *Protecting Indigenous knowledge and heritage: A global challenge*. Saskatoon: Purich.

Berger, T., 1977. *Northern frontier, northern homeland: Mackenzie Valley pipeline inquiry*, vol. 1. Ottawa: Minister of Supply and Services Canada.Ottawa: Minister of Supply and Services Canada.

Bombay, A., Matheson, K. and Anisman, H., 2009. Intergenerational trauma: Convergence of multiple processes among First Nations peoples in Canada. *International Journal of Indigenous Health*, 5(3), pp. 6–47.

Boyer, Y., 2003. No. 1: Aboriginal health: A constitutional rights analysis, discussion paper. Saskatoon: Native Law Centre, University of Saskatchewan and National Aboriginal Health Organization.

Brondolo, E., Gallo, L.C. and Myers, H.F., 2009a. Race, racism and health: Disparities, mechanisms, and interventions. *Journal of Behavioral Medicine*, 32(1), pp. 1–8.

Brondolo, E., ver Halen, N.B., Pencille, M., Beatty, D. and Contrada, R.J., 2009b. Coping with racism: A selective review of the literature and a theoretical and methodological critique. *Journal of Behavioral Medicine*, 32(1), pp. 64–88.

Browne, A. and Fiske, J., 2001. First Nations women's encounters with mainstream health care services. *Western Journal of Nursing Research*, 23(2), pp. 126–47.

Browne, A.J., MacDonald, H. and Elliott, D., 2009. First Nations urban Aboriginal health research discussion paper: A report for the First Nations Centre, National Aboriginal Health Organization. Ottawa: National Aboriginal Health Organization.

Canadian Institutes of Health Research, Natural Sciences and Engineering Research Council of Canada, and Social Sciences and Humanities Research Council of Canada, 1998. *Tri-Council policy statement: Ethical conduct for research involving humans*. Ottawa: Public Works and Government Services Canada.

Canadian Institutes of Health Research, Natural Sciences and Engineering Research Council of Canada, and Social Sciences and Humanities Research Council of Canada, 2010. *Tri-Council policy statement: Ethical conduct for research involving humans.* Available online at www.pre.ethics.gc.ca/pdf/eng/tcps2/TCPS_2_FINAL_Web.pdf (accessed January 5, 2015).

Cajete, G., 2000. *Native science: Natural laws of interdependence.* Santa Fe, NM: Clear Light Publishers.

Cajete, G.A. and Pueblo, S.C., 2010. Contemporary Indigenous education: A nature-centered American Indian philosophy for a 21st century world. *Futures,* 42(10), pp. 1126–32.

Cannon, M. and Sunseri, L. eds., 2011. *Racism, colonialism, and Indigeneity in Canada: A reader.* Don Mills, ON: Oxford University Press.

Cardinal, H., 2011. Nation-building as process: Reflections from a Nihiyow (Cree). *Canadian Review of Comparative Literature,* 34(1), pp. 65–77.

Castellano, M.B. and Archibald, L. 2007. Healing historic trauma: A report from the Aboriginal healing foundation. In: J. White, S. Wingert, D. Beavon and P. Maxim, eds. *Aboriginal policy research: Moving forward, making a difference,* vol. 4. Toronto: Thompson Educational Publishing, pp. 69–92.

Castleden, H., Garvin, T. and Huu-ay-aht First Nation, 2009. "Hishuk Tsawak" ["Everything is one/connected"]: A Huu-ay-aht worldview for seeing forestry in British Columbia, Canada. *Society & Natural Resources,* 22(9), pp. 789–804.

Castleden, H., Crooks, V.A., Hanlon, N. and Shuurman, N., 2010. Providers' perceptions of Aboriginal palliative care in British Columbia's rural interior. *Health and Social Care in the Community,* 18(5), pp. 483–91.

CBC News, 2016. Canada discriminates against children on reserves, tribunal rules, January 26. Available online at www.cbc.ca/news/aboriginal/canada-discriminates-against-children-on-reserves-tribunal-rules-1.3419480 (accessed January 26, 2016).

Cunsolo Willox, A., Harper, S., Edge, V., Landman, K., Houle, K., Ford, J. and Rigolet Inuit Community Government, 2013. The land enriches the soul: On climatic and environmental change, affect, and emotional health and well-being in Rigolet, Nunatsiavut, Canada. *Emotion, Space and Society,* 6, pp. 14–24.

Czyzewski, K., 2011. Colonialism as a broader social determinant of health. *International Indigenous Policy Journal,* 2(1), pp. 1–16.

D'Auria, G., Kimmett, C. and Smith, R., 2013. The summer BC's woods roared back. *The Tyee,* August 10. Available online at http://thetyee.ca/Life/2013/08/10/BC-Woods-Roar-Back/ (accessed January 30, 2016).

Deloria, V., 1995. *Red earth, white lies: Native Americans and the myth of scientific fact.* Golden, CO: Fulcrum Publishing.

First Nations Health Authority, 2014. *Our history, our health.* Available online at www.fnha.ca/wellness/our-history-our-health (accessed October 1, 2014).

Frohlich, K., Ross, N. and Richmond, C., 2006. Health disparities in Canada today: Some evidence and a theoretical framework. *Health Policy,* 79, pp. 132–43.

Gesler, W. and Kearns, R., 2002. *Culture/place/health.* London: Routledge.

Godlewska, A., Moore, J. and Bednasek, C.D., 2010. Cultivating ignorance of Aboriginal realities. *Canadian Geographer/Le Géographe canadien,* 54(4), pp. 417–40.

Government of Canada, 1996. *Royal Commission on Aboriginal Peoples* (5 vols). Ottawa: Government of Canada.

Government of Canada, 2015a. *Constitution Acts 1867 to 1982: Part II – Rights of Aboriginal Peoples of Canada*. Available online at http://laws-lois.justice.gc.ca/eng/Const/page-16.html#h-52 (accessed January 30, 2016).

Government of Canada, 2015b. *National inquiry into missing and murdered indigenous women and girls*. Available online at www.aadnc-aandc.gc.ca/eng/1448633299414/1448633350146 (accessed January 30, 2016).

Greenwood, M. and de Leeuw, S., 2007. Teachings from the land: Indigenous people, our health, our land, and our children. *Canadian Journal of Native Education*, 30(1), pp. 48–53.

Guilfoyle, J., Kelly, L. and St. Pierre-Hansen, N., 2008. Prejudice in medicine: Our role in creating health care disparities. *Canadian Family Physician*, 54(11), pp. 1511–18.

Gunn Allen, P., 1986. *The sacred hoop: Recovering the feminine in American Indian traditions*. Boston, MA: Beacon Press.

Harper, S.L., Edge, V.L., Cunsolo Willox, A. and Rigolet Inuit Community Government, 2012. Changing climate, changing health, changing stories' profile: Using an ecoHealth approach to explore impacts of climate change on Inuit health. *EcoHealth*, 9(1), pp. 89–101.

Harrison, P., 2009. Dispelling ignorance of residential schools. In: G. Younging, J. Dewar and M. Degagné, eds. *Response, responsibility and renewal: Canada's truth and reconciliation journey*. Ottawa: Aboriginal Healing Foundation, pp. 137–44.

Helfield, J. and Naiman, R., 2006. Keystone interactions: Salmon and bear in riparian forests of Alaska. *Ecosystems*, 9(2), pp. 167–80.

Houston, C.S. and Houston, S., 2000. The first smallpox epidemic on the Canadian Plains: In the fur-traders' words. *The Canadian Journal of Infectious Diseases*, 11(2), pp. 112–15.

Jackson, J.S., Knight, K.M. and Rafferty, J.A., 2010. Race and unhealthy behaviors: Chronic stress, the HPA axis, and physical and mental health disparities over the life course. *American Journal of Public Health*, 100(5), pp. 933–9.

James, C., Thomas Bernard, W., Este, D., Benjamin, J., Lloyd, B. and Turner, T., 2010. *Race & well-being: The lives, hopes and activism of African Canadians*. Halifax: Fernwood Publishing.

Jones, L., 2008. The distinctive characteristics and needs of domestic violence victims in a Native American community. *Journal of Family Violence*, 23(2), pp. 113–18.

Kalland, A., 2003. Environmentalism and images of the other. In: H. Selin and A. Kalland, eds. *Nature across cultures*. Norwell, MA: Kluwer Academic Publishers. pp. 1–18.

King, M., Smith, A. and Gracey, M., 2009. Indigenous health part 2: The underlying causes of the health gap. *The Lancet*, 374(9683), pp. 76–85.

King, T., 2012. *The inconvenient Indian: A curious account of Native people in North America*. Toronto: Doubleday Canada.

Kovach, M.E., 2010. *Indigenous methodologies: Characteristics, conversations, and contexts*. Toronto: University of Toronto Press.

Krieger, N., 2000. Discrimination and health. In: L. Berkman and I. Kawachi, eds. *Social epidemiology*. New York: Oxford University Press, pp. 36–75.

Latimer, M., Young, S., Dell, C. and Finley, G.A., 2012. Aboriginal children and physical pain: What do we know? *International Journal of Indigenous Health*, 9(1), pp. 7–14.

Long, K. 2014. The relationship between traditional cultural engagement and health: Data from Miawpukek First Nations regional health survey. Unpublished Master's thesis. Halifax: Dalhousie University.

Loppie, C., 2007. Learning from the grandmothers: Incorporating Indigenous principles in qualitative research. *Qualitative Health Research*, 14(2), pp. 276–84.

McEwen, B.S. and Gianaros, P.J., 2010. Central role of the brain in stress and adaptation: Links to socioeconomic status, health, and disease. *Annals of the New York Academy of Sciences*, 1186(1), pp. 190–222.

McGregor, D., 2005. Coming full circle: Indigenous knowledge, environment, and our future. *American Indian Quarterly*, 28(3), pp. 385–410.

Mehta, D., 2014. Family of Aboriginal girl with cancer can opt for traditional medicine: Judge. Macleans, November 15. Available online at www.macleans.ca/society/health/family-of-aboriginal-girl-with-cancer-can-opt-for-traditional-medicine-judge/ (accessed January 30, 2016).

Miller, J.R. ed., 1991. *Sweet promises: A reader on Indian–White relations in Canada.* Toronto: University of Toronto Press.

National Aboriginal Health Organization, 2014. *Ownership, Control, Access, and Possession (OCAP) or self-determination applied to research: A critical analysis of contemporary First Nations research and some options for First Nation communities.* Available online at www.naho.ca/documents/fnc/english/FNC_OCAPCriticalAnalysis.pdf (accessed November 25, 2014).

Palmater, P.D., 2011. Stretched beyond human limits: Death by poverty in First Nations. *Canadian Review of Social Policy*, 65–66, pp. 112–27.

Paradies, Y.C., 2006a. Beyond black and white essentialism, hybridity and indigeneity. *Journal of Sociology*, 42(4), pp. 355–67.

Paradies, Y.C., 2006b. A systematic review of empirical research on self-reported racism and health. *International Journal of Epidemiology*, 35(4), pp. 888–901.

Patterson, B., Bartlett, C., Moore, C., Roberts, A., Sock, L., Wien, F., Francis, S., Reading, C., Sark, R. and Wall, D., 2011. *Talking with their feet: Non-attendance of Aboriginal people at diabetes clinics.* Halifax: Atlantic Aboriginal Health Research Program.

Peters, F.J., 2004. Three myths about Aboriginals in Canadian cities. Presentation to the Centre for Aboriginal Economic Policy Research, Australia National University. Available online at http://caepr.anu.edu.au/sites/default/files/Seminars/presentations/Three%20Myths.pdf (accessed November 30, 2014).

Place, J., 2012. *The health of Aboriginal people residing in urban areas.* Prince George: National Collaborating Centre for Aboriginal Health.

Prosper, K., McMillan, L.J., Davis, A.A. and Moffitt, M., 2011. Returning to Netukulimk: Mi'kmaq cultural and spiritual connections with resource stewardship and self-governance. *International Indigenous Policy Journal*, 2(4). Available online at http://ir.lib.uwo.ca/cgi/viewcontent.cgi?article=1037&context=iipj (accessed January 30, 2016).

Provincial Court of Manitoba, 2014. In the matter of the Fatality Inquiries Act, and in the matter of Brian Lloyd Sinclair, deceased, December 12. Available online at www.manitobacourts.mb.ca/site/assets/files/1051/brian_sinclair_inquest_-_dec_14.pdf (accessed January 30, 2016).

Radkau, J., 2008. *Nature and power: A global history of the environment.* New York: Cambridge University Press.

Reading, J., 2003. A global model and national network for Aboriginal health research excellence. *Canadian Journal of Public Health*, 94(3), pp. 185–9.

Reading, J. and Nowgesic, E., 2002. Improving the health of future generations: The Canadian Institutes of Health Research Institute of Aboriginal Peoples' Health. *American Journal of Public Health*, 92(9), pp. 1396–400.

Reading, C. and Wien, F., 2009. *Health inequalities and social determinants of Aboriginal People's health*. Prince George, BC: National Collaborating Centre for Aboriginal Health. Available online at www.nccah-ccnsa.ca/Publications/Lists/Publications/Attachments/46/health_inequalities_EN_web.pdf (accessed January 30, 2016).

Rice, B and Snyder, A., 2008. Reconciliation in the context of a settler society: Healing the legacy of colonialism in Canada. In: M.B. Castellano, L. Archibald and M. Degagné, eds. *From truth to reconciliation: Transforming the legacy of residential schools*. Ottawa: Aboriginal Healing Foundation. pp. 45–65.

Richmond, C. and Ross, N., 2009. The determinants of First Nation and Inuit health: A critical population health approach. *Health & Place*, 15(2), pp. 403–11.

Richmond, C., Martin, D., Dean, L., Castleden, H. and Marsden, N., 2013. *Transforming networks: How ACADRE/NEAHR support for graduate students has impacted Aboriginal health research in Canada*. London, ON: Western University.

Royal Commission on Aboriginal Peoples, 1996. *People to people, nation to nation: Highlights from the report of the Royal Commission on Aboriginal Peoples*. Ottawa: Minister of Supply and Services Canada, Government of Canada.

Senese, L. and Wilson, K., 2013. Aboriginal urbanization and rights in Canada: Examining implications for health. *Social Science & Medicine*, 91, pp. 219–28.

Simpson, L., 2004. Listening to our ancestors: Rebuilding indigenous nations in the face of environmental destruction. In: J.A. Wainwright, ed. *Every grain of sand: Canadian perspectives on ecology and environment*. Waterloo, ON: Wilfred Laurier University Press. pp. 121–34.

Smith, L., 1999. *Decolonizing methodologies: Research and indigenous peoples*. London: Zed Books.

Spears, W., 2014. *Full circle: The Aboriginal Healing Foundation and the unfinished work of hope, healing, and reconciliation*. Ottawa: Aboriginal Healing Foundation.

Tang, S.Y. and Browne, A.J., 2008. "Race" matters: Racialization and egalitarian discourses involving Aboriginal people in the Canadian health care context. *Ethnicity & Health*, 13(2), pp. 109–27.

Tjepkema, M., 2002. The health of the off-reserve Aboriginal population. *Supplements to Health Reports*, 3, pp. 1–17. Available online at www.statcan.gc.ca/pub/82-003-s/2002001/pdf/82-003-s2002004-eng.pdf (accessed January 30, 2016).

Tobias, J.K. and Richmond, C.A., 2014. "That land means everything to us as Anishinaabe....": Environmental dispossession and resilience on the North Shore of Lake Superior. *Health & Place*, 29, pp. 26–33.

Truth and Reconciliation Commission of Canada, 2015. *Honouring the truth, reconciling for the future: Summary of the final report of the Truth and Reconciliation Commission of Canada*. Winnipeg: Truth and Reconciliation Commission of Canada.

Union of Nova Scotia Indians, 2013. *The health of the Nova Scotia Mi'kmaq population: Results from the 2008–10 survey for the on-reserve population*. Sydney, NSW: Union of Nova Scotia Indians.

United Nations, 2007. *United Nations Declaration on the Rights of Indigenous Peoples.* New York: United Nations.

Waldram, J., Herring, D. and Young, T., 2006. *Aboriginal health in Canada: Historical, cultural, and epidemiological perspectives*, 2nd ed. Toronto: University of Toronto Press.

Walters, K.L., Beltran, R., Huh, D. and Evans-Campbell, T., 2011. Dis-placement and dis-ease: Land, place, and health among American Indians and Alaska natives. In: L.M. Burton, S.P. Kemp, M. Leung, S.A. Matthews and D.T. Takeuchi, eds. *Communities, neighborhoods, and health.* New York: Springer. pp. 163–99.

Waziyatawin, 2009. *You can't un-ring a bell: Demonstrating contrition through action.* Ottawa: Aboriginal Healing Foundation. pp. 137–44.

Wesley-Esquimaux, C., 2007. The intergenerational transmission of historic trauma and grief. *Indigenous Affairs*, 4(6), pp. 6–11.

Wilson, K., 2003. Therapeutic landscapes and First Nations peoples: An exploration of culture, health, and place. *Health & Place*, 9(2), pp. 83–93.

Wilson, S., 2008. *Research is ceremony: Indigenous research methods.* Halifax: Fernwood Publishing.

World Health Organization. 2012. *Frequently asked questions.* Available online at www.who.int/suggestions/faq/en/index.html (accessed January 30, 2016).

Wylie, J., 2012. *Suicide prevention and Two-Spirited people.* Ottawa: National Aboriginal Health Organization.

4 Exploring the Intersections Between Violence, Place, and Mental Health in the Lives of Trans and Gender Nonconforming People in Canada

Cindy Holmes

Transgender and gender nonconforming (T/GNC) people represent some of the most creative, resilient, courageous, diverse, and beautiful people in Canada. They also represent one of the most marginalized groups in our society, and experience a variety of intersecting health inequities (Bauer et al., 2009). Although there is very limited Canadian-specific research, existing North American studies reveal that T/GNC people are more vulnerable to violence across their life span than the general population, experiencing multiple and pervasive forms of violence in various public and private places (White and Goldberg, 2006; Stotzer, 2009, 2014; Grant et al, 2011; Scheim et al., 2014). It also has been noted that gender surveillance, harassment, and violence may occur and be experienced differently by different T/GNC people, and in some places more than others (Namaste, 2000; Stotzer, 2014). As such, geography can provide a valuable lens for gaining a better understanding of violence, mental health, and emotional well-being within the lives of T/GNC individuals, particularly as different spaces and places can shape experiences of belonging, safety, exclusion, harassment, and violence.

Numerous mental health conditions have been associated with experiencing violence for all survivors (not only T/GNC people), including post-traumatic stress disorder, anxiety, depression, and suicide. Recent studies show extremely high rates of depression and suicide for T/GNC people who have experienced social injustice, including anti-trans stigma, harassment, as well as physical and sexual assault (Scanlon et al., 2010; Grant et al., 2011; Rotondi et al., 2011a, 2011b; Bauer et al., 2013). Furthermore, T/GNC individuals experience multiple barriers to accessing health care (Bauer et al., 2009; Heinz and MacFarlane, 2013) and violence intervention support (Namaste, 2000; White and Goldberg, 2006; National Coalition of Anti-Violence Programs, 2014). T/GNC people who are Indigenous, of color, sex workers, and/or living in poverty face some of the highest levels of discrimination and violence due to a combination of racism, poverty, and anti-transgender and/or sex worker stigma, discrimination, and injustice (Grant et al., 2011; Longman Marcellin et al., 2013a, 2013b; Scheim et al., 2013; World Health Organization et al., 2013).

In this chapter I provide an overview of some themes emerging in the literature about violence, place, and mental health in the lives of T/GNC people.

I bring together literature from geography, trans studies, social work, psychology, and health studies while identifying the benefit of an intersectional and interdisciplinary approach to understanding health equity issues in the lives of T/GNC people in Canada (for an introduction to intersectionality in health research, see Chapter 2). While there are many urgent health equity issues facing T/GNC youth, this chapter focuses on literature about the experiences of adults. Given the dominant social and cultural context that perpetuates harmful stereotypes about T/GNC people and privileges cisgender (non-trans) identities and expressions, I begin this chapter by discussing some key concepts and terms.

Understanding the Terminology

A person's identity is made up of many parts, including their gender identity, gender expression, biological sex, and sexual orientation. However, it is commonly believed that humans are either male or female, and that gender and sex are the same and unchangeable (For Ourselves: Reworking Gender Expression [FORGE], 2012a). These are harmful misconceptions, as gender is a spectrum and not determined by biology (chromosomes) and anatomy (genitals) (FORGE, 2012a).

Gender identity can be understood as a person's deeply felt sense of themselves as male, female, both, neither, something in-between, or beyond (FORGE, 2012a). As such, a person's sex can be different from their gender identity. Transgender, or trans, is an umbrella term that describes a wide range of diverse people whose gender identity and/or gender expression differs from what they were assigned at birth. It may include those who identify as transsexual, "Two-Spirit," bigender, genderqueer, cross-dressers, gender variant, gender fluid, or simply man or woman (Grant et al., 2011). Sometimes, an asterisk is included (trans*) to actively include non-binary and/or non-static gender identities such as genderqueer (National Film Board of Canada, 2014). (As mentioned in Chapter 3, the term "Two-Spirit" is used by some Indigenous people to describe the diverse roles and identities of lesbian, gay, bisexual, trans, queer, and/or gender-diverse Indigenous people in North America.) "Gender nonconforming" refers to individuals who express their gender in ways that differ from societal expectations and/or stereotypes related to gender (Grant et al., 2011). Some gender nonconforming people identify with the broad umbrella category of "trans," while others do not.

"LGBTQ2S" is another umbrella category to represent lesbian, gay, bisexual, transgender, queer and Two-Spirit people of diverse sexual orientations and gender identities. Although commonly used, this umbrella term can have a homogenizing effect, blurring the differences between gender identity and sexual orientation.

Importantly, these terms and definitions do not include all of the many identities or lived experiences of T/GNC people. For example, some trans people choose to transition medically by taking hormones and/or having surgery, while others do not. Some choose to socially and legally transition by changing their name, clothing, hairstyle, mannerisms, and/or social roles, while others do not (National Film Board of Canada, 2014). In other words, identifying as trans, transgender, or other terms within this umbrella category does not depend on criteria such as surgery or hormone treatment status, but can be decided upon only by individuals themselves (National Film Board of Canada, 2014).

Transphobia is an "irrational fear of, aversion to, or discrimination against people whose gendered identities, appearances, or behaviors deviate from societal norms" (Serano, 2007, p. 12), and is produced through multiple forms of social exclusion and violence. It exists within a context of cisnormativity, which refers to the expectation that all people are – and should be – cisgender, and the belief that transgender identities or bodies are less "authentic" or "normal" than cisgender identities and bodies (Bauer et al., 2009). Cisgender refers to someone who identifies with the gender they were assigned at birth, and is the term used to acknowledge the societal privilege of those people who are not T/GNC (National Film Board of Canada, 2014). Considering this, transphobia and cisnormativity can be understood as social determinants of health. (These specific social determinants were not outlined in Chapter 2 when this approach was introduced. However, they are highly relevant and influential in shaping the lives of T/GNC people.)

What We Know About Canadian Trans People

Our knowledge about the social demographics of T/GNC people in Canada is very limited. Much of the data we rely on in our research, education, and service delivery with T/GNC people are based on communities in the USA (Bauer et al., 2012; Heinz and MacFarlane, 2013). However, some recent research in Canada does provide a glimpse of who trans people are in different regions of the country. The Trans PULSE Project – a community-based research project investigating the impact of social exclusion and discrimination on the health of trans people in Ontario, Canada – conducted a survey of 433 trans people aged 16 or over in Ontario. This project revealed that while most trans people had either a male/masculine or female/feminine identity, about one in five identified in some way as both, neither, or gender fluid (Coleman et al., 2011), and that the "participants identified across a broad range of sexual orientation identities" (Bauer et al., 2010, p. 1). This survey also found that geographically, trans people live in communities across the province, and "despite the fact that the majority of trans services are located in Metropolitan Toronto, 68 percent of trans Ontarians live outside that postal code area" (2010, p. 2). The majority of respondents (88 percent) identified as white Canadian, American or European, while 7 percent identified as First Nations, Métis and Inuit, and 22 percent indicated a range of other ethnoracial identities including East Asian, South Asian, Southeast Asian, black Canadian, black American, black African, Latin American, Middle Eastern and "other" (Longman Marcellin et al., 2013b; Scheim et al., 2013).

In a recent community needs assessment with 54 trans respondents on Vancouver Island, British Columbia, 43 percent identified as female-to-male (FTM), 39 percent identified as male-to-female (MTF), while 18 percent described their gender identity as either transgender, bigender, mixed gender, or genderqueer, and did not select a gender-specific referent (Heinz and MacFarlane, 2013, p. 4). Most respondents lived in the Greater Victoria area (68 percent), while others were located throughout the island including remote rural locations, as well as neighboring islands. In terms of ethnicity, 67 percent were of British descent, 47 percent of other European descent, 13 percent of Aboriginal descent, and 9 percent of East Asian or South Asian descent (2013, p. 4).

This brief description of survey results is not meant to provide comprehensive or representative sociodemographic statistics about the diverse identities of T/GNC people in Canada, but rather to share some of the recent data collected by trans-Canadian community research projects seeking to learn more about the sociodemographics and lived experiences of T/GNC people in Canada.

Setting the Context

It is important to place this research topic within the past and present context of the regulatory power of psychiatric discourses. As Canadian scholars Nick Mulé, Andrea Daley, and the Rainbow Health Network state, "the continued classification of diverse sexual and gender identities and expressions as clinical disorders constitutes the ongoing surveillance, pathologizing and regulating of otherwise variant expressions of sexuality and gender" (2010, p. 11; see also Daley and Mulé, 2014).

Transgender identities first appeared in the Diagnostic and Statistical Manual of Mental Disorders (DSM) of the American Psychiatric Association in 1980, and were categorized as "gender identity disorder" until the most recent revision (DSM-5), which replaced "Gender Identity Disorder" with the term "Gender Dysphoria" – with the stated intention to avoid stigma for people whose gender at birth is contrary to the one with which they identify (American Psychiatric Association, 2013). The dominant discourse surrounding the DSM suggests that it provides mental health clinicians with a common language, or "diagnostic criteria," for accurate and consistent diagnosis of mental health "disorders." However, many reject the DSM's pathology and contest its legitimacy, arguing it is a power-laden classification system that institutionalizes arbitrary constructions of normalcy or abnormalcy, and reflects the interests and assumptions of dominant social groups. In this way, the DSM reproduces hegemonic notions of gender, race, ethnicity, class, (dis)ability, and sexuality (Cermele et al., 2001; LeFrancoise et al., 2013), ultimately contributing to stigma towards diverse gender expressions and trans identities.

Erasure

Unfortunately, a legacy of negative academic research conducted on T/GNC people also exists, as well as the erasure of trans people from knowledge production (Namaste, 2000). Montreal-based activist scholar Viviane K. Namaste (2000) first proposed the framework of erasure to describe "the conceptual and institutional relations through which transsexual and transgender people disappear from view" (p. 137). She defines erasure as the "defining condition of how transsexuality is managed in culture and institutions, a condition that ultimately inscribes transsexuality as impossible" (pp. 4–5). Namaste's work has been critically important for theorizing and documenting the way trans people are made invisible through discourse and institutionalized practices, and excluded from social service and health care agencies, and anti-violence organizing.

Researchers from the Trans PULSE Project argue that transphobia is an insufficient explanatory framework for understanding the processes that exclude trans people from accessible and appropriate health services (Bauer et al., 2009). Informed by Namaste's work, they state that

> while transphobia may be a useful concept in understanding the motivations underlying the actions of individuals, its use as an explanation has obscured the more systematic nature of trans marginalization by isolating the particular problem to acts rather than embedding the problem in broader cultural and political contexts. (Bauer et al., 2009, p. 350)

Based on qualitative data from focus groups with 85 trans community members, Bauer and colleagues' (2009) health research documented how the systemic erasure of trans people occurs in many ways, both through informational and institutional contexts. They identified two key sites of erasure in health care contexts (which can be applied to other contexts as well):

1) informational erasure – which is evident in the lack of knowledge, research, and knowledge synthesis about trans people's lives, and in the minimization of the importance of trans-related research; and
2) institutional erasure – which occurs through policies and practices that impose cisnormative gender binaries.

Bauer et al. (2009) also found that erasure could be both active and passive, with active erasure including visible discomfort by service providers, refusal of service, and violent responses with the intent to harm or intimidate. Passive erasure involves a lack of knowledge about trans people and their health needs, and the assumption that their lives and health needs are not relevant or important (Bauer et al., 2009). The main finding from this research is that trans people experience profound social exclusion in their daily lives (Bauer et al., 2009).

Kwakwaka'wakw activist and scholar Sarah Hunt (2015) draws on both Indigenous and decolonial theorizing about the disappearance of Indigenous people through settler colonialism, and Namaste's work on erasure, to address the way that colonial gender binaries function as key tools of settler colonialism. As she explains:

> At the heart of the colonization of Turtle Island lies the settler colonial project of native disappearance, which is necessary for the development of a prosperous settler society. Colonial laws and ideologies have entailed the imposition of gendered and racialized categories, which have been used to ensure fewer and fewer natives over time. (105)

She notes that the "erasure and invisibility of those we now call Two-Spirit and transgender people was accomplished through ... combined ideological, socio-legal and spatialized enforcements of colonial gender norms for 'Indians'" (106). Importantly, Hunt (2015) points out that some Indigenous self-determination frameworks and Indigenous women's organizations in Canada have also relied on these colonial gender categories, and as a result their frameworks and approaches often fail to account for Indigenous trans and Two-Spirit people's lives.

While T/GNC communities have been erased in knowledge production and generally understudied, research which *has* included trans people often has been conducted through processes that are stigmatizing and alienating, most being conducted in university or clinical settings without community input (Bauer et al., 2009). This is also combined with a history of research about trans people by cisgender researchers in Canada and around the globe that has been paternalistic, voyeuristic, pathologizing, and unethical – such as collecting data without consent, frequently neglecting to report research findings back to communities, and failing to disseminate the research in meaningful ways that are useful for trans communities (see the discussion in Bauer et al., 2009; Travers et al., 2013; Pyne, 2014). Similar harmful health research practices have been widely practiced on other marginalized communities, including Indigenous people (see Chapter 3), low-income and poor people (see Chapter 7), sex workers, and people of color. Consequently, this has produced skepticism and mistrust towards academic, cisgender researchers, as well as those who are white and middle class. Being aware of this context of erasure and harmful research practices with T/GNC people is important for understanding the lack of research about their lives, as well as the implications for current research in the area of mental health, violence, and place.

Violence in the Lives of T/GNC People

Research has shown that violence in the lives of T/GNC people across the globe takes many forms, including hate or bias-motivated violence, intimate partner violence and/or domestic violence, and sexual assault (National Coalition of Anti-Violence Programs, 2014; Stotzer, 2014). These forms of violence often include transphobic elements, and may be combined with sexist, racist, economic or classist, ableist and homophobic tactics, including for example:

> [A]ssault, mutilation or denigration of body parts such as chest, genitals, and hair that signify specific cultural notions of gender ... withdrawal of financial support for trans-specific care (e.g. electrolysis, hormones, surgeries) ... ridicule of cross-gendered behaviour or appearance; [trans-specific] threats to limit or prohibit access to children or services ... and threats to reveal the victim's gender identity to employers, financial aid workers, health care workers, immigration personnel, or anyone else with possible influence or control over the survivor's well being. (White and Goldberg, 2006, p. 126)

Many challenges exist in accurately determining the rates and scope of violence due to a lack of reliable data sources, underreporting, problematic tracking mechanisms, sampling research methodologies, inconsistent data analysis methods, the conflation of gender and sexual orientation, and diverse definitions of violence used among researchers and organizations (White and Goldberg, 2006; Goldberg and White, 2011; Ristock, 2011; FORGE, 2012b; Greenberg, 2012; Stotzer, 2014). For example, a lack of data due to underreporting is a result of many T/GNC individuals' fear of transphobic and racist responses from police, victim assistance programs, health care providers, and crisis counseling support services (White and Goldberg, 2006; Grant et al., 2011; FORGE, 2012a; National Coalition of Anti-Violence Programs, 2014; Stotzer, 2014). In addition, in a transphobic social context, many people are not out as trans, making it difficult to identify a large random sample and demonstrate a clear and accurate prevalence rate.

Regardless of difficulties in determining actual prevalence rates, it has been shown that violence in the lives of T/GNC individuals is pervasive, ongoing, and severe across the globe (Stotzer, 2014, p. 51). Stotzer (2014) notes that the first quantitative study of transphobic bias crimes across the European Union (see Turner et al., 2009) found that in a sample of more than 2,500 transgender people, 70 percent reported experiencing some type of verbal or physical violence because of their gender identity. More specifically, it is anti-trans or hate-motivated violence that is the most frequently recorded form of violence experienced by T/GNC people. For example, it has been found that reports from T/GNC people of hate violence in the USA have increased by 21 percent since 2012 (National Coalition of Anti-Violence Programs, 2014), while another US-based study on hate-motivated violence against T/GNC people found that 60 percent of all trans people had experienced it (Moran and Sharpe, 2004).

Research has documented various forms of hate-motivated violence against T/GNC individuals including:

- threats and harassment;
- hate speech (via letter, e-mail, telephone, or in person);
- vandalism;
- physical attacks;
- assault with a weapon;
- sexual violence; and
- murder.

Transphobic violence also intersects with other forms of systemic oppression and violence such as colonialism, racism, classism, ableism, and state and police violence. For example, studies in the USA (Stotzer, 2009) and Europe (Turner et al., 2009) suggest that trans women (MTF transgender individuals), as opposed to trans men (FTM individuals) may be more at risk of experiencing transphobic violence (White and Goldberg, 2006; National Coalition of Anti-Violence Programs, 2014; Stotzer, 2014). Although most studies of anti-LGBTQ2S violence have tended to overlook the intersectional nature of race, class, gender, ability, and sexuality in the experiences of victims or perpetrators of hate-motivated violence, some research suggests that trans women of color and trans Indigenous and Two-Spirit women are more at risk of violence than other LGBTQ people – with a large percentage of transgender murder victims internationally being trans women of color (White and Goldberg, 2006, p. 125; National Coalition of Anti-Violence Programs, 2014).

Violence against T/GNC individuals may be perpetrated by strangers, but more often it is perpetrated by those who are known to the victim, including co-workers, neighbors, employers, acquaintances, ex-lovers, community members, and even friends (White and Goldberg, 2006; Grant et al., 2011; Stotzer, 2014). The National Transgender Discrimination Survey (Grant et al., 2011) in the USA found that 50 percent of respondents had experienced sexual assault, with the majority being perpetrated by intimate partners, family members, and others known to the individual. These findings disrupt common understandings of trans-specific violence, as some "reports indicate that a significant number of trans survivors knew the perpetrator ... which challenges conventional understandings of hate crimes as 'public' and distinct from family and relationship violence" (White and Goldberg, 2006, p. 125; also see Stotzer, 2014). Research conducted through the Transgender Sexual Violence Project by FORGE (an American national education, advocacy, and support umbrella organization for trans people and significant others, family, friends, and allies), found that 29 percent of respondents had been sexually assaulted by an intimate partner (Munson and Cook-Daniels, 2015). Another US study conducted by The Survivor Project (a volunteer-run organization addressing the needs of intersex and trans survivors of domestic and sexual violence in Portland, Oregon), found that 50 percent of respondents had been raped or assaulted by an intimate partner; yet as commonly found among this population, only 62 percent (31 percent of the total sample) of those raped or assaulted actually identified as being survivors of domestic violence when asked directly (Courvant and Cook-Daniels, 1998, p. 2). Overall, there are very few empirical studies which have explicitly examined intimate partner violence or domestic violence in the lives of T/GNC people, and none of these have taken place in Canada (Courvant and Cook-Daniels, 1998; Brown, 2011; Grant et al., 2011; National Coalition of Anti-Violence Programs, 2014). Nicola Brown (2007, 2011) explores the experiences of trans people living in Canada and the USA who have been abused and/or abusive in their intimate relationships. She argues that the traditional gender-based heterosexual model is insufficient for understanding violence perpetrated by, or against, trans people in intimate relationships. She calls for community initiatives to raise awareness by discussing the complexities of power, privilege, marginalization, and dynamics of abuse.

Within Canada and beyond, very little research has examined intimate partner violence in the lives of Indigenous trans and Two-Spirit people. However, some Canadian literature has included general discussion of trans and Two-Spirit experiences of intimate partner violence or domestic violence (for example, see White and Goldberg, 2006; Brown, 2007, 2011; Ristock et al. 2010; Goldberg and White, 2011; Ristock, 2011; Taylor and Ristock, 2011). Catherine Taylor and Janice Ristock (2011) reviewed studies which have looked at intimate partner violence experienced by Indigenous LGBTQ and Two-Spirit people, showing that these studies have documented experiences of multiple forms of physical and sexual violence, historical trauma, and state violence. Research conducted by the Canadian Aboriginal Two-Spirit and LGBTQ Migration, Mobility, and Health Research Project revealed that 23 out of 25 participants in Vancouver, British Columbia indicated that they had experienced domestic violence, while 19 out of 24 participants in Winnipeg, Manitoba reported they had experienced some form of violence in a same-sex relationship (Ristock et al., 2010, 2011). As Taylor and Ristock (2011) describe, this context of violence is "linked to and supported by larger social structures that create and sustain inequalities and disadvantages" (p. 309), and as a result, anti-violence efforts must be allied with anti-colonial Indigenous strategies to oppose state violence.

Research conducted by trans people and their allies has addressed more often the intersections between multiple forms of interpersonal, hate-motivated, institutional, police, and state violence (Namaste, 2000; Goldberg and White, 2011). For example, Joshua Goldberg and Caroline White (2011) note that the history of trans anti-violence organizing in North America has been different from the dominant feminist anti-violence movement in a number of ways:

> Trans activism was led in large part by racialized working poor and working class sex trade workers and night club entertainers, many of whom identified as male-to-female (MTF). As a consequence, the ways that

"violence" and "safety" were tackled by trans activists were not limited in the same ways as dominant feminism; police violence, prison violence, violence against sex trade workers and people living on the street, violence in the psychiatric system, deaths resulting from refusal of emergency services, and other manifestations of systemic as well as interpersonal class–race–gender violence were high priorities for many early transgender organizers in urban areas throughout North America. (2011, p. 57)

Although not widespread, some research has acknowledged the interconnections between racialization and anti-transgender stigma, and some scholars and activists have applied an intersectional approach, an Indigenous gender-based analysis and/or a decolonial approach (White and Goldberg, 2006; Taylor, 2009; Ristock et al., 2010, 2011; Goldberg and White, 2011; Grant et al., 2011; Taylor and Ristock, 2011; Longman Marcellin et al., 2013a; Scheim et al., 2013; Hunt, 2015). Such approaches not only hold the potential to shed much-needed light on the diverse experiences of violence among a diverse community of T/GNC individuals, but they also encourage us to critique hegemonic framings and expand our theorizing and politics to account for the interlocking nature of the different forms and spaces of violence.

Trans Health Geographies: The Significance of Place

Health geography "considers the significance for physical and mental health of *interactions between people and their environment*. It investigates why *space* and *place* are important for health variation in human populations" (Curtis, 2010, p. 3; emphasis in original). A health geographic perspective can provide a unique understanding regarding the ways that various social and spatial contexts, landscapes, and environments enhance or harm T/GNC people's emotional well-being or mental health. For example, it is important to understand and identify the places where T/GNC people experience transphobic discrimination, harassment, and violence, and the places they avoid to maintain their safety; as well as those places where they do experience a sense of belonging, well-being, and safety. Although a geographic perspective can be valuable in addressing social, health, and spatial inequities among T/GNC populations, no health geographic work exists per se in Canada or elsewhere that explicitly explores theorizing and/or the lived experiences of T/GNC people.

Although the focus on health is not explicit, some geographers have begun to explore the relationships between space, place, and T/GNC people. Namaste's (1996) article is one of the most important in the field of geography, which examines the issue of gender and regulation of public space. Drawing on Namaste's work, Kath Browne (2004) was one of the first queer geographers to examine the violent regulation of gender nonconformity in public spaces such as bathrooms. Catherine Nash (2010) and Petra Doan (2007, 2010) are two other geographers who have written about gender, trans people, and place. In examining the regulation of public space, Doan (2010) has looked at how individuals who "transgress gender norms experience a tyranny of gender that shapes nearly every aspect of their public and private lives" (2010, p. 635). Cisgender looks of disapproval, whispers, and long stares work to create an environment of discomfort and make T/GNC people feel out of place in everyday spaces. As such, Doan calls for more geographers to "explore the parameters of the tyranny of gender as it *constrains* behavior in a spectrum of spaces and localities" (2010, p. 649, emphasis added). A pivotal special issue on "Trans Geographies" published in *Gender, Place & Culture* (Browne et al., 2010) points out that despite a few important exceptions (Namaste, 2000; Browne, 2004, 2005; Doan, 2007; Nash, 2007), geographical inquiry in general has assumed male/female and man/woman binaries, and has not fully engaged with queer and trans theorizing about gender diversity; neither has it addressed the lives and experiences of T/GNC people (Browne et al., 2010, p. 573). While the articles in this special issue contribute significantly to the field of trans geographies, few geography researchers have explored these issues further since its publication.

Other researchers have pointed to the importance of studying how T/GNC people change their behavior and avoid certain public places in response to transphobic harassment and/or violence (see Taylor, 2009; Scheim et al., 2013; Stotzer, 2014). Jody Herman's (2013) research surveyed 93 T/GNC people in Washington, DC about their experiences in gendered public restrooms, and found that 70 percent of survey respondents reported being denied access, and had been verbally harassed or physically assaulted in public restrooms (Herman, 2013). She argues that we have "built minority stressors for transgender and gender non-conforming people into our very environment due to our reliance on gender segregation in public facilities" (Herman, 2013, p. 67).

Clearly, gender segregation, place, and a fear of harassment and violence impact the health and well-being of T/GNC people. Through examining the relationship between trans people's avoidance of public spaces, transition status, and past experiences of violence, the Trans PULSE Project (Scheim et al., 2013) found that the majority of participants avoided using public washrooms for fear of transphobic harassment or violence. Among those who had begun or completed transition, 83 percent had avoided at least one space, compared to one-quarter of those who had not begun medical or social transition (Scheim et al., 2013). Bathroom avoidance has serious implications for physical health and emotional well-being, as it can lead T/GNC people to avoid a wide range of public spaces (such as schools, recreation facilities, stores, health care settings), simply because the bathrooms are unsafe (Scheim et al., 2013).

Emphasizing the important connection between health and place, the Aboriginal Two-Spirit and LGBTQ Migration, Mobility, and Health Research Project conducted in Winnipeg and Vancouver examined the impacts of moving on health and well-being as well as the use of, and recommendations for, services for Aboriginal Two-Spirit and LGBTQ people (Ristock et al., 2010, 2011). In addition to social exclusion resulting from homophobia and transphobia (including from some Aboriginal communities and within housing programs), the participants in this study also described experiences of racism (when looking for housing, employment, and health services) as being among the negative impacts of moving (Ristock et al., 2010).

Although some participants from this project indicated that they had experienced suicidal feelings because of having little opportunity for housing or employment, many of those moving to Vancouver described positive outcomes, including increased well-being due to reduced social isolation, and opportunities to connect with other Two-Spirit people. Importantly, the study noted that "the resilience in the transgender community was enormous, not only did they physically change their living environments, they also changed their physical selves; some going on this journey without family support" (Ristock et al., 2011, p. 18). The research highlights the importance of a sense of community belonging and its connection to the health and well-being of Aboriginal Two-Spirit and LGBTQ people. In both Vancouver and Winnipeg, "participants moved in search of something and in order to create community and a feeling of belonging" (Ristock et al., 2010, p. 34). In sum, the researchers identified two key themes regarding how moving impacted the health and well-being of the participants:

1) moving in search of a "home" – described as being a "sense of belonging that can come with finding a safe, accepting community ... rooted in relationships ... that people have with each other and with geography"; and
2) disconnection – as a result of the impact of forced mobility through colonization, adoption or foster care, and/or residential schools which are also "connected to experiences of homophobia and transphobia in home communities and experiences of racism in LGBTQ communities" (2011, p. 19).

Mental Health and Well-being

The World Health Organization (WHO) (2014) defines mental health as:

a state of well-being in which the individual realizes his or her own abilities, can cope with the normal stresses of life, can work productively and fruitfully, and is able to make a contribution to his or her community. (n.p.)

It also stresses that:

a climate that respects and protects basic civil, political, socio-economic and cultural rights is fundamental to mental health promotion. Without the security and freedom provided by these rights, it is very difficult to maintain a high level of mental health. (n.p.)

For T/GNC people, the social and spatial contexts of injustice, discrimination, and violence seriously erode mental health and well-being (Grant et al., 2011; Bauer et al., 2013).

Mental health issues emerging as a result of systemic oppression and marginalization, accumulated stigma, and discrimination can be referred to as "minority stress" (Meyer, 2003; Herman, 2013). Often, mental health issues arising from minority stress are misinterpreted by mental health service providers as resulting from an individual's gender identity or expression (McIntyre et al., 2011). Qualitative research conducted by the Trans PULSE Project found that trans participants reported

> a "double bind," in which health care providers were not able to see mental health issues as distinct from gender identity, and tended to either attribute mental health conditions to a client's gender identity or to attribute their gender identity to their mental health condition. (Rotondi et al., 2011b, p. 151)

McIntyre et al. (2011) note that, "the medical model typically neither accounts for nor responds to the impact of the social context of an individual's life and social determinants of health and well-being" (p. 182). Their research with mental health service providers in the Greater Toronto Area of Ontario found a tendency to rely on mental health practices and interventions governed by the medical model, which often results in mental health providers overlooking the social contexts of T/GNC people's lives (McIntyre et al., 2011).

T/GNC people experience poorer mental health outcomes compared with cisgender people, and this is directly related to experiences of discrimination associated with living in a transphobic and cisnormative environment (Bauer et al., 2013). Research has consistently shown that trans people experience high levels of depression, suicidal ideation, and suicide attempts (Scanlon et al., 2010; Rotondi et al., 2011a, 2011b; McNeil et al., 2012; Bauer et al., 2013; Heinz and MacFarlane, 2013; Scheim et al., 2013). Importantly, Bauer et al. (2013) in the Trans PULSE Project have pointed out that while most literature acknowledges these high levels of depression and suicide within trans communities, there has been limited examination of the relationship between experiences of trans-related social injustice and suicide. The findings from their research highlight a number of protective factors that have been shown to reduce depression, the risk of suicide for trans people, and improve their mental health. Some of these include:

- timely, accessible, and affordable transition-related health care;
- social and family support;
- strong parental support for T/GNC youth;
- having one's gender affirmed, in the case of trans women; and
- sexual satisfaction for trans men (Bauer et al., 2013).

Clear correlations exist between experiences of violence and various forms of mental health distress, including depression, post-traumatic stress disorder, increased anxiety, suicidal ideation, suicide attempts, and substance misuse (Stotzer, 2014). Recent studies in Canada and the USA have found extremely high rates of suicide for those who have experienced transphobic-related harassment, physical, and sexual assault (Scanlon et al., 2010; Bauer et al., 2013). The Trans PULSE Project found that "those who had experienced transphobic physical or sexual violence were seven times more likely to have attempted suicide in the past year" (Bauer et al., 2013, p. 42). The National Transgender Discrimination Survey in the USA found that visual noncon-formers (44 percent), and those who are generally out about their transgender status (44 percent), were two groups at higher risk for attempted suicide (Grant et al., 2011).

Access to needed health and social services is another issue related to T/GNC peoples' mental health, particularly barriers in accessing substance use and addiction services, homeless shelters, transition houses, and sexual assault services, as well as mental health, harm reduction, and HIV intervention services (Lombardi and van Servellen, 2000; Namaste, 2000; White and Goldberg, 2006; Bauer et al., 2009; McNeil et al., 2012). In many cases, this has included an actual *denial* of health care, as well as a *refusal* to approve gender-affirming medical procedures (Namaste, 2000; McNeil et al., 2012; Rutherford et al., 2012). These barriers in accessing health and mental health support services have been discussed in recent literature, generally focusing on the relationship between access to transition-related health needs, mental health system gatekeeping, and T/GNC people's mental health; and a lack of trans-competent mental health service providers and discrimination in the delivery of services. Both of these themes are a result of systemic, institutional transphobia, and cisnormativity in health service contexts that contribute to the invisibility of T/GNC people and lack of provider knowledge (Bauer et al., 2009; McIntyre et al., 2011; Heinz and MacFarlane, 2013; Taylor, 2013).

Mental health service utilization rates in trans communities have not been widely documented in Canada. Some have suggested that this might be a result of the "complex relationship between medical service providers and trans individuals, who may be accessing mental health services for medical (transition-related) reasons rather than for mental health concerns" (McIntyre et al., 2011, p. 174). One Canadian study – the Vancouver Island Trans* Needs Assessment – documented whether respondents identified a need for mental health services, as well as their experiences with accessing mental health care (Heinz and MacFarlane, 2013). When asked to identify their personal top health care need, few prioritized mental health care access, instead citing general health care, social support, and public education and acceptance as the top needs (Heinz and MacFarlane, 2013, p. 4). Significantly, those who identified these top needs discussed specific priorities for quick, affordable access to surgeries within the province; local, speedy access to trans-specific medical expertise; and information about long-term hormone use (Heinz and MacFarlane, 2013). This finding is interesting, as other studies have documented the relationship between a lack of access to supportive gender affirming or transition-related health care, and depression and suicide – as well as the correlation between societal acceptance and social inclusion, social support, and mental health or well-being (Bauer et al., 2009; Rotondi et al., 2011a, 2011b; MacNeil et al., 2012; Bauer et al., 2013).

In their survey, the researchers with the Vancouver Island Trans* Needs Assessment distinguished between mental health care needed for reasons related to gender identity, and mental health care needed for other reasons. Most of the respondents (69 percent) indicated that they had accessed mental health care related to gender identity (Heinz and MacFarlane, 2013), and of these respondents, 49 percent said that they had to educate a mental health provider about trans issues. Some individuals explained that it was only because this is a requirement for access to gender-affirming surgeries or hormones. Only 24 percent of the respondents in this study indicated that they had mental health issues, but the majority (63 percent) reported having either considered (35 percent) or attempted (28 percent) suicide. So, while mental health care access was not prioritized as a top need, and the majority of respondents did not identify as living with mental health issues, their experiences of considering and attempting suicide reveal a more complex story about trans people's mental health and well-being. This finding suggests that the language or category of *mental health* and *mental health care* may not be meaningful or helpful for understanding the true lived experiences of emotional distress and well-being in trans communities, given their association with pathologizing psychiatric and biomedical discourses.

Significantly, 72 percent of respondents in the Trans* Needs Assessment study had to travel away from their home to obtain gender-affirming, trans-related care (primarily for surgical care), which included traveling to the mainland of British Columbia, other provinces in Canada, and other countries (Heinz and MacFarlane, 2013, p. 5). This lack of access to gender-affirming medical procedures is a significant part of the context of social injustice in the lives of T/GNC people in Canada – one which has significant harmful effects on psychological health and well-being (Bauer et al., 2013).

The dominant discourses within psychiatry and psychology continue to have a profoundly negative impact on T/GNC people's lives. They have pathologized gender diversity and constructed T/GNC people as "disordered" and "ill." Moreover, media discourses have perpetuated these stereotypes. This context presents a burden for T/GNC people and their loved ones, and affects our ability to speak openly about the mental health and well-being of T/GNC people. In addition, within the academic health literature there has been minimal research and writing about trans resiliency, and few studies to date have examined what factors promote resilience (Testa et al., 2014). In response to these harmful dominant framings of trans people as "miserable and full of rejection, depression and despair," in 2008 and 2009 a volunteer group of trans people and allies in Vancouver decided to organize two community events for T/GNC people "based on the radical concept that trans people can be happy" (Neo Eamas and MacFarlane. 2014, p. 137). As Tien Neo Eamas and Devon MacFarlane (2014) describe, the organizers sought to "inspire others to find ways to promote the revolutionary idea of celebrating trans people" (137) and promote trans happiness, through organizing a "Happy Tranny Day" in 2008 and "Gender Euphoria Day" in 2009. These kinds of creative, grassroots community strategies are rarely included in discussions about community mental health interventions, yet it is critically important to make them visible and highlight the way that socially marginalized groups creatively address health, well-being, and resiliency outside of professionalized and institutionalized mental health services.

Frameworks: Intersectionality and Critical Trans Politics

An approach informed by intersectional, critical trans, and anti-colonial theories challenges us to think critically about what counts as a health issue or form of violence, and how cisnormative and colonial gender norms limit our imaginations, research strategies, and health prevention and intervention initiatives. These approaches also challenge de-raced and de-classed understandings of social exclusion and inclusion, belonging, health, well-being, and safety in the lives of T/GNC people. We can apply intersectional theory (see Chapter 2) to examine the way that interlocking oppressions may interact to increase health inequities or vulnerabilities to illness or violence. We can draw on intersectional theorizing, critical trans, and anti-colonial theorizing to look more in-depth at how these health inequities are socially and spatially produced, how they are interlocking, how we are connected to these systems, and what can be done to change them.

From the previous discussion of the existing literature, we can begin to see that to understand the connections between violence, mental health, and place in the lives of T/GNC people, and how these conditions of marginalization are produced, scholars and activists need to take up an interdisciplinary approach that acknowledges various social determinants of health in trans communities. Here, intersectionality, informed by critical trans and anti-colonial theories, supports us to resist universalist models of identity and "one-size-fits-all" approaches to health promotion, anti-violence organizing, health and trauma support service provision, and research. It moves away from additive approaches, and helps us to see how the conditions and spaces of violence and marginalization are produced simultaneously.

Critical trans politics call for an intersectional framework that places the lived experiences of poor, working-class, trans people of color and Indigenous people at the center of theorizing and organizing (particularly racialized poor trans women) (Namaste, 2000; Spade, 2011; Johnson, 2013). Trans legal scholar Dean Spade (2011) has called for a critical trans approach that draws from the insights of critical race feminist and intersectional theo-ries, but extends beyond by centering on resistance to systems that are most harmful to trans people. This "raises demands like an end to wealth and pov-erty, an end to immigration enforcement, and the abolition of all forms of imprisonment (immigration, criminal punishment, medical, and psychiatric)" (Nicols, 2012, n.p.). Spade suggests that a critical trans politics offers social justice movements "a particular frame for understanding how processes of gendered racialization are congealed in violent institutions" (Nicols, 2012, n.p.). Such approaches and frameworks would generate valuable knowledge regarding the injustices experienced by T/GNC individuals, as well as on the complex interconnections between violence, place, and mental health among this diverse community.

Directions for Health Geographers

The contexts of erasure and harmful research about T/GNC and Two-Spirit people conducted by cisgender researchers clearly indicate that future research by health geographers must begin with a critical examination of cisnormativ-ity as a social determinant of health, and one that is produced simultane-ously with other systems of oppression. It is important for health geographers to understand that cisnormativity, and the societal enforcement of gender norms and related violence, impacts the health of *all* Canadians, not only T/GNC Canadians. Most research published in health geography (and geog-raphy more broadly) assumes a gender and sex binary, and cisgender iden-tity as the most natural and normal. Health geographers must acknowledge gender diversity, and resist these problematic cisnormative assumptions as part of a wider commitment to investigating the sociospatial conditions that produce health inequities in Canada.

Drawing on the work by Namaste (2000), Trans PULSE (Bauer et al., 2009), and Hunt (2015), researchers can take up the concept of erasure as a framework for understanding the systematic nature of trans marginalization. The past and present context of harmful research with T/GNC communities, and negative experiences with health care providers, highlight the importance of collaborative, community-based participatory research that is controlled by T/GNC communities. Community-engaged and controlled research meth-odologies are well suited for marginalized populations whom historically have been left out of research processes, or whom have experienced discrimination or barriers to health care access.

Research is needed that examines the intersections between different forms of social marginalization, violence, place, and health in the lives of differ-ent T/GNC people. All T/GNC people are not at the same risk for violence, neither do they all experience violence in the same way, in the same places. It is important to acknowledge these differences: for example, the high rates of violence experienced by racialized T/GNC people living in poverty, who are working class and/or sex workers (especially trans women). More research is urgently needed that explicitly centers on the interlocking contexts of racism, poverty, and transphobia in particular places, and their impact on mental health and well-being. Such research also must employ community-engaged and collaborative research approaches which highlight sociospatial factors that promote resiliency and safety. Research is also needed that draws on T/GNC community knowledge to develop best practices for trauma-informed health care (including mental health care), by drawing on insights from intersectional, critical trans, and anti-colonial theories.

Drawing on previous work in health geography, researchers can look at the relationship between minority stress and place in the lives of T/GNC people, or what has been called "place-based minority stress" (Lewis, 2014). Recent research has suggested that minority stress may be informed by various geographical factors (Lewis, 2014). Researchers can examine the impact of this stress across the life course for T/GNC people, and the ways that such stress shapes mental health and well-being, social inclusion, and resilience. Similarly, recent work on gay, lesbian, queer and Two-Spirit people's mobility and migration in the fields of geography and health studies may be useful in providing insights for future research in trans health geography, and in health geography more broadly.

Health geographers in Canada must acknowledge colonialism as a social determinant of health that is spatially produced, and examine the way that colonial and cisnormative gender norms are enforced through colonial practices (Scheim et al., 2013; Hunt, 2015). Research discussed earlier from the Aboriginal Two-Spirit and LGBTQ Migration, Mobility, and Health Research Project highlights the combined health effects of historical trauma, colonialism, and anti-Aboriginal racism on Two-Spirit/Aboriginal trans and gender diverse people, as well as the importance of a sense of community belonging for Two-Spirit people. Research is needed that explores in-depth, how and where Aboriginal T/GNC and Two-Spirit people experience belonging, the impact on their mental health and well-being, as well as how forms of social exclusion and marginalization such as racism, classism, and ableism operate *within* T/GNC communities to create barriers to inclusion and a sense of belonging.

Health geography researchers need to be aware of the negative impact of cisnormative and transphobic psychiatric and mental health discourses on T/GNC people, and how this context influences what language is meaningful (or not) when talking about emotional and psychological well-being. For example, "mental health" may not be a term that resonates for T/GNC people. Researchers also need to be aware of the critiques of psychiatric frameworks for understanding psychological distress, and to explore new language and ways of conceptualizing psychological or emotional distress or well-being. Similarly, researchers need to unpack and critically examine the assumptions surrounding the language of "violence" (including intimate partner violence, domestic violence, hate-motivated violence) and "place," and examine the exclusions produced through cisnormativity. Researchers can draw on existing work in mental health geography to explore how different contexts and places undermine or enhance safety, belonging, resiliency, mental health, and well-being for T/GNC people. It would be useful to examine the mental and physical health impacts of transphobic policies and the relationship to place: for example, being forced to travel or move as a result of transphobic institutionalized policies and laws. This also could extend work in the area of geography of health care access in rural and urban spaces.

Future research is needed also to examine the relationship between place and belonging by drawing on findings from previous studies that have indicated that for some T/GNC people, a "connection with a trans community may be a determinant of resilience" (Testa et al., 2014, p. 33). T/GNC communities have stressed the importance of highlighting and studying individual and collective resilience and strength, not only experiences of marginalization, violence, emotional distress, or mental health challenges. It is important to take direction from T/GNC communities, and to not assume that studies on resilience in other communities will necessarily translate to T/GNC communities. Despite a historical and ongoing lack of Canadian and trans-positive research, important new research is being conducted or led by trans communities. Trans activism and organizing in Canada continues to drive important new research, inform policy decisions, advance new understandings about violence, health, and place, while setting out new directions for best practice for trans-affirming health services. Importantly, this work on resilience also needs to acknowledge the diversity and inequalities that exist *within* this community, and the ways that race, class, ability, age, sexual orientation, and gender complexly intersect to shape the everyday lives of T/GNC people.

References

American Psychiatric Association, 2013. Gender dysphoria. Available online at http://www.dsm5.org/Documents/Gender%20Dysphoria%20Fact%20Sheet.pdf (accessed October 3, 2014).

Bauer, G.R., Hammond, R., Travers, R., Kaay, M., Hohenadel, K. and Boyce, M., 2009. "I don't think this is theoretical; this is our lives": How erasure impacts health care for transgender people. *Journal of the Association of Nurses in AIDS Care*, 20(5), pp. 348–61.

Bauer, G.R., Boyce, M., Coleman, T., Kaay, M., Scanlon K. and Travers, T., 2010. Who are trans people in Ontario? *Trans PULSE E-Bulletin*, 1(1). Available online at http://transpulseproject.ca/wp-content/uploads/2010/07/E1English.pdf (accessed October 3, 2014).

Bauer, G.R., Travers, R. Scanlon, K. and Coleman, T.A., 2012. High heterogeneity of HIV-related sexual risk among transgender people in Ontario, Canada: A province-wide respondent-driven sampling survey. *BMC Public Health*, 12. Available online at www.biomedcentral.com/1471-2458/12/292 (accessed October 3, 2014).

Bauer, G.R, Pyne, J., Francino, M.C. and Hammond, R., 2013. Suicidality among trans people in Ontario: Implications for social work and social justice. *Service Social*, 59(1), pp. 35–62.

Brown, N., 2011. Holding tensions of victimization and perpetration: Partner abuse in trans communities. In: J. Ristock, ed. *Intimate partner violence in LGBTQ lives.* New York: Routledge. pp. 153–68.

Brown, N.R., 2007. Stories from outside the frame: Intimate partner abuse in sexual-minority women's relationships with transsexual men. *Feminism & Psychology,* 17(3), pp. 373–93.

Browne, K., 2004. Genderism and the bathroom problem: (Re)materializing sexed sites, (re)creating sexed bodies. *Gender, Place & Culture,* 11(3), pp. 331–46.

Browne, K., 2005. Stages and streets: Reading and misreading female masculinities. In: B. Van Hoven and K. Horschelmann, eds. *Spaces of masculinities.* London: Routledge, pp. 237–48

Browne, K., Nash, C.J. and Hines, S., 2010. Introduction: Towards trans geographies. *Gender, Place & Culture,* 17(5), pp. 573–77.

Cermele, J., Daniels, S. and Anderson K., 2001. Defining normal: Constructions of race and gender in the DSM-IV casebook. *Feminism & Psychology,* 11(2), pp. 229–47.

Coleman, T., Bauer, G., Scanlon, K., Travers, R., Kaay, M. and Francino, M., 2011. Challenging the binary: Gender characteristics of trans Ontarians. *Trans PULSE E-Bulletin,* 2(2), pp/. 1–3. Available online at http://transpulseproject.ca/wp-content/uploads/2011/12/E4English.pdf (accessed February 3, 2016).

Courvant, D. and Cook-Daniels, L., 1998. *Trans and intersex survivors of domestic violence: Defining terms, barriers & responsibilities.* Portland, OR: Survivor Project. Available online at www.survivorproject.org/defbarresp.html (accessed October 3, 2014).

Curtis, S., 2010. *Space, place, and mental health.* Farnham: Ashgate.

Daley, A. and Mulé, N.J., 2014. LGBTQs and the DSM-5: A critical queer response. *Journal of Homosexuality,* 61(9), pp. 1288–312.

Doan, P.L., 2007. Queers in the American city: Transgendered perceptions of urban space. *Gender, Place & Culture,* 14(1), pp. 57–74.

Doan, P.L., 2010. The tyranny of gendered spaces: Reflections from beyond the gender dichotomy. *Gender, Place & Culture,* 17(5), pp. 635–54.

FORGE (For Ourselves: Reworking Gender Expression), 2012a. Who are transgender people? Victim service providers' fact sheet #1. Available online at http://forge-forward.org/wp-content/docs/FAQ-05-2012-trans101.pdf (accessed October 3, 2014).

FORGE (For Ourselves: Reworking Gender Expression), 2012b. Transgender rates of violence. Victim service providers' fact sheet #6. Available online at http://forge-forward.org/wp-content/docs/FAQ-10-2012-rates-of-violence.pdf (accessed February 3, 2016).

Goldberg, J.M. and White, C., 2011. Reflections on approaches to trans anti-violence education. In: J. Ristock, ed. *Intimate partner violence in LGBTQ lives.* New York: Routledge. pp. 56–77.

Grant, J., Mottet, L., Tanis, J., Harrison, J., Herman, J. and Keisling, M., 2011. *Injustice at every turn: A report of the National Transgender Discrimination Survey.* Washington, DC: National Center for Transgender Equality and National Gay and Lesbian Task Force.

Greenberg, K., 2012. Still hidden in the closet: Trans women and domestic violence. *Berkeley Journey of Gender, Law & Justice,* 27(3), pp. 198–251.

Heinz, M. and MacFarlane, D., 2013. Island lives: A trans community needs assessment for Vancouver Island. *SAGE Open,* 3(3), pp. 1–13.

Herman, J.L., 2013. Gendered restrooms and minority stress: The public regulation of gender and its impact on transgender people's lives. *Journal of Public Management & Social Policy*, 19(1), pp. 65–80.

Hunt, S., 2015. The embodiment of self-determination: Beyond the gender binary. In: M. Greenwood, C. Reading and S. de Leeuw, eds. *Determinants of Indigenous peoples' health in Canada*. Canadian Scholars' Press, pp. 104–19.

Johnson, J., 2013. Cisgender privilege, intersectionality, and the criminalization of CeCe McDonald: Why intercultural communication needs transgender studies. *Journal of International and Intercultural Communication*, 6(2), pp. 135–44.

LeFrancoise, B.A., Menzies, R. and Reaume, G., 2013. *Mad matters: A critical reader in Canadian mad studies*. Toronto: Canadian Scholars' Press Inc.

Lewis, N., 2014. Rupture, resilience, and risk: Relationships between mental health and migration among gay-identified men in North America. *Health and Place*, 27, pp. 212–19.

Longman Marcellin R., Scheim A., Bauer G. and Redman N., 2013a. Experiences of racism among trans people in Ontario. *Trans PULSE E-Bulletin*, 3(1), pp. 1–2. Available online at http://transpulseproject.ca/research/experiences-of-racism-among-trans-people-in-ontario/ (accessed October 3, 2014).

Longman Marcellin R., Bauer, G.R. and Scheim, A.I., 2013b. Intersecting impacts of transphobia and racism on HIV risk among trans persons of colour in Ontario, Canada. *Ethnicity and Inequalities in Health and Social Care*, 6(4), pp. 97–107.

Lombardi, E. and van Servellen, G., 2000. Building culturally sensitive substance use prevention and treatment programs for transgendered populations. *Journal of Substance Abuse Treatment*, 19(3), pp. 291–6.

McIntyre, J., Daley, A., Rutherford, K. and Ross, L., 2011. Systems-level barriers in accessing supportive mental health services for sexual and gender minorities: Insights from the provider's perspective. *Canadian Journal of Community Mental Health*, 30(2), pp. 173–86.

McNeil, J., Bailey, L., Ellis, S., Morton, J. and Regan, M., 2012. *Trans mental health study* 2012. Edinburgh: Equality Network. Available online at www.scottishtrans. org/Uploads/Resources/trans_mh_study.pdf (accessed October 3, 2014).

Meyer, I.H., 2003. Prejudice, social stress, and mental health in lesbian, gay, and bisexual populations: Conceptual issues and research evidence. *Psychological Bulletin*, 129(5), pp. 674–97.

Moran, L. and Sharpe, A., 2004. Violence, identity and policing: The case of violence against transgender people. *Criminology and Criminal Justice*, 4(4), pp. 395–417.

Mulé, N., Daley, A. and The Rainbow Health Network, 2010. Queer lens of resistance: A critical anti-oppressive response to the DSM-V. In: Ontario Studies in Education (OISE), *PsychOut: A Conference for Organizing Resistance Against Psychiatry*. Toronto: OISE. Available online at http://individual.utoronto.ca/ psychout/papers/mule-etal_paper.pdf (accessed October 3, 2014).

Munson, M. and Cook-Daniels, L., 2015. Transgender sexual violence survivors: A self-help guide to healing and understanding. FORGE Transgender Sexual Violence Project. Available online at http://forge-forward.org/wp-content/docs/self-help-guide-to-healing-2015-FINAL.pdf (accessed February 2, 2016).

Namaste, K., 1996. Genderbashing: Sexuality, gender, and the regulation of public spaces. *Environment and Planning D*, 14, pp. 221–40.

Namaste, V.K., 2000. *Invisible lives: The erasure of transsexual and transgender people*. Chicago, IL: University of Chicago Press.

Nash, C., 2007. Material entanglements: Queer geographies and trans experience and embodiment. Paper presented at the Association of American Geographers, Washington, DC, April.

Nash, C., 2010. Trans geographies, embodiment and experience. *Gender, Place & Culture*, 17(5), pp. 579–95.

National Coalition of Anti-Violence Programs, 2014. *Lesbian, gay, bisexual, transgender, queer and HIV-affected hate violence 2013*. New York: National Coalition of Anti-Violence Programs.

Neo Eamas, T. and MacFarlane, D., 2014. Happy Tranny Day. In: D. Irving, and R. Raj, eds. *Trans activism in Canada: A reader*. Toronto: Canadian Scholars' Press, pp. 137–46.

Nicols, R., 2012. Toward a critical trans politics: An interview with Dean Spade. *Upping the Anti*, 14. Available online at http://uppingtheanti.org/journal/article/14-dean-spade/ (accessed November 28, 2014).

National Film Board of Canada, 2014. Educator's guide for *My Prairie Home, A documentary-musical featuring Rae Spoon: A film by Chelsea McMullan*. Available online at www3.nfb.ca/sg/100749.pdf (accessed October 3, 2014).

Pyne, J., 2014. The governing of gender non-conforming children: A dangerous enclosure. *Annual Review of Critical Psychology*, 11, pp. 79–96.

Ristock, J., ed. 2011. *Intimate partner violence in LGBTQ lives*. New York: Routledge.

Ristock, J., Zoccole, A. and Passante, L., 2010. Aboriginal Two-Spirit and LGBTQ Migration, Mobility, and Health Research Project: Winnipeg final report. Available online at www.2spirits.com/PDFolder/MMHReport.pdf (accessed October 3, 2014).

Ristock, J., ed. 2011. *Intimate partner violence in LGBTQ lives*. New York: Routledge.

Ristock, J., Zoccole, A. and Potskin, J., 2011. Aboriginal Two-Spirit and LGBTQ Migration, Mobility, and Health Research Project: Vancouver, final report. Available online at www.2spirits.com/PDFolder/2011%20Vancouver%20full%20report%20final.pdf (accessed October 3, 2014).

Rotondi, N.K., Bauer G., Travers R., Travers A., Scanlon K. and Kaay M., 2011a. Depression in male-to-female transgender Ontarians: Results from the Trans PULSE Project. *Canadian Journal of Community Mental Health*, 30(2), pp. 113–33.

Rotondi, N.K., Bauer, G., Scanlon, K., Kaay, M., Travers, R. and Travers, A., 2011b. Prevalence of and risk and protective factors for depression in female-to-male transgender Ontarians: Trans PULSE Project. *Canadian Journal of Community Mental Health*. 30(2), pp. 135–55.

Rutherford, K., MacIntyre, J., Daley, A. and Ross, L.E., 2012. Development of expertise in mental health service provision for lesbian, gay, bisexual and transgender communities. *Medical Education*, 46(9), pp. 903–13.

Scanlon, K., Travers, R., Coleman, T., Bauer, G. and Boyce, M., 2010. Ontario's Trans communities and suicide: Transphobia is bad for our health. *Trans PULSE E-Bulletin*, 1(2). Available online at http://transpulseproject.ca/research/ontarios-trans-communities-and-suicide/ (accessed October 3, 2014).

Scheim, A.I, Jackson, R., James, L., Dopler, T.S., Pyne, J. and Bauer, G.R., 2013. Barriers to well-being for Aboriginal gender-diverse people: Results from the Trans PULSE Project in Ontario, Canada. *Ethnicity and Inequalities in Health and Social Care*, 6(4), pp. 108–20.

Scheim, A.I., Bauer, G.R, Pyne, J., 2014. Avoidance of public spaces by trans Ontarians: The impact of transphobia on daily life. *Trans PULSE E-Bulletin*, 4(1). Available online at http://transpulseproject.ca/research/avoidance-of-public-spaces-by-trans-ontarians-the-impact-of-transphobia-on-daily-life/ (accessed October 3, 2014).

Serano, J., 2007. *Whipping girl: A transsexual woman on sexism and the scapegoating of femininity*. Emeryville, CA: Seal Press.

Stotzer, R. L., 2009. Violence against transgender people: A review of United States data. *Aggression and Violent Behavior*, 14, pp. 170–9.

Stotzer, R. L., 2014. Bias crimes based on sexual orientation and gender identity: Global prevalence, impacts and causes. In: D. Peterson and V. R. Panfil, eds. *Handbook of LGBT Communities, Crime, and Justice*. New York: Springer, pp. 45–64.

Spade, D., 2011. *Normal life: Administrative violence, critical trans politics and the limits of law*. New York: South End Press.

Taylor, C., 2009. Health and safety issues for Aboriginal transgender/Two-Spirit people in Manitoba. *Canadian Journal of Aboriginal Community-Based HIV/AIDS Research*, 2, pp. 63–84. Available online at www.caan.ca/wp-content/uploads/2012/05/Health-and-Safety-Issues-for-Aboriginal-TransgenderTwo-Spirit-People-in-Manitoba.pdf (accessed October 3, 2014).

Taylor, C., and Ristock, J.L. 2011. "We are all treaty people": An anti-oppressive research ethics of solidarity with Indigenous LGBTQ people living with partner violence. In: J.L. Ristock, ed. *Intimate partner violence in LGBTQ lives*. New York: Routledge. pp. 301–19.

Taylor, E., 2013. Trans men's health care experiences: Ethical social work practice beyond the binary. *Journal of Gay & Lesbian Social Services*, 25(1), pp. 102–20.

Testa, R., Jimenez, C., and Rankin, S. 2014. Risk and resilience during transgender identity development: The effects of awareness and engagement with other transgender people on affect. *Journal of Gay and Lesbian Mental Health*, 18(1), pp. 31–46.

Travers, R., Pyne, J., Bauer, G., Munro, L., Giambrone, B., Hammond, R., and Scanlon, K., 2013. "Community control" in CBPR: Challenges experienced and questions raised from the Trans PULSE project. *Action Research*, 11(4), pp. 403–22.

Turner, L., Whittle, S. and Combs, R., 2009. *Transphobic hate crime in the European Union: Press for change*. Available online at http://transgenderinfo.be/wp-content/uploads/transphobic_hate_crime_in_eu.pdf (accessed February 3, 2016).

White, C. and Goldberg, J.M., 2006. Expanding our understanding of gendered violence: Violence against trans people and their loved ones. *Canadian Women's Studies Journal*, 25(1–2), pp. 124–8.

World Health Organization (WHO), 2014. Mental health: Strengthening our response, Factsheet no. 220. Available online at www.who.int/mediacentre/factsheets/fs220/en (accessed October 3, 2014).

World Health Organization, United Nations Population Fund, Joint United Nations Programme on HIV/AIDS, Global Network of Sex Work Projects, The World Bank, 2013. *Implementing comprehensive HIV/STI programmes with sex workers: Practical approaches from collaborative interventions*. Geneva: World Health Organization. Available online at www.who.int/hiv/pub/sti/sex_worker_implementation/en/ (accessed October 3, 2014).

5 "I'm a Better Person When I'm Working"

Supportive Workplaces, Mental Illness, and Recovery

Joshua Evans and Robert Wilton

Today, the concept of mental health recovery is a central focus of mental health services. Conceptually speaking, mental health recovery is conceived as a deeply personal journey towards redefinition, self-determination, and participation in the community occurring in the context of ongoing, everyday transactions between an individual and his/her world (Onken et al., 2007; Borg and Davidson, 2008). In this context, recovery is situated in relation to a person's past experiences, current circumstances, and future goals, rather than the curing of a person's disease, disorder, or deficiency. Therefore, recovery is not a clinical phenomenon, but rather a personal journey orientated towards living well in the community, despite the restrictions imposed by illness (Davidson and Roe, 2007). Key elements of recovery include social connectedness, hope and optimism about the future, rebuilding positive identities, finding meaning in life, and personal empowerment (Leamy et al., 2011). In Canada, as in countries such as Australia, England, Ireland, New Zealand, and the USA (Slade et al., 2008), personal recovery is the prevailing framework organizing formal and informal mental health services in the community (Mental Health Commission of Canada, 2009).

In practice, the experience of personal recovery is complex. While the shift to community modes of care was intended, in part, to end the dehumanizing practice of isolating psychiatric patients within asylums away from mainstream society, the personal experience of people living with serious mental illness (herein referred to as people with psychiatric disabilities) recovering in community settings has been far from inclusive (Knowles, 2000; see Chapter 12 for discussion of the implications of a shift to a community model of care for informal caregiving). The ubiquity of "psychiatric ghettoes" – an urban phenomenon common to most large North American cities – reflects the continued spatial concentration of community-based mental health services in low-quality, inner-city neighborhoods, reproducing in effect an asylum without walls in the city (DeVerteuil and Evans, 2010). To a large extent this pattern of sociospatial marginalization can be attributed to the persistent exclusion of disabled people from mainstream places, coupled with ongoing restructuring of the welfare state, including its provisions for people with work-limiting disabilities. This sociospatial exclusion and welfare state retrenchment has contributed to pervasive patterns of chronic poverty among people with psychiatric disabilities (Wilton, 2003). As a result, community-based recovery remains an elusive ideal for many Canadians.

In response to these challenges, people with psychiatric disabilities – in many cases, allied with mental health advocates and professionals – have long been working to establish arenas of recovery (Sells et al., 2006) within mainstream settings that engage people with psychiatric disabilities in so-called "normal" activities (see also Hall, 2005; Parr, 2008). Given the economic precariousness faced by many with psychiatric disabilities (Wilton, 2003), one mainstream setting of particular significance is the workplace. In Canada, the labor participation rate of people with disabilities (57.2 percent) ranks lower than Aboriginal peoples living off-reserve (75 percent), recent immigrants (77.1 percent), and individuals with a high school education (79 percent). Moreover, 20 percent of the 2.5 million working-age adults with disabilities lived below the poverty line in 2006, compared to only 10 percent of people without disabilities (Prince, 2014). The rates for people with psychiatric disabilities are believed to be much worse (Fawcett and Marshall, 2014). These disproportionate rates of unemployment and underemployment speak to the many barriers that exist in mainstream employment settings.

For several decades, psychiatric consumer and survivor groups and other social economy organizations have been working to overcome barriers to employment by developing alternative workplaces for people with psychiatric disabilities recovering in the community. Generally, these social enterprises are distinguished from mainstream businesses by the type of accommodation and support offered to workers. Such support and accommodation can include more flexible work schedules, increased job security, and openness regarding mental health problems. These supportive workplaces make work possible – a type of activity that has been positively associated with mental health recovery (Berjerholm and Eklun, 2007). However, little research has examined the role of these unique settings in the process of personal recovery (Williams et al., 2012).

In this chapter, we focus our attention on the recovery-related benefits of supportive workplaces for Canadians with psychiatric disabilities recovering in the community. More specifically, we examine their potential for addressing the chronic poverty experienced by many such individuals. In so doing, this chapter considers one place-based dimension of mental difference (the workplace) and its role in the recovery process. Such an analysis draws attention to the everyday lived experiences of those with psychiatric disabilities recovering in the community, particularly those experiences situated at the intersection of low income, unemployment, and inaccessible workplaces. Income, employment, and working conditions are fundamental determinants of health which shape living conditions, psychological functioning, health-related behavior (Mikkonen and Raphael, 2010) and, as we aim to show, personal recovery from serious mental illness.

We begin by reviewing the relationship between poverty and serious mental illness, highlighting the implications of poverty traps in the day-to-day lives of people with psychiatric disabilities. We then examine more closely the significance of work for the recovery process, including the barriers that exist in mainstream employment settings, before examining the experiences of workers employed in three social enterprises operating in the southwestern region of the province of Ontario. We conclude the chapter by discussing the significance of these enterprises as sites of engagement linked to individuals' ability to achieve their full potential in the community. As sites of occupational, social, and symbolic engagement, these supportive workplaces mediate forms of material and social deprivation, as well as the symbolic exclusion of people with psychiatric disabilities from mainstream society.

Poverty and Mental Health

The linkage between poverty and mental illness is widely known. Decades worth of social epidemiological studies have confirmed a negative relationship between socioeconomic conditions and the risk of serious mental disorder in adults and adolescents (Muntaner et al., 2004; Lund et al., 2010). For example, there is a higher risk for conditions such as schizophrenia, anxiety disorders, bipolar disorder, major depression, and psychiatric hospitalization among individuals of lower socioeconomic status (Muntaner et al., 2004; Hudson, 2005) and social class (Tiikkaja et al., 2013). However, the direction of causality is less clear when it comes to specific disorders and their relation to socioeconomic status or class position. For example, more prevalent conditions such as major depression and anxiety disorders likely reflect social causation (the impact of socioeconomic status on individual risk), whereas less prevalent conditions such as schizophrenia likely reflect social selection (the impact of mental illness on socioeconomic status) (Muntaner et al., 2004). These relationships, whether stressful experiences associated with material deprivation that induce mental suffering, or the symptoms of particular disorders that induce downward social drift, point to a reciprocal and synergistic relationship between poverty and worsening mental health (Hanandita and Tampubolon, 2014).

This synergistic relationship between material deprivation, social exclusion, and enduring mental health problems ensnares people in poverty. To make matters worse, social welfare policies in many Western countries have done little to address these poverty traps (Manderscheid, 2013). Neoliberally-inspired welfare policy reforms in countries such as Canada have exacerbated the economic hardship faced by people with psychiatric disabilities (Wilton, 2004). In Canada, welfare income among people unable to work due to physical and mental disability (see Table 5.1) generally has not increased on a par with inflation – and in some provinces it has remained frozen for years, resulting in growing poverty gaps (Tweddle et al., 2013).

Table 5.1 Comparison of 2012 welfare income for a single person with disability with after-tax low income cut-offs (LICO)

Province	Total welfare income (C$)	LICO (C$)	Poverty gap (C$)	Welfare income (% of LICO)
Newfoundland and Labrador	10,846	16,573	−5,727	65.4
Prince Edward Island	9,416	16,366	−6,950	57.5
Nova Scotia	9,970	16,573	−6,603	60.2
New Brunswick	8,837	16,573	−7,736	53.3
Quebec	11,957	19,597	−7,640	61
Ontario	13,772	19,597	−5,825	70.3
Manitoba	9,640	19,597	−9,957	49.2
Saskatchewan	11,263	16,573	−5,310	68
Alberta	18,228	19,597	−1,369	93
British Columbia	22,386	37,052	−14,666	60.4

Source: Based on Tweddle et al. (2013).

As a result, low-income people with psychiatric disabilities – who depend on safety net programs such as government disability benefits – face tremendous difficulty accessing the material and social resources required to live well in the community. This poverty has significant and profound impacts on the quality of life available to these groups, inhibiting their ability to participate in society in meaningful ways. For example, Wilton (2003) has documented how chronic poverty negatively impacted fundamental life domains such as living situations, family relations, and social standing among people with psychiatric disabilities who relied on insufficient disability benefits as a primary source of income. A majority of the respondents had difficulty meeting their basic needs with regard to food and clothing, felt constrained in terms of their ability to reciprocate in relationships with family members and friends, could not participate in leisure activities to the extent that they wished, and felt doubly stigmatized by community members due to their psychiatric diagnosis and visible poverty.

The everyday hardship of poverty, coupled with the social stigma attached to mental illness, raises a host of barriers to successful recovery from mental health problems (Onken et al., 2007). These poverty traps deny individuals the opportunity to live well in the community, and participate in Canadian society in a meaningful and fulfilling way. Employment represents one potential avenue to combat poverty, yet people with serious mental health problems face significant obstacles accessing employment. These obstacles, as well as the significance of employment for recovery, are examined next.

Employment, Unsupportive Workplaces, and Personal Recovery

The centrality of employment for health and well-being in the general population is well documented: it is a vital source of income, social status, and belonging, and as such an important social determinant of health (Mikkonen and Raphael, 2010). In light of the social stigma and exclusion experienced by people with psychiatric disabilities, employment stands as a valued but complex domain of life. Employment has been shown to be a positive and motivating source of financial independence, structure and routine, self-esteem, and self-worth (Saunders and Nedelec, 2014). Being employed is associated with a wide range of benefits, including a sense of purpose as well as greater autonomy, status, and acceptance in society. Moreover, employment is associated often with improved social relationships, hope for the future, and generally better well-being (Fossey and Harvey, 2010; Blank et al., 2011).

Acquiring employment and remaining gainfully employed can be seen as a meaningful yardstick in the process of personal recovery (Onken et al., 2007). Borg and Kristiansen (2008) examined the impact of employment on the recovery process, noting the significance of work participation in experiencing a sense of normality and social inclusion. They found that engagement in work and the work setting itself to be particularly significant for recovery. Work situations provided an opportunity to distance oneself from problematic areas of life, and to engage with others on tasks unrelated to illness. Work as an activity provided a sense of belonging tied to socially valued roles rather than diagnostic categories and individualized pathology. These roles and responsibilities helped engender routine, regularity, and predictability in everyday life. Integral to maintaining these roles were flexible work environments characterized by sympathetic managers and co-workers, trustful and positive interactions, as well as a sense of openness regarding the patterns and realities of illness.

While employment is widely recognized to be an important factor in personal recovery, many people with psychiatric disabilities living in the community face various barriers accessing employment (Fossey and Harvey, 2010; Blank et al., 2011). It is important to recognize that serious mental illnesses vary in terms of their symptomology, and that not all illness experiences are the same. For some forms of mental illness such as schizophrenia, the first episode of psychosis typically occurs in early adulthood, which disrupts young adults' efforts to pursue educational and vocational goals, and hinders educational achievement and employment in early life (Rinaldi et al., 2010). Those who do secure employment in the competitive job market often experience difficulties sustaining it due to the effects of medication, work-related stress, and time away from work due to illness (Fossey and Harvey, 2010; Kinn et al., 2014). In this regard, disclosing illness is often a source of great anxiety, given the stigma associated with different types of mental health conditions; however, disclosing an illness is necessary in many cases to secure the accommodations required to remain employed (Marwaha and Johnson, 2005). Moreover, for low-income individuals who receive social assistance from the state, earning too much income can put state benefits in jeopardy. The threat of losing benefits often encourages individuals to work less, or not at all. This reflects how the workplace itself is a complex and stressful environment for people with psychiatric disabilities. Not surprisingly, high levels of unemployment persist for these groups, further complicating their abilities to recover a meaningful and fulfilling life (Waghorn and Lloyd, 2005).

Taking these benefits and barriers into consideration, it follows that in order to access sustained employment, people with psychiatric disabilities may require assistance in finding and maintaining employment (Fossey and Harvey, 2010; Kinn et al., 2014). Recent examinations of workplace experiences have shed light on the types of workplace accommodations and support which can promote sustained employment. This includes pragmatic forms of support such as empathetic and emotionally supportive relationships between supervisors and employees, openness about mental health problems and conditions, and flexibility regarding tasks and schedules (Borg and Kristiansen, 2008; Blank et al., 2011; Kinn et al., 2014). A fundamental principle in the case of workplace accommodations and support is that an individual's capabilities and needs may change over the course of his/her recovery journey (Blank et al., 2011).

Sensitivity to such realities is relatively rare in mainstream employment settings, leading people with psychiatric disabilities to experience them as stressful and exclusive spaces. In this employment landscape, the social enterprise model has been identified as a key mechanism for establishing pathways to gainful employment (Prince, 2014). Social enterprises are organizations that use business practice to pursue social goals. They have an entrepreneurial orientation, and "their prime interest does not lie in profit-maximization, but in building social capacity (e.g. through employing or training socially disadvantaged groups) and responding to under-met needs ... and in the process creating new forms of work" (Amin et al., 2002, p. 1). Social enterprise organizations are part of a larger social economy that exists between the public and private sectors. Many of these organizations are non-profit, while others are for-profit enterprises with strong social missions.

There has been little research to date on the efficacy of the social enterprise model in providing people with psychiatric disabilities with supportive and sustainable employment. One exception is a study by Williams et al. (2012), which examined the experiences of workers employed within a social enterprise in Australia. They identified a number of features in the workplace that promoted workers' performance, job satisfaction, and sense of well-being. These included:

- adequate pay, supportive benefits, and job security;
- assignment of challenging yet achievable tasks;
- having regular part-time hours on different days of the week, and flexibility in scheduling; and
- positive relationships with supervisors and managers.

In this chapter we examine the role of these types of accommodations and support offered by social enterprises in southwestern Ontario, Canada, while paying particular attention to the relationship between work experiences and personal recovery. We ask: how are these accommodating and supportive workplaces implicated in the process of personal recovery, particularly in the capacity of low-income people with psychiatric disabilities to escape the poverty trap?

Method

Study Overview

This chapter is drawn from a qualitative study examining how social enterprises attempt to create accommodating and supportive work environments for people with psychiatric disabilities. Before detailing the study, we provide a note on the terminology adopted in this chapter. Recent social science scholarship has tended to adopt one of three different discursive frames. First, there is a language of mental illness that corresponds more or less closely to the diagnostic categories used in psychiatry. Here, people are defined in relation to specific disorders – e.g. psychoses, mood or anxiety disorders – with attention given to the seriousness of these disorders specified in terms of the impact on people's ability to function, and duration (see Ruggeri et al., 2000).

Second, some scholars deliberately have adopted a language of madness to shift focus to the lived experience of mental health in settings and spaces where these diagnostic categories have less meaning and relevance (Knowles, 2000; Parr, 2008). Third, there is a language of disability, where the conceptual distinction drawn between the impairment effects of mental ill-health, and the disabling effects of the surrounding social environment, has offered an important analytical tool with which to highlight the material and discursive processes that work against people's social participation.

In this chapter we use the language of disability, because it allows us to focus attention on the characteristics of the social enterprise workplace as one arena of recovery. This focus does not preclude acknowledgment of the impacts of mental ill-health on people's everyday lives. Indeed, many of the people we spoke with were living with illnesses which had – and continued to have – significant impacts on their ability to function at work, and in other spheres of daily life. Nevertheless, it is the character of the social enterprise, and its potential to contribute to a recovery journey, that is our principal focus.

Participants and Data Collection

In the following we consider the experiences of workers employed by social enterprises operating in three different cities located in southwestern Ontario. The first study site (Site A) was an enterprise established in 1997 as vocational training program. Today, the enterprise encompasses a number of businesses providing a range of services including grounds maintenance and landscaping; eaves-trough cleaning; painting, deck restoration and cleaning; janitorial and clean-up; sewing; and flyer services. The enterprise is subsidized partly through funds received by a local hospital, is governed by a board of directors, and employs four to five full-time employees, approximately 21 part-time workers, and another 20 seasonal workers. Salaries range from minimum wage of C$10.25/hour to C$15.75/hour, depending on the position.

The second study site (Site B) was a janitorial services enterprise. Established in 1989, the enterprise began as a consumer/survivor organization, and today is still governed by a board elected in part from the enterprise workforce. The enterprise's main focus is cleaning buildings but also includes extreme cleaning, landscaping, lawn care, and snow removal. The janitorial work primarily consists of contract work with social housing organizations. These contracts entail cleaning bathrooms and common areas in group homes, transitional housing, and office buildings. When it comes to cleaning, job descriptions are distinguished between supervisors who are paid slightly more, and cleaners. Typically, two to three cleaners and a supervisor complete a job at each building. Approximately 66 people are employed, which includes approximately 55 members and 11 administrative staff. During winter the membership grows, as approximately 20 seasonal workers are needed. Salaries range from C$10.50/hour to C$30/hour, depending on the position.

The third study site (Site C) was a catering enterprise that began as a consumer/survivor initiative in the early 1990s, but later became part of a larger mental health service organization. The enterprise employs anywhere from nine to 12 people on an ongoing basis, the majority of whom work part-time. The enterprise provides catering for non-profit and municipal clients in the local area, as well as catering for private functions such as weddings. The enterprise aims to help individuals learn useful skills through employment in a variety of roles related to food services, including food preparation, delivery, and dining service. Salaries ranged from C$10.25/hour to C$18/hour, depending on the position.

All three enterprises were characterized by a strong commitment to workplace accommodation in terms of flexible scheduling, job security, openness about mental illness, and social support both on and off the job. Twenty-six workers across the three social enterprises were interviewed (Site A, $n = 7$; Site B, $n = 14$; Site C, $n = 5$). The mental health experiences varied among the interview respondents and included conditions such as schizophrenia, multiple personality disorder, severe depression, bipolar disorder, and anxiety disorder. The average age of respondents was 50 years (three respondents declined to give their age). The youngest respondent in the sample was 32 years, and the oldest respondent was 73 years. The sample included 11 women and 15 men. Two women from Site A, five women from Site B and four women from Site C were interviewed. The sample of respondents encompassed a number of long-term employees and new employees. The average length of time working at the businesses was seven years. The respondent with the most seniority had worked at the business for nearly 21 years, whereas the respondent with the least seniority had been working for only three months when interviewed.

Data Analysis

Digital recordings of the interviews were transcribed in full and subsequently entered into a qualitative data management software package (NVivo 10™). The analysis began by sorting the interview content into the broad themes developed to organize the interview guide. This included experiences tied to the hiring process, the typical workday, wages, work environment, benefits of work, challenges of work, accommodations, health, as well as demographic information. More detailed coding was then developed within and across these themes with a focus on income security, the significance of workplace accommodations in maintaining employment, and the relationship between work and personal recovery.

In the following section we examine the significance of these workplaces in the process of personal recovery, particularly in relation to the abilities of low-income people with psychiatric disabilities to escape the poverty trap.

Findings

Poverty, Mental Illness and Supportive Workplaces

Our interviews provided numerous insights into the significance of supportive workplaces in respondents' recovery journeys. In the cases examined, workplaces opened up a space of engagement between self and world where positive embodied experiences and identities beyond mental illness were found and developed. In so doing, these workplaces afforded important psychological and social benefits linked to elements of recovery (Leamy et al., 2011). First, they provided the opportunity to get out of the house and do something with a purpose. For example, Jay (Site A) felt that he was functionally at his best when he was "keeping busy" and away from home:

> It's important to me, it gets me out of my home. I got an apartment, a one bedroom apartment. It gets me out of my house, I make a couple of bucks, I get the extra hundred from disability. I like keeping busy, I want to work – that's my main, main thing. Everything about work is just, I'm a better person when I'm working: I sleep better, you know? I function better when I'm working. Everyone here says ... "Jay you're at your best when you're working".

Spending time in ordinary environments with nondisabled and minded people has been linked to processes of recovery (Borg and Davidson, 2008), and here this type of occupational engagement resonated strongly with respondents' desires to get out and do something productive. Through this engagement with the surrounding world, the respondents related differently with the here and now, as well as with their place in society.

Second, workplaces provided opportunities to see and interact with other people. A majority of the respondents described how they valued working at the social enterprise because of the social contact that it fostered. At the most basic level, respondents valued working simply because it encouraged social contact with other people. For example, Jason (Site B) had been working as a cleaner for 14 years. Like many other respondents, he referenced the importance of socializing with other people:

> It's more of a social thing to me too because, just to chill and hang out and talk with the staff, or hang out with the staff ... I don't like being at home, kind of just sitting there. So I think it's just the motivation to get out and do something, whatever – the purpose, it gives me a purpose, whether I'm working or not I'll come in basically, and they seem pretty good with that [...] and it feels pretty good when you do a good job and you get to make a bit of money. You feel like you are a bit more connected with society ... 'cause usually it is the other way round.

Moving from social withdrawal and spatial isolation to social engagement and connectedness is associated with recovery processes (Leamy et al., 2011). The respondents' narratives clearly demonstrated how the workplace functioned as a meaningful site of social interaction and peer support. The quality of this social engagement was linked commonly to the openness of the enterprise's social environment with regard to mental illness – a characteristic unique to social enterprises such as the ones considered here.

However, while undoubtedly these workplaces were supportive of elements of recovery, their prospects for addressing the chronic poverty faced by many of the respondents were less straightforward. We examine their role in mediating the everyday material and symbolic challenges of poverty in the following.

Working but Poor

On the one hand, it was clear that the extra income earned through employment made a significant difference in the lives of many of the respondents. For example, Charlene (Site B) was in her late fifties: she had been hospitalized several times as a result of severe depression over the course of her life. She had worked at the cleaning business for nearly 15 years, having started there after answering a newspaper advert seeking applicants for cleaning positions; since then, she had moved into a supervisory role. When asked why working was important, she responded:

> Well, I was thinking about that the other day, you know. I can buy some things that I wouldn't normally be able to buy on ODSP [Ontario Disability Support Program]. I feel normal, even though I'm not; I feel like I could sit in Tim Horton's and order a soup and sandwich, like the normal people do. If on ODSP, it would probably be food bank and whatever I could get from any of the social drop-ins. This way I can go and buy a pair of new socks. If I wasn't working, would probably have to depend on goodwill [thrift store] and things like that.

Here, the extra money acquired through cleaning afforded Charlene more choice in where she could eat and shop, as well as a new sense of self. On the other hand, the earned income did not challenge the broader material constraints facing people. As noted earlier, poverty, unemployment, and mental illness are bound together in a mutually reinforcing and synergistic relationship. Typically, individuals receiving disability benefits in Ontario through ODSP are living below the poverty line: a trend only exacerbated by the difficulty in accessing employment in mainstream work settings. This poverty and exclusion from paid work is a major barrier to personal recovery.

All but four of the respondents considered in this analysis received income from ODSP. The annual ODSP benefit during the period of data collection was C$13,772 (approximately C$1,147.67 per month). As a form of social assistance, ODSP is a means-tested safety net program of last resort. To qualify for ODSP, individuals must have a substantial, continuous, and recurrent mental or physical impairment that substantially restricts participation in work and the community, and which has been verified by an approved health care professional. (Province of Ontario, 2016).

In addition, an individual's or household's liquid assets (i.e. cash on hand and in a bank account, as well as stocks, bonds, and securities) must fall below C$5,000. As with other social assistance programs, any earned income obtained through employment reduces the amount of the disability benefit dollar-for-dollar. At the time of the study interviews, the rules stated that individuals could keep the first C$200 of earned income, above which 50 percent of their earnings were to be subtracted from their ODSP benefit.

In this regard, Ontario's ODSP reflects the familiar welfare principle of least-eligibility common to liberal welfare regimes (Esping-Anderson, 1993). Means-tested social assistance programs function not only as a social safety net of last resort, but also serve to regulate the working poor by deflecting – due to either the stinginess of benefit levels or the stringency of eligibility rules – nondisabled individuals to the job market. Social assistance exists not only to support but also to regulate the poor (Piven and Cloward, 1993). Following this logic, social assistance programs, including disability benefit programs such as Ontario's ODSP, set benefit levels capriciously low – well beneath the poverty line. For example, the low income cut-off (LICO) point in Ontario in the year prior to the study's interviews (2012) was C$19,597 annually, whereas the annual ODSP benefit was C$13,772, a difference of C$5,825 (Tweddle et al., 2013). Assuming no other sources of income, and taking into consideration the rules on earned income, respondents receiving ODSP would have to earn at least C$773 a month in extra income to reach the LICO poverty line. At Ontario's minimum wage in 2012–13 (C$10.25/hour), this was the equivalent of 18 hours of work per week.

In the study sample, many respondents had experienced sustained employment for several years. The average number of years employed was seven. The number of hours worked in a given week varied from respondent to respondent; however, a majority of the respondents did not work 18 hours per week: the average number was 11 hours. Reported hours ranged from a minimum of two hours to a maximum of 37.5 hours per week. The information collected regarding the number of hours worked, wage levels, and other sources of income revealed that only six respondents earned enough income to pull themselves above the poverty line. Of these six individuals, two were not currently receiving ODSP, and two occupied supervisory positions. We estimated the average annual salary for the sample to be C$18,338 – C$1,259 below the 2012 LICO for Ontario.

Charlene was one respondent who had managed to work her way up into a supervisory position, which awarded her a higher salary and more economic security. Yet she repeatedly emphasized the struggle that the average cleaner experiences in the face of mental illness, chronic poverty and societal pressure to work:

Charlene: but what society doesn't understand, even now in the year 2013, is that they think people on ODSP or welfare are just lazy good-for-nothing nothings. But you know what? They need to come work at [the business] and see the struggle people are going through to learn the cleaning ... it's a struggle, because when I grew up in the 1950s, it was looked down upon if you were on family benefits and all that – but you know, some people need to be on it ... It's a struggle for them, like getting their shoes on, their shirt, but for people at [the business] to come out and try and work, society doesn't even know the struggle we go through.

Interviewer: Right – there is a lot of courage involved in just kind of, coming out to just try?

Charlene: Oh yeah, you wouldn't believe the struggle. You might not be feeling good, you know, not everybody is going to be making the money a supervisor does – like the cleaners don't make that much. Let's say they want to buy a winter coat that might set them back a bit, they might have to go to the food bank ... I know what some of the cleaners are going through. It's a struggle.

A major challenge experienced by the respondents was simply balancing the fluctuating symptoms of their illness and work. When feeling well enough to work a full schedule, several respondents noted difficulty securing additional shifts. This was a tension also identified by supervisors and managers, who were aware of the benefits of working, and were trying to distribute hours equitably among a pool of workers.

For example, Tammy was in her late fifties and had worked at the catering business (Site C) for almost five years. She noted how shifts were now split between morning and afternoon. In addition, some weeks required more or fewer workers to handle the orders, depending on how busy the kitchen was:

There's no favorites and I receive about at least one day a week. Some weeks there's no work at all occasionally, and that's not anybody's fault – it's just [that] we don't have the customers calling […] and I receive I'd say, in a good week lately now for the last few months, it's been two shifts a week – and a shift can only be maybe three hours, three and a half hours, there's no long shifts anymore. When I first started working here we stayed the whole day. […] Now it's understood somehow, there's a morning shift and there's an afternoon shift.

Others experienced the opposite problem: having to turn down shifts so as not to lose their disability benefits. For example, Jay had worked at the landscaping business (Site A) for roughly three years. He described how, in his case, it was not worth working more than three days a week:

Jay: I was working four days a week, or something like that. I was making something like C$200 to $300 [every week].
Interviewer: Wow, well that was good, right?
Jay: So they cut my disability [ODSP] off.
Interviewer: So how was that – was that ok, or was that difficult?
Jay: No, that was a little difficult – I had to give up a shift. I had to give up one of my days at [the enterprise] so I could get my disability back … they literally took it away from me because I was making too much money.

Given the nature of the business, particularly lawn care and catering, demand for workers fluctuated. For the respondents, their ODSP benefit as a base income was a critical form of economic security. The imperative to stay within the earned income rules influenced some respondents' decisions regarding how many shifts to seek out or accept: in some cases, discouraging respondents from working more, despite their financial challenges and other benefits of work (summarized previously).

This situation reflects the benefit trap faced by many working people receiving disability assistance (Marwaha and Johnson, 2005). However, for a majority of the respondents, the extra earned income – no matter how big or small – was seen as significant in terms of their quality of life. This speaks to the economic precariousness that many respondents navigated. While these economic benefits were prominent in the respondents' narratives, for a majority of them, the benefits of work also extended beyond money to symbolic dimensions.

Poor, but Better Off than Before

At the time of interview, Maria, a cleaner in her early fifties, had been in post a few years with the social enterprise. She disclosed the impact of having a job on her emotional well-being and sense of belonging:

It's only been the last three, four years, and with the help of the company, that has really pulled me off the corner and off the streets, and changed my way of thinking. Every now and then I still go back down there, but I'm more at home now, and now I can actually see like, I realize that I'm not a brick in the city, I'm actually part of society. Even though it's only four hours of work, it makes me feel good to work.

When discussing the importance of employment, and the social contact that it afforded, it was common for the respondents to connect their participation in paid work to feeling "part of society." This sense of belonging appeared to buffer the social stigma of mental illness and welfare dependency. For this reason, participation in paid employment was an important element in a larger process of re-identification. For example, feeling part of society was linked by the respondents to an ability to assume an everyday, "normal" life, like a "regular" person. When asked why it was important to work, Dorothy responded:

It just gets you out of the house – keeps you going, just like a regular person, and the only thing you're not doing is 40 hours a week, you['re] just trying to get back to a regular person lifestyle.

Dorothy worked on average only four hours a week, yet her wages and what they could buy were symbolically important. As she explained in the following exchange, it allowed her to "walk like a regular person":

Dorothy: Yes, it's important so I can get extra things. I can get a different type of food, I can get expensive food or expensive clothing.
Interviewer: Right – so it's important in that, right?
Dorothy: It's important to go to work to gain something, because you can walk like a regular person, you can shop like a regular person in the store – if you buy just one piece for a month, you still will get something.
Interviewer: Right, it makes you feel –
Dorothy: You still get something, to go out like a regular person.
Interviewer: It's interesting, other people have said that same thing about feeling like a regular person – you know, when you got some money to spend?
Dorothy: Yeah it's like a regular person. You go to work, you come home, you do your grocery, you pay your bills.

Charlene, a cleaner at Site B, echoed Dorothy's perspective:

Charlene: Yeah, nobody knows I'm mentally ill unless they know me personally. Not like I walk around, dragging my leg saying, "I'm mentally ill". You just line up in the store like everybody else does, and you get your stuff, right? You know if you have a newer coat on, or it was just goodwill living over in that ditch, you know?
Interviewer: So it's kind of partly about feeling better about yourself?
Charlene: Yeah, and I'm able to buy some things, and I just feel part of society.

Ben, a worker at Site B, described how he had previously felt "forgotten," whereas now, after acquiring employment he felt "useful." Moreover, Ben explained that because the work was standard, "regular" waged employment as opposed to charity or volunteer work, it had greater potential to change perceptions about the mentally ill among the general public:

Ben: It gives people a chance to do something and don't judge them, and they're probably going to come back and work again, right? So that's why.
Interviewer: And feel good about doing it, which is what you're saying, right?
Ben: And these aren't people in organizations that aren't appreciating your work, you know, like people at the hospital or the court system or police. These are ... people that would normally judge you if you weren't working for them, because of your illnesses. Like, if they saw you on a bus talking to yourself, they think: "Oh my God, oh, I wouldn't want that guy around me!" But yet we got him working in our backyard, so it's also good that it's not a charity thing. They think, "You know what? We're giving them the money, these are normal people, average people in the community" ... When they see that person on the bus they don't say, "Oh look, he's talking to himself," because they may think, "You know what? Somebody was like that in my backyard, and they did a better job than most landscaping companies would do."

For respondents such as Dorothy, Charlene, and Ben, the social affirmation of undertaking paid work helped repel the social stigma of mental illness and poverty.

In this regard, a sense of being a productive member of Canadian society was prominent in the respondents' accounts. Achieving normality was a common thread connecting all of the interviews. In the mental health recovery literature, recovery is conceived as a multifaceted process involving transactions between individuals and their community, and society at large (Onken et al., 2007). This dimension of symbolic engagement, reflected above, demonstrates how workplaces provided a basis from which to confront the stigma of mental illness and welfare dependency and, by extension, to feel part of society. In this way, these workplaces were integral to the respondents' attempts to rebuild a positive self-identity. In the following section, the relevance of these findings for understanding the significance of these supportive workplaces for low-income people with psychiatric disabilities is discussed further.

Discussion

Halfway Points: Supportive Workplaces and the Recovery Landscape

As discussed, this chapter has examined the recovery-related benefits of the social enterprise model, and the supportive workplaces that they make available, from the perspective of workers with psychiatric disabilities in Ontario, Canada. This examination has revealed these enterprises to be significant sites of engagement linked to individuals' ability to achieve their full potential in the community, despite the restrictions of their illness. As sites of occupational, social, and symbolic engagement, these supportive workplaces mediated forms of material and social deprivation, as well as the symbolic exclusion of people with psychiatric disabilities from mainstream society.

The workplaces examined here allowed many of the respondents to acquire years of sustained employment: a significant achievement in light of the dismal labor participation rates among people with psychiatric disabilities in Canada. For the respondents these workplaces were a critical source of money, which was essential, given the chronic poverty experienced by most. Importantly, these workplaces also functioned as vital "arenas of recovery." Sells et al. (2006, p. 15) define these arenas as community settings that: "Promote recovery to the extent that they foster an interplay between being with others who are supportive and/or receptive to support, and doing things that feel meaningful, ultimately kindling – and over time building – a favorable redefinition of self."

By encouraging meaningful routines, social interaction, peer support, and re-identification with socially valued identities, these workplaces helped respondents rescript the meaning of their illness, combat social isolation, and confront the social stigma associated with their mental health conditions. They provided the opportunity to occupy active and dignified roles and to develop a different understanding of the self *within the community*, rather than within enclosed or sheltered settings operating within the medical system.

Keeping these important benefits in mind, it was also apparent in the cases examined that a significant number of respondents – many of whom were working as much as they could handle, or as much as the enterprise made available – were still struggling financially. While this struggle was due in part to the limited number of available hours and the low wage rates of much of the social enterprise work, several respondents also felt constrained by earned income rules in terms of how much they could work. These benefit traps, coupled with the deficiency of existing disability benefit rates, suggest that the poverty trap continues to be a reality for those engaged in paid employment in supportive workplaces. This holds implications for individuals' ability to sustain recovery. Without adequate financial resources, individuals cannot expect to participate fully in society. While paid employment offers some financial benefit, a serious mental illness limits the degree to which a person can participate, irrespective of the level of accommodation and support. The findings point to the fact that in Canada, breaking the synergistic link between poverty and mental ill-health will require significant reworking of disability assistance programs, with a focus on both increasing benefit rates and relaxing the rules governing earned income. Therefore, supportive workplaces are in no way a panacea for the chronic poverty faced by people with serious and enduring mental health problems.

If not a panacea, what are they? Supportive workplaces operating within the social economy occupy a middle ground between sheltered settings within the mental health care system, and mainstream employment settings that often are experienced as stressful and unaccommodating. As such, they offer a critical pathway for social repositioning in the recovery landscape. This function reflects one important practical reality of community-based recovery: individuals do not occupy absolute positions (i.e. psychiatric patient); rather, they negotiate an "evolving middle-ground between isolation and integration, between states of dependency and ones of independence" (Pinfold, 2000, p. 210). In this regard, supportive workplaces operating in the social economy may be seen as what Yates et al. describe as "halfway points": "places which have an ethos of inclusivity but are not located in a mental healthcare setting or solely attended by mental healthcare recipients" (2012, p. 110). By operating beyond the spaces of medicine, halfway points such as social enterprises are essential in an ongoing process of community inclusion (Parr, 2008). While in fact sites such as the workplaces examined here might only buffer the health-damaging effects of poverty, they do provide an opportunity to occupy a different social location in the community, despite the restrictions and stigma of illness.

Conclusion

This chapter has examined how, by enabling accommodating and sustainable employment, supportive workplaces assist the recovery process of people with psychiatric disabilities in significant and profound ways. In so doing, it has considered one place-based dimension of mental difference (the workplace), and its role in the recovery process. Our analysis draws attention to the intersection of three health determinants – poverty, employment, and workplace conditions – and their implications for community inclusion of people with psychiatric disabilities. This nexus has significant ramifications for the recovery hopes of such people: when barriers in the workplace limit employment opportunities, their income potential is detrimentally impacted, affecting living conditions, psychological functioning, and health-related behavior. In the case of people with psychiatric disabilities, both the poverty trap and the benefit trap can be read as experiential dimensions of this particular intersectionality. While not a panacea for the chronic poverty faced by this group, the supportive workplaces made available by social economy organizations intervene at this point of intersection. They function as critical halfway points in the recovery landscape. As such, they are experienced as important arenas of recovery by individuals seeking out meaning, purpose, and belonging in the context of everyday life. These geographies are a reminder of the centrality of one's place-in-the-world in shaping health and health inequalities (Kearns, 1993).

Acknowledgments

We extend our sincere thanks to the staff and workers of the social enterprises which agreed to participate in the interviews. We also thank the editors of the collection for constructive criticism on an earlier draft of the chapter. This chapter is based on research funded by the Social Sciences and Humanities Research Council of Canada (SSHRC).

References

Amin, A., Cameron, A. and Hudson, R., 2002. *Placing the social economy*. New York: Routledge.

Bejerholm, U. and Eklund, M., 2007. Occupational engagement in persons with schizophrenia: Relationships to self-related variables, psychopathology, and quality of life. *American Journal of Occupational Therapy*, 61(1), pp. 21–32.

Blank, A., Harries, P. and Reynolds, F., 2011. Mental health service users' perspectives of work: A review of the literature. *British Journal of Occupational Therapy*, 74(4), pp. 191–9.

Borg, M. and Davidson, L., 2008. The nature of recovery as lived in everyday experience. *Journal of Mental Health*, 17(2), pp. 129–40.

Borg, M. and Kristiansen, K., 2008. Working on the edge: The meaning of work for people recovering from severe mental distress in Norway. *Disability & Society*, 23(5), pp. 511–23.

Davidson, L. and Roe, D., 2007. Recovery from versus recovery in serious mental illness: One strategy for lessening confusion plaguing recovery. *Journal of Mental Health*, 16(4), pp. 459–70.

DeVerteuil, G. and Evans, J., 2010. Landscape of despair. In: T. Brown, S. McLafferty and G. Moon, eds. *A companion to health and medical geography*. London: Wiley-Blackwell, pp. 278–300.

Esping-Andersen, G., 1993. *The three worlds of welfare capitalism*. Princeton, NJ: Princeton University Press.

Fawcett, G. and Marshall, C., 2014. People with mental/psychological disabilities: Results from the 2012 Canadian Survey on Disability. Paper presented at Canadian Disability Studies Association meeting, Brock University, St Catherine's, Ontario, May 28.

Fossey, E. and Harvey, C., 2010. Finding and sustaining employment: A qualitative meta-synthesis of mental health consumer views. *Canadian Journal of Occupational Therapy*, 77(5), pp. 303–14.

Hall, E., 2005. The entangled geographies of social exclusion/inclusion for people with learning disabilities. *Health & Place*, 11(2), pp. 107–15.

Hanandita, W. and Tampubolon, G., 2014. Does poverty reduce mental health? An instrumental variable analysis. *Social Science & Medicine*, 113, pp. 59–67.

Hudson, C., 2005. Socioeconomic status and mental illness: Tests of the social causation and selection hypothesis. *American Journal of Orthopsychiatry*, 75(1), pp. 3–18.

Kearns, R.A., 1993. Place and health: Towards a reformed medical geography. *Professional Geographer*, 45(2), pp. 139–47.

Kinn, L., Holgersen, H., Randi, A. and Davidson, L., 2014. "Balancing on skates on the icy surface of work": A metasynthesis of work participation for persons with psychiatric disabilities. *Journal of Occupational Rehabilitation*, 24(1), pp. 125–38.

Knowles, C., 2000. *Bedlam on the streets*. New York: Routledge.

Leamy, M., Bird, V., Le Boutillier, C., Williams, J. and Slade, M., 2011. Conceptual framework for personal recovery in mental health: Systematic review and narrative synthesis. *British Journal of Psychiatry*, 199(6), pp. 445–52.

Lund, C., Breen, A., Flisher, A., Kakuma, R., Corrigall, J., Joska, J., Swartz, L. and Patel, V., 2010: Poverty and common mental disorders in low and middle income countries: A systematic review. *Social Science & Medicine*, 71(3), pp. 517–28.

Manderscheid, R., 2013. Escaping the "poverty trap." *Behavioral Healthcare*, July/August, pp. 49–50.

Marwaha, S. and Johnson, S., 2005. Views and experiences of employment among people with psychosis: A qualitative descriptive study. *International Journal of Social Psychiatry*, 51(4), pp. 302–16.

Mental Health Commission of Canada, 2009. *Toward recovery and well-being: A framework for a mental health strategy for Canada*. Ottawa: Mental Health Commission of Canada.

Mikkonen, J. and Raphael, D., 2010. *Social determinants of health: The Canadian facts*. Toronto: York University School of Health Policy and Management.

Muntaner, C., Eaton, W.W., Miech, R. and O'Campo, P., 2004. Socioeconomic position and major mental disorders. *Epidemiologic Reviews*, 26(1), pp. 53–62.

Onken, S.J., Craig, C.M., Ridgeway, P., Ralph, R. and Cook, J., 2007. An analysis of the definitions and elements of recovery: A review of the literature. *Psychiatric Rehabilitation Journal*, 31(1), pp. 9–22.

Parr, H., 2008. *Mental health and social space: Towards inclusionary geographies?* Malden, MA: Blackwell Publishing.

Pinfold, V., 2000. "Building up safe havens ... all around the world": users' experiences of living in the community with mental health problems. *Health & Place*, 6(3), pp. 201–12.

Piven, F. and Cloward, R., 1993. *Regulating the poor: The functions of public welfare*. New York: Vintage.

Prince, M.J., 2014. Locating a window of opportunity in the social economy: Canadians with disabilities and labour market challenges. *Canadian Journal of Nonprofit and Social Economy Research*, 5(1), pp. 6–20.

Province of Ontario, 2016. *Eligibility for ODSP income support*. Available online at www.mcss.gov.on.ca/en/mcss/programs/social/odsp/income_support/IS_Eligibility.aspx (accessed February 4, 2016).

Rinaldi, M., Killackey, E., Smith, J., Shepherd, G., Singh, S. and Craig, T., 2010. First episode psychosis and employment: A review. *International Review of Psychiatry*, 22(2), pp. 148–62.

Ruggeri, M., Leese, M., Thornicroft, G., Bisoffi, G. and Tansella, M. 2000. Definition and prevalence of severe and persistent mental illness. *British Journal of Psychiatry*, 177, pp. 149–55.

Saunders, S.L. and Nedelec, B., 2014. What work means to people with work disability: A scoping review. *Journal of Occupational Rehabilitation*, 24(1), pp. 100–10.

Sells, D., Stayner, D. and Davidson, L., 2004. Recovering the self in schizophrenia: An integrative review of qualitative studies. *Psychological Quarterly*, 75(1), pp. 87–97.

Sells, D., Borg, M., Marin, I., Mezzina, R., Topor, A. and Davidson, L., 2006. Arenas of recovery for persons with severe mental illness. *American Journal of Psychiatric Rehabilitation*, 9(2), pp. 3–16.

Slade, M., Amering, M. and Oades, L., 2008. Recovery: An international perspective. *Epidemiologia e Psichiatria Sociale* [*Epidemiology and Social Psychiatry*], 17(2), pp. 128–37.

Tiikkaja, S., Sandin, S., Malki, N., Modin, B., Sparen, P. and Hultman, C., 2013. Social class, social mobility and risk of psychiatric disorder: A population-based longitudinal study. *PLOS ONE*, 8(11), pp. 1–9.

Tweddle, A., Battle, K. and Torjman, S., 2013. *Welfare in Canada 2012*. Ottawa: Caledon Institute of Social Policy.

Waghorn G. and Lloyd C., 2005. The employment of people with mental illness. *Australian e-Journal for the Advancement of Mental Health*, 4(2), pp. 1–43. Available online at www.tandfonline.com/doi/abs/10.5172/jamh.4.2.129 (accessed February 4, 2016).

Williams, A., Fossey, E. and Harvey, C., 2012. Social firms: Sustainable employment for people with mental illness. *Work*, 43(1), pp. 53–62.

Wilton, R., 2003. Poverty and mental health: A qualitative study of residential care facility tenants. *Community Mental Health Journal*, 39(2), pp. 139–56.

Wilton, R., 2004. More responsibility, less control: Psychiatric survivors and welfare state restructuring. *Disability & Society*, 19(4), pp. 371–85.

Yates, I., Holmes, G. and Priest, H., 2012. Recovery, place and community mental health services. *Journal of Mental Health*, 21(2), pp. 104–13.

6   Spaces and Places

Engaging a Mixed-methods Approach for Exploring the Multiple Geographies of Pedestrian Injury

Jonathan Cinnamon and Daniel Z. Sui

Injury transcends boundaries: it is a scourge in every part of the world and in all sectors of society. Injury is a leading cause of mortality in children and working-age adults in most countries (Mock et al., 2004; World Health Organization, 2010), a sobering fact incongruous with the conventional belief that injuries are the consequence of accident or events that are not controllable (Krug et al., 2000). The Global Burden of Disease study, a comprehensive study of global mortality and morbidity for all causes, estimated that in 2010 injury was responsible for more than 5 million global deaths annually (9.6 percent of total mortality), representing an increase from 4.1 million in 1990 (8.8 percent of total mortality) (Lozano et al., 2012). Interestingly, these 2010 injury mortality estimates are substantially higher than the approximate 3.8 million deaths caused by HIV/AIDS, malaria, and tuberculosis combined (Lozano et al., 2012). Despite this massive burden of morbidity and mortality, injury continues to be largely overlooked as a public health issue by all sectors of society, including governments, health organizations, health funders, and by the public itself (Mock et al., 2004).

Although injury transcends socioeconomic status, age, sex, and other dimensions of difference, it is not evenly experienced across a homogenous population; rather, analysis of injury data demonstrates that particular age groups, social classes, and geographic locations are disproportionately burdened by injury. In Canada, rates of injury vary widely among different population groups which tend to be at increased risk. Particularly, a relationship exists between age and injury, especially when sex is also considered. For all causes combined, injury is the leading cause of death for both females and males in the 1–34 age groups; however, in males this statistic expands to include those aged 1–44 (Statistics Canada, 2012). Looking at specific injury types, such as road traffic injuries, it is evident that all young people are disproportionately at risk; however, males are particularly overrepresented (Emery et al., 2008). Internationally, this overrepresentation of males is related to factors such as lack of experience and increased risk-taking behaviors (MacDonald et al., 2007). Within Canada, these risks are likely amplified by winter weather and the culture of youth driving. Conversely, a recent troubling rise in overall rates of severe injuries in Canada has been attributed to a notable increase in fall injuries in older Canadians (Hill et al.,

2014): a trend that may be expected to rise even further as Canada's population continues to age. In addition, some minority ethnic and cultural groups in Canada are overrepresented in injury statistics. For example, high rates of self-harm injuries and suicide in Aboriginal youth are well documented (Kirmayer et al., 2007) (for an overview of Indigenous peoples' health, see Chapter 3). Moreover, a study in Montreal suggests that occupational injuries are likely to be higher in immigrant, ethnic, and linguistic minority groups (especially among women) due to their overrepresentation in higher-risk jobs (Premji et al., 2010).

By identifying specific population groups which are disproportionately at risk of injury through population and geographic analyses, evidence-based injury prevention efforts can be implemented to target specific groups. Potentially, this has the double impact of addressing the social consequences of injury while at the same time reducing massive economic consequences. Although figures on the economic costs of injury are estimates only, a Canadian study came up with a total figure of C$26.8 billion for all injuries in 2010, including the direct costs (C$15.9 billion) of patient care and rehabilitation to the national health system, and the indirect costs (C$10.9 billion) to the economy through decreased productivity (Parachute, 2015).

In many high-income countries including Canada, evidence-based injury-prevention efforts have been successful in reducing the burden of injury. Yet when injury is broken down into its various causes or mechanisms, it becomes clear that some injury-prevention efforts still have a long way to go. Most notable are road traffic injuries, which remain a major problem in the urban areas of many countries, regardless of their development status. Although the 2010 version of the Global Burden of Disease study notes that age-standardized mortality rates for all injury types combined have dipped since 1990, some injury subtypes have risen dramatically in this time frame: for example, pedestrian injury, which rose almost 18 percent; as well as road traffic injuries, where a rise of more than 6 percent was found (Lozano et al., 2012). Road traffic injuries have been predicted to become the fifth largest cause of death for all age groups by 2030, while already today it is the leading cause of death worldwide for those aged 15–29 (World Health Organization, 2010).

Within Canada, pedestrian injury is one mechanism of overall road traffic injuries that continues to rise, despite existing concerns and consistent ongoing data collection. Between 2003 and 2013, pedestrian injury as a percentage of total road traffic injuries increased each year from 9.8 percent to 14.5 percent, while pedestrian fatalities rose from 13.6 to 15.6 percent over that time period (Transport Canada, 2004, 2015). As such, improving pedestrian safety should be a primary concern for urban planners and traffic engineers due to the significant public health burden, but it is often overlooked. Furthermore, with active transportation such as cycling and walking becoming increasingly promoted for urban livability, environmental, and personal health reasons, pedestrian safety will only become a more serious concern.

In this chapter we aim to explore the diversity of population groups and geographic contexts implicated in pedestrian injury risk, while considering the role of a mixed-methods approach for so doing. Through its focus on scalar and methodological diversity, we begin by exploring the range of knowledge produced by intersecting qualitative and quantitative approaches to understanding pedestrian injury in Vancouver, Canada. Building from this evidence, we then introduce the emerging area of qualitative geographic information systems (GIS): a rapidly developing range of approaches that combine spatial analysis and place-based qualitative methods and data. Here, we claim that such an approach may be useful for geographic health research that requires methodological diversity in order to understand better the diversity within and between population groups. Examples are provided from our work in Cape Town, South Africa, and Columbus, Ohio. The main contention of this chapter is that harnessing diversity in method, at both aggregated spatial scales and the level of individual places, is necessary for developing effective pedestrian safety interventions that address the needs of diverse local populations. This argument derives its basis from an increasing recognition of the heterogeneity of places, and the folly of the "one-size-fits-all" approach to health promotion and prevention. The following section provides a brief overview on the current use of methodological diversity in health and pedestrian injury research.

Understanding Pedestrian Injury through Methodological Diversity

The use of mixed methods has enjoyed steady growth in the sciences and social sciences in recent years. Tashakkori and Teddlie (2003) have described this period as the "third methodological movement," which itself is a synthesis of the quantitative movement that became dominant in the 1950s, and the qualitative movement that superceded it in more recent decades. Specifically, mixed methods is an approach to research that combines both qualitative and quantitative data, methods, and/or analysis in a single study. Rebuffing the incompatibility thesis (Howe, 1988) – the notion that qualitative and quantitative approaches are discordant – proponents of mixed methods have helped to deconstruct the binary thinking responsible for such paradigm wars that has long pitted proponents of one side against the other: positivist versus interpretivist (Johnson and Onwuegbuzie, 2004). While the reasons for employing mixed methods are multitudinous, typically such an approach is used for the purposes of confirming, complementing, or triangulating knowledge.

Given the different types of knowledge that qualitative and quantitative approaches each can produce, mixed methods have the ability to illustrate a deeper, more comprehensive, and nuanced picture of a particular issue than one method used alone, or each approach conducted in parallel rather than together (Creswell, 2009). A meta-analysis by Collins et al. (2006) distilled four broad reasons for carrying out mixed methods:

1) participant enrichment – for example, a quantitative analysis may be conducted first to inform a sampling strategy for a subsequent qualitative ethnography;
2) instrument fidelity – for example, a quantitative analysis could be employed to determine the utility and appropriateness of a qualitative interview method, thereby improving the study's validity, credibility, or transferability;
3) treatment integrity – mixing methods to assess the fidelity of interventions, treatments, or programs; and
4) significance enhancement – for example, using qualitative data and analysis to enhance the interpretation of meaning derived from quantitative data and analysis.

Health geography may be one of the more diverse subdisciplines of human geography in terms of research foci and topics, and certainly in terms of the data, analysis techniques, and methods employed (Rosenberg, 1998). The shift from medical to health geography beginning in the 1990s purportedly marked a shift away from quantitative, positivist approaches emblematic of a biomedical model of health towards the interpretivism or social constructivism of qualitative methods (Kearns, 1993; Kearns and Moon, 2002). Concomitantly, we have witnessed the subtle shift from space to place perspectives in health geography studies. Yet quantitative methods have remained a significant part of an expansive contemporary health geography, despite the increasingly rare use of the medical geography epithet. A recent review article (Andrews et al., 2012) identified a range of current methodological approaches in global health geographical inquiry, from quantitative approaches such as spatial analysis and GIS and multilevel statistical modeling, to qualitative methods including oral history, participatory methods, and narrative analysis. In Canada specifically, a review of recent research themes in Canadian health geography identified – in addition to conventional methods – a number of novel research methods being used in the country, including photovoice, digital storytelling, and autoethnography (Giesbrecht et al., 2014). These recent reviews of the subdiscipline characterize a healthy and diverse field able to produce diverse knowledge using a range of tested and cutting-edge methods, both qualitative and quantitative.

Knowledge of the particular groups at risk of pedestrian injury has been greatly enhanced through geographic analysis by health geographers and public health researchers. In recent years, due to the wider availability of location data in health datasets and the rapid expansion of GIS, quantitative methods have been extensively used in pedestrian injury research to illustrate spatial distributions and uncover its range of social determinants (e.g. Braddock et al., 1994;

Lightstone et al., 2001; Yiannakoulias et al., 2002; Sciortino et al., 2005). A study by LaScala et al. (2000) provides an early example of the value of this approach. The authors used a GIS-based, spatial analysis approach to map pedestrian injury locations and statistically associate the locations with socioeconomic and demographic risk factors. The findings suggested that pedestrian injuries are disproportionate in areas with greater unemployment and areas that have lower levels of education. The value in this type of spatial analysis of pedestrian injury lies in the ability to identify specific hotspot (high incident) locations, as well as specific demographic and socioeconomic groups that should be targeted for injury prevention.

Although less common than statistical and spatially informed analyses, geographic approaches to pedestrian injury have been enhanced also through qualitative data, methods, and analysis. For example, Butchart et al. (2000) reported on the qualitative responses to a survey that asked residents of a Johannesburg township about their perceptions of the causes of pedestrian injuries (and other mechanisms) in the local area. The findings from this study provided valuable place-specific evidence to address pedestrian safety in local neighborhoods. For example, in informal settlement areas, the respondents suggested that environmental and infrastructure improvements would be most successful for addressing pedestrian safety; while in areas with more formal housing, the respondents pointed to a need for more police and enforcement. While, for example, this difference in opinion might be reflective of socioeconomic differences between residents of the two neighborhoods, the point is that qualitative methods are particularly valuable for eliciting nuanced, locally-specific evidence compared to the more generalizable, large-scale evidence of spatial analysis methods. (This view is also shared in Chapter 7.)

Despite the value of both quantitative and qualitative geographic analyses of pedestrian injury, few studies combine them – particularly those that aim to design effective injury prevention interventions (Heinonen and Eck, 2007). One research project conducted in Mexico highlights the deeper and more thorough evidence that can be generated by mixing methods in a single study (Híjar et al., 2003). Híjar and colleagues conducted a statistical analysis of pedestrian mortality records to calculate death rates, and a spatial analysis to understand injury patterns at the aggregate level (neighborhoods). Since those methods could not describe traffic characteristics, the presence of safety infrastructure, attitudes towards safety, or other similar determinants of pedestrian safety, they employed two other types of qualitative methods. An observational survey of the built environment uncovered place-specific contextual information about pedestrian injury risk, as did in-depth interviews with drivers and pedestrians. Notably, given the lack of data on survivors inherent in the mortality records used in the statistical analysis, the interviews were valuable for eliciting evidence of the demographic and socioeconomic status of pedestrian injury survivors. Interestingly, this qualitative aspect of the study suggested that groups with lower levels of education may be disproportionately at risk of pedestrian injury because they are less likely to drive, and therefore may be less aware of traffic speeds, road rules, and safety.

Similarly, a study in Los Angeles, California attempted to understand the diverse contexts and populations at risk of pedestrian injury by using both quantitative and qualitative methods, although in a slightly different way (Loukaitou-Sideris et al., 2007). Rather than conduct the various methods in parallel, Loukaitou-Sideris and colleagues first conducted a statistical and spatial analysis to provide preliminary evidence of the relationships between pedestrian–motor vehicle collisions and aggregate sociodemographic and land use characteristics at census tract level, then used this information to design a qualitative, detailed case study analysis of specific hotspot locations. Combined, these approaches identified how pedestrian injury is associated with specific segments of society – notably, lower income and Hispanic populations. This example is emblematic of Collins et al.'s (2006) significance enhancement rationale for mixed methods, since they used qualitative methods to enhance the interpretation of meaning from the initial quantitative methods. As Loukaitou-Sideris and colleagues (2007) describe, this approach allowed them to understand the bigger picture in the first phase, then to drill down and uncover deeper meaning at ground level by conducting observational studies of hotspots identified in the first phase, together providing robust evidence for strategies and policies that could produce a safer pedestrian environment. For example, one hotspot location examined in the qualitative phase of the study was observed to have many elderly residents crossing the street at a slower pace, which did not allow them to complete crossing before the light turned red. This place-specific knowledge is valuable for pedestrian safety at this location (e.g. a longer pedestrian crossing phase could be implemented), and would not have been identified using macro-level spatial or statistical methods.

Pedestrian Injury in Vancouver: A Mixed-methods Approach

Our research uses a range of methods and approaches to understand pedestrian injury in Vancouver, BC (Schuurman et al., 2009; Cinnamon et al., 2011). Vancouver is an important site for pedestrian injury research, given its high rates of pedestrian injuries coupled with a diverse population and heterogeneous urban neighborhoods. Vancouver is a city with a large degree of diversity along ethnic, linguistic, and cultural lines, with almost 50 percent of the population in 2011 indicating that English was not their native tongue (Statistics Canada, 2011). Vancouver is also a city of socioeconomic diversity, evident in the range of incomes and levels of education of its residents. For example, some neighborhoods such as Point Grey and West Vancouver primarily comprise residents with very high average incomes and levels of education, compared to those residents of several eastside neighborhoods including the Downtown Eastside, and suburban areas including Whalley in Surrey (Bell et al., 2007).

As identified in the previous section, pedestrian injury is frequently observed in higher rates in populations and areas of lower socioeconomic status, which often include minority, lower income, and less educated groups. One of the goals of this research project was to identify this diversity in the Vancouver context. More specifically, this project was designed to provide evidence of the diverse social, environmental, and behavioral issues that intersect to create safe environments for pedestrians, with the ultimate goal of providing a comprehensive collection of knowledge for evidence-based decision-making on pedestrian injury prevention. Given the variety of factors that are believed to contribute to pedestrian injury risk, this project utilized a mixed-method study design to tease out both macro-level and micro-level factors at play.

Method

Procedure

The first step in the project was to conduct a spatial analysis, in order to understand the spatial distribution of pedestrian injury in the City of Vancouver (Schuurman et al., 2009). As in the studies mentioned in the previous section, GIS and spatial analysis methods have been shown to be highly valuable for making sense of pedestrian injury data. The use of GIS in this field, and in public health research more generally, has grown substantially now that relevant databases often have location information available (e.g. location of injury event) which is frequently collected in trauma registry databases, emergency medical services reports, police records, and insurance reports. For this study, a pedestrian injury database was created that merged six years of records kept by the Insurance Corporation of British Columbia for all crash claim reports, and data from the British Columbia Trauma Registry for patients admitted to hospital with a severe injury. It was believed that the two datasets combined would capture most of the pedestrian injuries that occurred in Vancouver. Not all pedestrian injury victims will be admitted to a hospital or make a claim to an insurance company; however, these are limitations inherent in many datasets. The locations were mapped to a midblock or intersection location, and analyzed using ArcGIS software to visualize the spatial pattern. Analysis of the dataset revealed that 2,358 pedestrian–motor vehicle collisions occurred in the six-year period from 2000–5. A majority of incidents occurred at intersections rather than midblock locations, while most happened on major arterial roads in the city. Kernel density maps were produced to identify high incident or hotspot locations throughout the city (see Figure 6.1). A number of high incident intersection and midblock locations were identified, with a vast majority found to be occurring on downtown core streets. More specifically, many of the most serious hotspots were found to be clustered in a small part of downtown Vancouver: the Downtown Eastside.

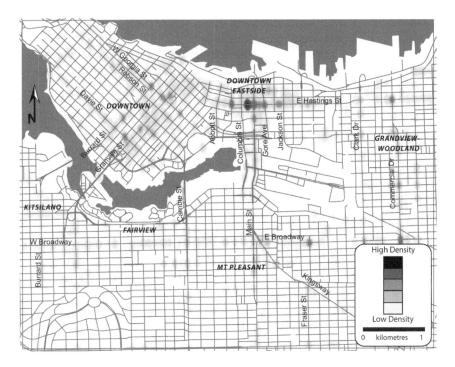

Figure 6.1 Pedestrian injury hotspots in Vancouver, 2000–5

Location

The Downtown Eastside is described infamously as Canada's poorest urban neighborhood – well known as a site of homelessness, drug use, and poor health, juxtaposed with strong community activism and social capital. This area is made up of a diverse population of approximately 18,000 people, although this number is likely higher due to underrepresentation of homeless and low-income residents of the area (City of Vancouver, 2012). The proportion of the Downtown Eastside population comprising low income is 53.3 percent (varying between different Downtown Eastside neighborhoods, from 38 percent in Strathcona to 80 percent in Victory Square), compared with just 19.2 percent for the City of Vancouver as a whole (City of Vancouver, 2012). An estimated 25 percent of the Downtown Eastside population are illicit drug users (Allford, 2008; Ley and Dobson, 2008). Similar to the findings of the studies in Mexico and Los Angeles described previously, it is likely that the social and material deprivation experienced by low-income populations in this area is a contributing factor in the high rate of pedestrian injury in the Downtown Eastside.

Because of the intriguing spatial pattern observed in the dataset and the large clustering of incidents in the Downtown Eastside, it was determined that a subsequent investigation should be undertaken to identify the specific factors at play at each of the hotspots. The hypothesis was that each individual hotspot might possess unique and diverse characteristics that produce an elevated risk of pedestrian injury, due in part to the socioeconomic diversity of residents living in proximity to the hotspots. As a result, it was determined that place-based methods would be most appropriate to paint a picture of each individual pedestrian injury hotspot in the city.

The spatial analysis provided the evidence to proceed with two observational place-based investigations to explore the risk factors for pedestrian injury at the identified hotspots. The first project focused on built environment risk factors that are known to be associated with a risk of pedestrian–motor vehicle collisions. A strategy was devised in which a team of observers would visit each of the hotspot locations and record the presence or absence of factors such as traffic calming measures, pedestrian safety infrastructure, roadway design choices (e.g. long blocks, visual obstructions, street parking), or land use associated with pedestrian injury (e.g. bars, retail, schools), which collectively form the uniqueness of each hotspot. The team of observers qualitatively rated the built environment according to the presence of these factors, in order to illustrate the local context at each hotspot and enable comparison between different locations.

The second hotspot survey was designed to uncover behavioral factors that might contribute to pedestrian injury risk, such as road rule infractions by pedestrians and motorists when navigating intersections. Using a method similar to the built environment survey, with the exception of collecting quantitative data, a team of researchers observed infractions by drivers (e.g. entering the intersection in the yellow/red light phase), and pedestrians (e.g. crossing outside of the markings or walk signal phase), and total vehicle and pedestrian volumes at intersection hotspots throughout the city.

Findings

The findings of both hotspot surveys suggested that each hotspot was unique in terms of the built environment, land use, and behavioral factors contributing to pedestrian injury risk. For example, the results of the survey identified great variation in the presence of bars and alcohol serving establishments in the immediate vicinity of different hotspots around the city – a known risk factor for pedestrian injuries. At all of the hotspots identified in the Downtown Eastside neighborhood, including the intersections of East Hastings and Main, Carrall, and Gore Streets, all locations were rated as having a high density of bars in their immediate vicinity. This differs from many hotspots in other areas of the city, such as Broadway and Commercial and Georgia and Burrard Streets, where alcohol establishments were not present in the immediate vicinity, but shopping and retail land use was ranked as high. The road-rule violations recorded also varied greatly between hotspots. For example, at Hastings and Commercial almost 40 percent of pedestrians committed one of the observed infractions while crossing the street, while only about

10 percent did at Georgia and Burrard Streets. For motorists, 7.5 percent committed one of the observed infractions at Broadway and Commercial, while only 3.2 percent did at Hastings and Commercial. These few examples are representative of the much larger amount of evidence collected on built environment, land use, and behavioral factors at each hotspot. The primary finding from this research is that great variation exists between the risk factors at each hotspot, which suggests that each specific place is unique with respect to the factors contributing to pedestrian injury.

The spatial and place-specific analyses described above provide a range of macro-level and micro-level evidence that proved to be valuable for decision-makers wanting to address the pedestrian injury problem in Vancouver. The spatial analysis and mapping revealed a distinct pattern that highlighted the downtown core – especially the Downtown Eastside – as the epicenter of pedestrian injury in the city. This finding provided the stimulus for a community-based research project: the Downtown Eastside Pedestrian Safety Project. This project brought together a range of stakeholders including Downtown Eastside residents, City of Vancouver employees, public health workers, and academic injury researchers to inform place-based data collection at the hotspots highlighted in the spatial analysis.

Education was also a key component of the Downtown Eastside Pedestrian Safety Project, particularly for drivers via on-street, online, and media campaigns. Since local residents were primarily pedestrians of lower socioeconomic means, a wider range of education campaigns were developed, including in-person, one-on-one discussions, leafleting, and community-based meetings in which residents were involved in discussions about the reasons for their greater risk of pedestrian injury. Furthermore, the Pedestrian Safety Project used and modified the observational survey methodologies described above to collect a range of social, environmental, and behavioral data at locations within the Downtown Eastside. This information was compiled into a report presented to the city council, along with a number of area-wide and site-specific recommendations to improve pedestrian safety in the neighborhood.

The final project report (Russwurm and Buchanan, 2010), along with evidence from the spatial and place-based academic analyses (Schuurman et al., 2009; Cinnamon et al., 2011), provided a range of evidence at various scales which helped to influence safety policy. On receiving this evidence, the City of Vancouver implemented a number of the recommendations, including a reduced speed zone (from 50 to 30 km/h) along a six-block stretch of Hastings Street from Abbott to Gore, countdown timers, increased crossing times, and mid-block crossings at individual sites.

This example of pedestrian injury research in Vancouver points to the value of taking a diverse approach to methods, including qualitative and quantitative, macro-level spatial analysis and micro-level place-based analysis. In this example, a quantitative spatial analysis was conducted first to illustrate the overall pattern, which then informed a place-based analysis using both qualitative and quantitative methods to illustrate local conditions at ground level. This could be described as an example of what Collins et al. (2006) describe as the significance enhancement rationale for mixed-methods, since the place-based analyses helped to enhance the interpretation of meaning pertaining to the observed spatial pattern. The spatial analysis identified the hotspots and the clustering in the Downtown Eastside, but the place-based methods probed deeper to reveal potential reasons for the existence of each individual hotspot.

Qualitative Geographic Information Systems

A promising new field of inquiry within a broader GIS science may prove to be valuable for conducting mixed methods and combining spatial and place-based approaches in pedestrian injury research, and in health geography more broadly. Qualitative GIS has appeared in the past several years as a collection of approaches that attempts to infuse the qualitative worldview into geospatially informed research projects; thus, it may be best described as a mixed-methods approach (Cope and Elwood, 2009) that attempts to position GIS outside of the positivist and quantitative by nurturing diversity in data, method, knowledge production, and representation (Elwood and Cope, 2009; Sui and DeLyser, 2012). With qualitative GIS and its siblings, feminist GIS and participatory GIS, geographic information technologies are being increasingly used in inductive and interpretive ways for exploratory purposes and to generate hypotheses – which is a major shift from its more conventional use as a tool for hypothesis testing and deductive forms of knowledge production. Qualitative GIS has emerged out of the shadow of two decades of critique of GIS, under the banner of *critical* GIS (Schuurman, 1999) which, among many other issues, focused on the inability of GIS to represent and foster diversity with respect to data, methods, and epistemology (Pickles, 1995; Sheppard, 2005; O'Sullivan, 2006). Furthermore, GIS was seen to be incongruent with geography-as-place, given its powerful capabilities to represent and analyze the spatial. These critiques were spearheaded from within human geography, a discipline which had become increasingly diverse in these respects over the past several decades. GIS was seen as a "Trojan Horse," representing a return to positivism and the reductionism and abstractness of spatiality – both of which represented the antithesis of the discipline's budding diversity. Qualitative GIS has since developed as a direct attempt to address GIS's shortcomings pertaining to data, methods, and knowledge production. As Wilson (2009) describes, qualitative GIS disrupts conventional ideas about GIS: it challenges what terms such as distance and location mean; it mixes the numeric with the non-numeric; it deconstructs the subject/object dualism of positivism; and entertains some of the central concerns of the qualitative worldview (e.g. positionality, plurality, partiality, and situated knowledge).

While not a specific method or approach in itself, qualitative GIS is more of an umbrella concept for a wide range of possibilities that combine geospatial approaches with the qualitative at various levels, including at the level of data, methods, analysis, or representation. As Jung and Elwood summarize, in some examples of qualitative GIS:

> "[T]he qualitative" means evidence gathered through qualitative methods, such as interview transcripts, field notes and observations, or sketches or photographs. For others, "the qualitative" is rendered through forms of analysis that are usually associated with qualitative methods, such as content, discourse, or narrative analysis, triangulation among multiple sources of evidence, or grounded theory. (2010, p.67)

Kwan and Ding's (2008) geo-narrative – an approach to visually represent ethnographic data pertaining to the daily lives of women – is a good example of the use of a mixed-methods, qualitative GIS approach that is enacted at the levels of analysis and representation. Knigge and Cope (2006) describe a qualitative GIS approach that they term "grounded visualization," which attempts to undertake mixed-methods research by integrating qualitative and quantitative data at the level of analysis. Knigge and Cope describe how the qualitative grounded theory approach and GIS-based visualization mutually support exploratory and iterative modes of knowledge production, as demonstrated through a case study of community gardens in Buffalo, New York. A range of methods was employed, including census data interpretation, GIS analysis and visualization, participant observation, and textual analysis. According to them:

> Although participant observation, fieldwork, and attendance of public meetings would have provided information about processes associated with creating community gardens, these methods alone would not have provided a complete picture of the neighborhood without the inclusion of quantitative data, and, conversely, an analysis solely consisting of census data, GIS and visualization, and other quantitative methods would not have revealed trends in community-based activities such as the creation of community gardens. (Knigge and Cope, 2006, p. 2034)

Jung and Elwood (2010) describe computer-aided qualitative GIS (CAQ-GIS) as a potentially powerful way to do qualitative GIS at the level of analysis. Rather than trying to conduct qualitative analysis from within GIS, they propose a parallel strategy for harnessing GIS alongside computer-aided qualitative data analysis (CAQDAS) software such as Atlas.ti, in which data are processed using qualitative coding and then analyzed in GIS and CAQDAS platforms. As they describe:

> [P]arallel queries are valuable for robust qualitative GIS because they open the door to a much richer exploration of *all* data related to a specific theme, and because they allow researchers to develop explanations about this theme through multiple modes of analysis. (Jung and Elwood, 2010, p. 82; emphasis in original)

The methods described above illustrate the somewhat complex examples of qualitative GIS for the purposes of analysis, yet there are also examples of qualitative GIS that are enacted at the more accessible levels of data production and representation. For example, the production and represen-tation of qualitative data in a GIS or mapping environment has become popular, especially due to the rise of geospatial Web technologies such as Google Earth and Google Maps, mobile technologies, social media, and volunteered geographic information. Qualitative and quantitative data can be produced using a qualitative GIS approach. Research that we have been involved with in Cape Town, South Africa is emblematic of this move-ment towards producing and representing spatial and place-related data using visual technologies and a mixed-methods approach (Cinnamon and Schuurman, 2013).

Cape Town, South Africa Project

Similar to Vancouver, Cape Town is an important field site for injury research due to its diversity and massive injury rates from interpersonal violence and motor vehicle collisions. As perhaps the most emblematic example of South Africa's "Rainbow Nation," Cape Town is a city comprising various ethnic groups from a range of socioeconomic classes, some of which are vastly over-represented in injury statistics. Despite the end of apartheid 20 years ago, this diversity is still rendered geographically, with a high degree of ethnic and socioeconomic homogeneity within specific areas of the city (Niekerk et al., 2006). Due to this reality, a key overall objective of this project was to iden-tify the spatial and place-based patterns of injury in Cape Town, which then would enable identification of specific ethnic and socioeconomic groups that could be specific targets for prevention.

This project emerged due to the lack of data available in Cape Town on the locations and local contributors to motor vehicle and pedestrian-related inju-ries. Our research team had been developing a number of hospital-based data collection strategies to collect data on injured patients, with a good deal of suc-cess (Cinnamon and Schuurman, 2010; Schuurman et al., 2011; Nicol et al., 2014; Zargaran et al., 2014). However, it was difficult to collect information on locations where injuries were sustained, as well as the range of social and environmental factors associated with injury at these locations. To address this particular gap in the data, a strategy was developed that would harness recent developments in GeoWeb technologies combined with a mixed-methods data collection strategy. A GeoWeb mapping interface was developed using the Google Maps JavaScript application programming interface (Google, 2011), as was an interview protocol to collect data about the specific locations in the city that are injury hotspots, and the circumstances by which they become high-incident locations. The data collection interface (Figure 6.2) consisted of a Google Map and a data collection form in which a participant could identify and geocode the locations they believed to be injury hotspots, and provide their

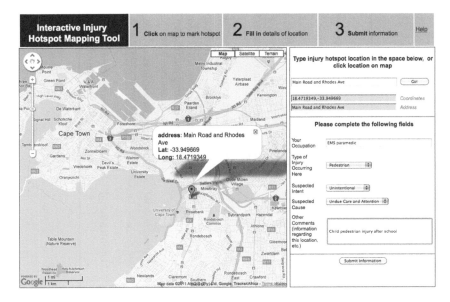

Figure 6.2 Injury hotspot mapping interface

opinion on the nature of the hotspot: for example, the factors they believed were responsible for it, and the specific population groups affected.

An informed participant group, emergency medical services (EMS) personnel, was selected for the informal interviews, given their knowledge of injury locations accrued as a key part of their duties retrieving patients from the site of the injury event. The interface was linked to an SQL database to store geocoded spatial location data, in addition to information about the type of injuries occurring at this location (e.g. violence, pedestrian), and the qualitative opinion of the participant as to the factors contributing to injuries at the hotspot. Table 6.1 and Figure 6.3 highlight examples of the location and contextual data that were produced using this approach.

This data collection approach was designed to fill a gap in the availability of information on the locations of injury hotspots in Cape Town, and the factors that contribute to their existence. The study used a qualitative research method and a Web mapping interface to produce both quantitative and qualitative information that could be valuable for injury prevention in this setting. The locations of injury hotspots could be further explored with regard to the comments made by the participants. Table 6.1 highlights a number of useful comments provided by the participants that are likely not to have been collected using conventional hospital-based quantitative data collection approaches. For example, the suggestion that one pedestrian hotspot was associated with the presence of children at the intersection on their way home after school provides evidence that could be used to educate at-risk children

Table 6.1 Qualitative and quantitative data about injury hotspots in Cape Town

X, Y coordinates	Location	Cause	Injury type	Intent	Comments and opinions
18.33585, -34.0519	Bay View Road	Violence	Assault	Intentional	This is a hotspot for violence between taxi drivers
18.5418641, -3.8176699	Dunoon	Violence	Assault	Intentional	Most victims here suffer from stab wounds
18.4031254, -33.900409	Mouille Point	Unknown	Self-harm	Intentional	Frequent self-harm victims in this affluent area
18.5835699, -33.935713	Elsie's River	Violence	Assault	Intentional	Recent increases in violence here
18.3925, -3.915277	Sea Point	Violence	Assault	Intentional	Post-club violence at this location
18.588621, -33.98356	Settlers Way	Violence	Vehicle occupant	Intentional	People from nearby KTC informal settlement causing intentional motor vehicle crashes here
18.4306419, -33.925057	Oswald Pirow Street	Undue care and attention	Pedestrian	Unintentional	Many pedestrian injuries here, especially on Wednesdays and Saturdays
18.4719349, -33.94669	Main Road and Rhodes Avenue	Undue care and attention	Pedestrian	Unintentional	Child pedestrian victims at this intersection after school lets out

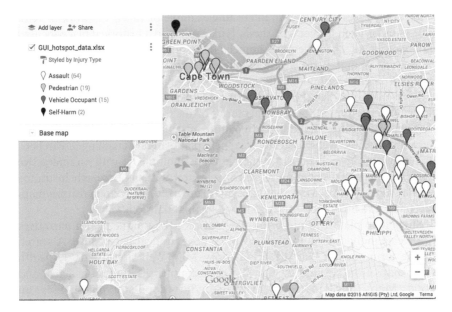

Figure 6.3 Injury hotspots by type, Cape Town, based on the opinions of emergency medical services personnel

in the local area. Similarly, the presence of violence-related injuries at another location was deemed to be associated with nearby nightclubs. If these suggestions could be further corroborated, decision-makers could develop interventions based on this evidence to address them.

Storymapping

It is now common practice and relatively simple to geotag photos, videos, audio, and text and visualize them on a map; this is widely seen on many commercial Web sites, and has been used as a representation approach in geographic research. Storymapping, a more recent addition to the qualitative GIS family, focuses particularly on the relationships between maps, spatial thinking, stories, and narratives (Caquard, 2013). Although maps, atlases, and other geographic visualizations always have been thought of as having the ability to tell a story, recent advances in Web technologies have made map-based narratives and storytelling an intriguing possibility for space- and place-based representation and inquiry. A particular example is the *New York Times* literary map of Manhattan, in which the user can navigate around a map interface, learning about the literary history of the city via text fragments from novels that describe their places and characters, images of local scenes, and the books' authors (see Cohen, 2005). For more research-oriented purposes, the hybridities of storymapping can simultaneously represent and draw out the macro-level spatial patterns at the same time as providing a platform to engage with the deeper personal experiences of place. An interesting example of this is the work of Kirk (2013) undertaken for her MA thesis. Kirk combined a historical place-focused ethnography of the Cherokee homeland as interpreted by James Mooney between 1887 and 1916, with the collective memory of the Cherokee nation using an interactive multimedia map. In so doing, Kirk (2013) demonstrates "what is possible when the Cherokee perspective is synthesized with geospatial technologies to present the ancient stories of the Cherokee homeland in a way that weaves traditional and modern culture into its components" (2013, p. iii). Several accessible Web-based storymapping platforms are enabling researchers, organizations, and citizens to combine online multimedia with an interactive mapping platform, including the Environmental Systems Research Institute's (ESRI) suite of Story Map apps (storymaps.arcgis.com/), Maptia (https://maptia.com/), and StoryMap[JS] (http://storymap.knightlab.com/).

Story map platforms are being used to trace the unique health narratives of diverse individuals and groups from a geographical perspective. A search of the term "health" on the ESRI Story Map Web site reveals 39 health story maps from around the world. One example, the Baltimore Farm and Food Map (http://mdfoodsystemmap.org/farm-food-storymap/) uses an ESRI Story Map platform to reveal the geographies of locally grown food. Navigating the interface reveals the spatial pattern of urban farms and the markets and restaurants where their food is available. Interacting with the photos, text, hyperlinks, and other multimedia reveals the local stories associated with each place. Together, both macro-level and micro-level information about the Baltimore food system is represented. Another example, entitled "Voices of the US Healthcare Safety Net" (www.directrelief.org/voices/) uses a story map interface to host qualitative data in the form of text, images, and audio interviews with non-profit health care providers, and quantitative data about the area including poverty level, the percentage of residents using Medicaid, and percentage of uninsured residents. The overall result simultaneously informs both the broader, overall picture and the specific, local particularities of nonprofit health care in a range of places across the USA.

For pedestrian injury, storymapping could help to construct a narrative that ties together macro-level spatial patterns with deeper contextual information of injury hotspot locations. Figure 6.4 is a screenshot of a story map that illustrates the pedestrian injury hotspots at intersections and midblock locations occurring between January 2009 and May 2014 on North High Street at Ohio State University (interactive version available at www.arcgis.com/apps/MapTour/?appid=ba206a43bfb04a788e3ce4ff38caec71). High Street is a primary commercial, retail, and nightlife corridor in Columbus, Ohio with high pedestrian activity. It is located at Ohio State University in the Short North area immediately south of campus, in downtown Columbus and in the German Village neighborhood. It is also a busy street for vehicles at all times of the day, since it is the major north–south thoroughfare that connects the campus and north Columbus neighborhoods with the downtown core

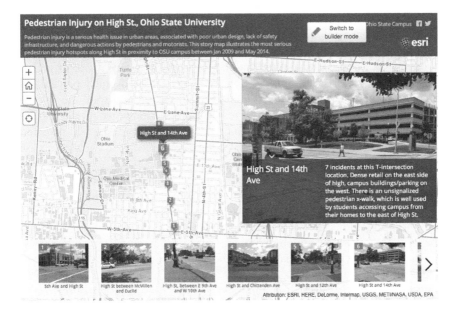

Figure 6.4 Screenshot of an interactive pedestrian injury story map, illustrating the spatial pattern and local characteristics of high incident locations on North High Street, Ohio State University campus

Source: www.arcgis.com/apps/MapTour/?appid=ba206a43bfb04a788e3ce4ff38caec71

and the neighborhoods to the south. The high numbers of incidents occurring on a short stretch of North High Street is cause for concern. The story map attempts to illustrate the spatial clustering along this short stretch of the street, along with local contextual information at each of the locations in terms of land use, pedestrian activity, and presence of safety infrastructure.

Returning to the Canadian health and health care context, a number of issues might be productively understood through qualitative GIS. For example, research on health care accessibility in rural areas of Canada often is explored either quantitatively or qualitatively. However, a mixed-method study focused on examining health care accessibility, and which acknowledges diversity among rural populations, could employ a qualitative GIS approach to merge spatial accessibility modeling with the visualized narratives and photographs of local residents. Such an approach would provide a nuanced understanding regarding how access to health care is experienced differently among various rural population groups.

Discussion and Conclusion

In this chapter we have illustrated the power of methodological diversity for producing a range of knowledge in health geography by using the specific example of research on the multiple geographies of pedestrian injury. We have demonstrated the valuable role that mixed-method approaches play in merging the spatial-analytical with the rich, unique, and contextual meanings bound up in place. Combining these perspectives can assist in identifying the specific locations and population groups that are disproportionately at risk of pedestrian injury, which is vital information for evidence-based injury prevention. A number of examples were provided that collectively illustrate the role of mixed-methods in pedestrian injury research. In so doing, we revisited existing research and attempted to illuminate the value that mixed qualitative and quantitative approaches have in contributing a comprehensive knowledge base that acknowledges the diverse spatial and place-based causes, consequences, and contingencies of pedestrian injury. Furthermore, we explored the potential value of qualitative GIS in contributing a nuanced understanding of pedestrian injury, which considers local behaviors and understandings among various populations, thus generating meaningful knowledge that could be used by various stakeholders interested in improving pedestrian safety.

Ultimately, we contend that the value of combining space and place knowledge via a mixed-methods approach allows research findings to be converted into actionable evidence for decision-makers. Many research topics of interest to health geographers demand instrumental knowledge for health promotion and prevention purposes. This is certainly the case for pedestrian injury, in which this type of knowledge can be directly applied to develop interventions that target the "three Es" of pedestrian safety: engineering, enforcement, and education. Pedestrian injuries cluster in specific locations, yet each location differs with respect to the factors at play that may be contributing to risk, including:

- road user behaviors;
- the unique characteristics of the local population, built environment and land use;
- pedestrian and driver volumes; and
- the presence or absence of traffic calming measures.

As such, it is critical to uncover the unique, local contributing factors and population groups at risk by conducting more in-depth, place-based research (qualitative or quantitative) in addition to broader spatial analyses. Such an approach is valuable since localized, place-specific interventions are often more effective than blanket, generalized safety campaigns (Duperrex et al., 2002; Heinonen and Eck, 2007). The example of the Downtown Eastside pedestrian safety collaboration illustrates the value in merging the *view from above* with the *view from below* – in other words, the spatial with place-specific knowledge production, education, and advocacy. The success that this project had in influencing pedestrian safety policy in the Downtown Eastside is due to combining the spatial knowledge of pedestrian injury (Schuurman et al., 2009) with the place-based knowledge produced in the subsequent study and the project's report (Russwurm and Buchanan, 2010).

While we argue for mixing methods through both spatial and place-based knowledge production, the potential difficulty in so doing must be acknowledged. This is particularly the case if diverse methods are run in parallel. However, a valid approach, as discussed throughout this chapter, is to allow the findings of one approach to inform the development of further research, using another suite of methods for the purposes of complementing, triangulating, or developing a more comprehensive body of knowledge. Thus, methodological diversity should be a priority for health geographers, particularly those who wish to develop a comprehensive account of health, well-being, and illness among diverse populations in diverse places.

References

Allford, J., 2008. *Letters from Hastings and Main: Signs of hope in Vancouver's Downtown Eastside*, Calgary: Canada West Foundation.

Andrews, G.J., Evans, J., Dunn, J.R. and Masuda, J.R., 2012. Arguments in health geography: On sub-disciplinary progress, observation, translation. *Geography Compass*, 6(6), pp. 351–83.

Bell, N., Schuurman, N., Oliver, L. and Hayes, M.V., 2007. Towards the construction of place-specific measures of deprivation: A case study from the Vancouver metropolitan area. *The Canadian Geographer*, 51(4), pp. 444–61.

Braddock, M., Lapidus, G., Cromley, E., Cromley, R., Burke, G. and Banco, L., 1994. Using a geographic information system to understand child pedestrian injury. *American Journal of Public Health*, 84(7), 1158–61.

Butchart, A., Kruger, J. and Lekoba, R., 2000. Perceptions of injury causes and solutions in a Johannesburg township: Implications for prevention. *Social Science and Medicine*, 50(3), pp. 331–44.

Caquard, S.B., 2013. Cartography I: Mapping narrative cartography. *Progress in Human Geography*, 37(1), pp. 135–44.

Cinnamon, J. and Schuurman, N., 2010. Injury surveillance in low-resource settings using Geospatial and Social web technologies. *International Journal of Health Geographics*, 9(1), pp. 1–13.

Cinnamon, J. and Schuurman, N., 2013. Confronting the data-divide in a time of spatial turns and volunteered geographic information. *GeoJournal*, 78(4), pp. 657–74.

Cinnamon, J., Schuurman, N. and Hameed, S.M., 2011. Pedestrian injury and human behaviour: Observing road-rule violations at high-incident intersections. *PLOS ONE*, 6(6), pp. 1–10.

City of Vancouver, 2012. Downtown Eastside DTES local area profile 2012. Vancouver: City of Vancouver.

Cohen, R. 2005. We'll Map Manhattan, New York Times, May 1. Available online at www.nytimes.com/2005/05/01/books/review/01COHENHO.html?ex=1272686400&en=f224304c75bc1469&ei=5088&partner=rssnyt&emc=rss&_r=0 (accessed July 8, 2014).

Collins, K.M., Onwuegbuzie, A.J. and Sutton, I.L., 2006. A model incorporating the rationale and purpose for conducting mixed methods research in special education and beyond. *Learning Disabilities: A Contemporary Journal*, 4(1), pp. 67–100.

Cope, M. and Elwood, S. eds, 2009. *Qualitative GIS: A mixed-methods approach.* London: Sage Publications.

Creswell, J.W., 2009. *Research design: Qualitative, quantitative, and mixed methods approaches.* Thousand Oaks, CA.: Sage Publications.

Duperrex, O., Bunn, F. and Roberts, I., 2002. Safety education of pedestrians for injury prevention: A systematic review of randomised controlled trials. *British Medical Journal*, 324, pp. 1129–33.

Elwood, S. and Cope, M., 2009. Introduction: Qualitative GIS: Forging mixed methods through representations, analytical innovations, and conceptual engagements. In: M. Cope and S. Elwood, eds. *Qualitative GIS: A mixed-methods approach.* London: Sage Publications, pp. 1–12.

Emery, P., Mayhew, D. and Simpson, H., 2008. *Youth and road crashes: Magnitude, characteristics, and trends.* Ottawa: Traffic Injury Research Foundation.

Giesbrecht, M., Cinnamon, J., Fritz, C. and Johnston, R., 2014. Themes in geographies of health and health care research: Reflections from the 2012 Canadian Association of Geographers annual meeting. *The Canadian Geographer*, 58(2), pp. 160–7.

Google 2011 Google Maps Javascript API. Available online at http://code.google.com/apis/maps/documentation/javascript/ (accessed May 21, 2011).

Heinonen, J.A. and Eck, J.E., 2007. Problem-oriented guides for Police: *Pedestrian injuries and fatalities.* Washington, DC: US Department of Justice.

Híjar, M., Trostle, J. and Bronfman, M., 2003. Pedestrian injuries in Mexico: A multi-method approach. *Social Science and Medicine*, 57(11), pp. 2149–59.

Hill, A.D., Pinto, R., Nathens, A.B. and Fowler, R.A., 2014. Age-related trends in severe injury hospitalization in Canada. *Journal of Trauma and Acute Care Surgery*, 77(4), pp. 608–13.

Howe, K.R., 1988. Against the quantitative–qualitative incompatibility thesis, or dogmas die hard. *Educational Researcher*, 17(8), pp. 10–16.

Johnson, R.B. and Onwuegbuzie, A.J., 2004. Mixed methods research: A research paradigm whose time has come. *Educational Researcher*, 33(7), pp. 14–26.

Jung, J.-K. and Elwood, S., 2010. Extending the qualitative capabilities of GIS: Computer-aided qualitative GIS. *Transactions in GIS*, 14(1), pp. 63–87.

Kearns, R.A., 1993. Place and health: Towards a reformed medical geography. *Professional Geographer*, 45(2), pp. 139–47.

Kearns, R. and Moon, G., 2002. From medical to health geography: Novelty, place and theory after a decade of change. *Progress in Human Geography*, 26(5), pp. 605–25.

Kirk, D.L., 2013. Visualizing the Cherokee Homeland through Indigenous historical GIS: An interactive map of James Mooney's ethnographic fieldwork and Cherokee collective memory. Lawrence, KS: Department of Geography, University of Kansas.

Kirmayer, L.J., Brass, G.M., Holton, T., Paul, K., Simpson, C. and Tait, C., 2007. *Suicide among Aboriginal People in Canada.* Ottawa: Aboriginal Healing Foundation.

Knigge, L. and Cope, M., 2006. Grounded visualization: Integrating the analysis of qualitative and quantitative data through grounded theory and visualization. *Environment and Planning A*, 38(11), pp. 2021–37.

Krug, E.G., Sharma, G.K. and Lozano, R., 2000. The global burden of injuries. *American Journal of Public Health*, 90(4), pp. 523–6.

Kwan, M.P. and Ding, G.X., 2008. Geo-narrative: Extending geographic information systems for narrative analysis in qualitative and mixed-method research. *Professional Geographer*, 60(4), pp. 443–65.

LaScala, E.A., Gerber, D. and Gruenewald, P.J., 2000. Demographic and environmental correlates of pedestrian injury collisions: A spatial analysis. *Accident Analysis and Prevention*, 32(5), pp. 651–8.

Ley, D. and Dobson, C., 2008. Are there limits to gentrification? The contexts of impeded gentrification in Vancouver. *Urban Studies*, 45(12), pp. 2471–98.

Lightstone, A.S., Dhillon, P.K., Peek-Asa, C. and Kraus, J.F., 2001. A geographic analysis of motor vehicle collisions with child pedestrians in Long Beach, California: Comparing intersection and midblock incident locations. *Injury Prevention*, 7(2), pp. 155–60.

Loukaitou-Sideris, A., Liggett, R. and Sung, H.-G., 2007. Death on the crosswalk: A study of pedestrian–automobile collisions in Los Angeles. *Journal of Planning Education and Research*, 26(3), pp. 338–51.

Lozano, R., Naghavi, M., Foreman, K., Lim, S., Shibuya, K., Aboyans, V., Abraham, J., Adair, T., Aggarwal, R., Ahn, S.Y., AlMazroa, M.A., Alvarado, M., Anderson, H.R., Anderson, L.M., Andrews, K.G., Atkinson, C., Baddour, L.M., Barker-Collo, S., Bartels, D.H., Bell, M. L., Benjamin, E. J., Bennett, D., Bhalla, K., Bikbov, B., Abdulhak, A.B., Birbeck, G., Blyth, F., Bolliger, I., Boufous, S., Bucello, C., Burch, M., Burney, P., Carapetis, J., Chen, H., Chou, D., Chugh, S.S., Coffeng, L.E., Colan, S.D., Colquhoun, S., Colson, K.E., Condon, J., Connor, M.D., Cooper, L. T., Corriere, M., Cortinovis, M., de Vaccaro, K.C., Couser, W., Cowie, B.C., Criqui, M. H., Cross, M., Dabhadkar, K.C., Dahodwala, N., De Leo, D., Degenhardt, L., Delossantos, A., Denenberg, J., Des Jarlais, D.C., Dharmaratne, S.D., Dorsey, E.R., Driscoll, T., Duber, H., Ebel, B., Erwin, P.J., Espindola, P., Ezzati, M., Feigin, V., Flaxman, A.D., Forouzanfar, M.H., Fowkes, F.G.R., Franklin, R., Fransen, M., Freeman, M.K., Gabriel, S.E., Gakidou, E., Gaspari, F., Gillum, R.F., Gonzalez-Medina, D., Halasa, Y.A., Haring, D., Harrison, J.E., Havmoeller, R., Hay, R.J., Hoen, B., Hotez, P.J., Hoy, D., Jacobsen, K.H., James, S.L., Jasrasaria, R., Jayaraman, S., Johns, N., Karthikeyan, G., Kassebaum, N., Keren, A., Khoo, J.-P., Knowlton, L.M., Kobusingye, O., Koranteng, A., Krishnamurthi, R., Lipnick, M., Lipshultz, S.E. et al., 2012. Global and regional mortality from 235 causes of death for 20 age groups in 1990 and 2010: A systematic analysis for the Global Burden of Disease Study 2010. *The Lancet*, 380, pp. 2095–2128.

MacDonald, N., Yanchar, N. and Hébert, P. C., 2007. What's killing and maiming Canada's youth? *Canadian Medical Association Journal*, 176, p.737.

Mock, C.N., Quansah, R.E., Krishnan, R., Arreola-Risa, C. and Rivara, F.P., 2004. Strengthening the prevention and care of injuries worldwide. *The Lancet*, 363(9427), pp. 2172–9.

Nicol, A., Knowlton, L.M., Schuurman, N., Matzopoulos, R., Zargaran, E., Cinnamon, J., Fawcett, V., Taulu, T. and Hameed, S.M., 2014. Trauma surveillance in Cape Town, South Africa: An analysis of 9236 consecutive trauma center admissions. *Journal of the American Medical Association Surgery*, 149(6), pp. 549–56.

Niekerk, A.V., Reimers, A. and Laflamme, L., 2006. Area characteristics and determinants of hospitalised childhood burn injury: A study in the city of Cape Town. *Public Health*, 120(2), pp. 115–24.

O'Sullivan, D., 2006. Geographical information science: Critical GIS. *Progress in Human Geography*, 30(6), pp. 783–91.

Parachute, 2015. The cost of injury in Canada. Toronto: Parachute.

Pickles, J., 1995. *Ground truth: The social implications of geographic information systems*. New York: Guilford Press.

Premji, S., Duguay, P., Messing, K. and Lippel, K., 2010. Are immigrants, ethnic and linguistic minorities over-represented in jobs with a high level of compensated risk?

Results from a Montréal, Canada study using census and workers' compensation data. *American Journal of Industrial Medicine*, 53(9), pp. 875–85.

Rosenberg, M.W., 1998. Medical or health geography? Populations, peoples and places. *International Journal of Population Geography*, 4(3), pp. 211–26.

Russwurm, L. and Buchanan, D., 2010. We're all pedestrians: Final report of the Downtown Eastside Pedestrian Safety Project. Vancouver: Vancouver Area Network of Drug Users.

Schuurman, N., 1999. Critical GIS: Theorizing an emerging discipline. *Cartographica*, 36, pp. 1–109.

Schuurman, N., Cinnamon, J., Crooks, V.A. and Hameed, S.M., 2009. Pedestrian injury and the built environment: An environmental scan of hotspots. *BMC Public Health*, 9(1), pp. 1–10. Available online at http://bmcpublichealth.biomedcentral. com/articles/10.1186/1471-2458-9-233 (accessed February 5, 2016).

Schuurman, N., Cinnamon, J., Matzopoulos, R., Fawcett, V., Nicol, A. and Hameed, S.M., 2011. Collecting injury surveillance data in low- and middle-income countries: The Cape Town Trauma Registry pilot. *Global Public Health*, 6(8), pp. 874–89.

Sciortino, S., Vassar, M., Radetsky, M. and Knudson, M.M., 2005. San Francisco pedestrian injury surveillance: Mapping, under-reporting, and injury severity in police and hospital records. *Accident Analysis and Prevention*, 37(6), pp. 1102–13.

Sheppard, E., 2005. Knowledge production through critical GIS: Genealogy and prospects. *Cartographica*, 40(4), pp. 5–21.

Statistics Canada, 2011. Population by Mother Tongue, by Census Metropolitan Area, Excluding Institutional Residents, 2011 Census. Available online at www.statcan. gc.ca/tables-tableaux/sum-som/l01/cst01/demo12g-eng.htm (accessed October 5, 2014).

Statistics Canada, 2012. Leading causes of death in Canada, 2009. Available online at www.statcan.gc.ca/pub/84-215-x/2012001/hl-fs-eng.htm (accessed October 5, 2014).

Sui, D.Z. and DeLyser, D., 2012. Crossing the qualitative–quantitative chasm I: Hybrid geographies, the spatial turn, and volunteered geographic information VGI. *Progress in Human Geography*, 36(1), pp. 111–24.

Tashakkori, A. and Teddlie, C., 2003. Preface. In: A. Tashakkori, and C. Teddlie, eds. *Handbook of mixed methods in social and behavioural research*. Thousand Oaks: Sage Publications. p.ix.

Transport Canada, 2004. Canadian motor vehicle traffic collision statistics: 2003. Ottawa: Road Safety and Motor Vehicle Regulation Directorate.

Transport Canada, 2015. Canadian Motor Vehicle Collision Statistics: 2013. Ottawa: Government of Canada.

Wilson, M.W., 2009. Towards a genealogy of qualitative GIS. In: M. Cope and S. Elwood, eds. *Qualitative GIS: A mixed methods approach*. London: Sage. pp. 156–70.

World Health Organization, 2010. Injuries and violence: The facts. Geneva: Department of Violence and Injury Prevention and Disability, World Health Organization.

Yiannakoulias, N., Smoyer-Tomic, K.E., Hodgson, J., Spady, D.W., Rowe, B.H. and Voaklander, D.C., 2002. The spatial and temporal dimensions of child pedestrian injury in Edmonton. *Canadian Journal of Public Health–Revue Canadienne de Sante Publique*, 93(6), pp. 447–51.

Zargaran, E., Schuurman, N., Nicol, A.J., Matzopoulos, R., Cinnamon, J., Taulu, T., Ricker, B., Garbutt Brown, D.R., Navsaria, P. and Hameed, S.M., 2014. The electronic trauma health record: Design and usability of a novel tablet-based tool for trauma care and injury surveillance in low resource settings. *Journal of the American College of Surgeons*, 218(1), pp. 41–50.

7 Countermapping Inner City "Deprivation" in Winnipeg, Canada

Jeffrey R. Masuda and Emily Skinner

A renewed enthusiasm for census-based deprivation indices, in conjunction with geographic information system (GIS) analysis, has given rise to a plethora of mapping efforts to visualize "problematic areas" aimed at informing policy prioritization and health intervention (Schuurman et al., 2007; Pampalon et al., 2012; Padilla et al., 2013; Morrison et al., 2014). With the increased popularity of GIS, deprivation maps have given new life to indexing methodologies that have been used since the 1970s to sort populations into categories on the basis of relative deprivation in social support, or the material resources needed to sustain health and quality of life (Carstairs, 1995). In essence, such indices are created from available measures of population diversity, usually from national censuses, with known relationships with (ill-)health (e.g. poverty, minority status, education levels) that theoretically align along an axis of additive deprivation. Often, such indices are validated through regression analysis against measures of morbidity and mortality, themselves usually derived from (other) secondary administrative data such as government health or mortality records (Padilla et al., 2013), or population surveys (e.g. Pampalon et al., 2007) to confirm the existence of social gradients in health. Further, because these data are provided in spatially aggregated forms (e.g. census tracts), they are readily translated into GIS, providing a spatial dimension to the social gradient and ostensibly reflecting the importance of *place effects* on health.

However, the mapping of statistically derived areal deprivation and its concomitant health effects is far from a benign process. Rather, maps have agency, often with unpredictable consequences. In this chapter we discuss the "deficit fixing" power of urban deprivation maps, insofar as their ability to reduce people's social identities and their health into stigmatizing representations of tainted urban bodies and places. While such maps can be useful for decision-makers, we suggest that problematic, often speculative, interpretations can lead to inappropriate interventions that may be detrimental to population health equity goals. We will argue for a more inclusionary interpretation of deprivation maps using participatory techniques, through the use of results from a mixed-method study undertaken in Winnipeg, Canada to illustrate our arguments. Through a novel mixed-method approach, we identify several ways in which such maps can be made to work at the scale of the whole city, in ways that shift the onus of intervention onto those that deny otherwise vibrant, inner-city communities their diverse ancestral, cultural, gender, and lifestage potential.

History and Critiques of Deprivation-based Approaches

The conceptual basis of deprivation-based indexing and mapping is that some social groups such as women, minorities, the young, the old, and material circumstances such as housing tenure, educational attainment, and poverty are known to have poorer-than-average health status at the population level. Numerous indices have been developed in Canada and elsewhere (Townsend et al., 1988; Morris and Carstairs, 1991; Frohlich and Mustard, 1996; Bell and Hayes, 2012), many of which are variations on a common theme adapted according to national census data constructs and aggregation units. At a theoretical level, all indices endeavor to confirm the same general hypothesis: those that lack social and/or material resources are likelier to be less healthy. Further, when visualized spatially, it is evident that such people tend to gravitate to particular locales, most likely on the basis of pull factors such as affordability, social support, or needed services targeted to particular social groups, as well as push factors such as socioeconomic exclusion or racial prejudice.

The aggregation of multiple dimensions of deprivation is meant to allow for more robust characterizations of the social gradient in health than previously employed maps employing single indicators. However, while we might praise deprivation mapping for its ability to confirm the *existence* of a social gradient in health (and outcome-driven hypothesis), accounting empirically for these push and pull factors requires a more sophisticated approach that is capable of explaining how such sociospatial gradients are produced (a process-driven hypothesis). To alleviate health inequities that coincide with spatial deprivation means that we must target not only health-related endpoints, but also deprivation processes, in order to identify and correct the so-called "causes of the causes" (Marmot, 2005). Failure to adopt equity-based approaches and to simply intervene in "health" is a socially palliative exercise: helping poor people to be healthy rather than less poor is intuitively a misdirected approach that represents an ongoing cost to the system, rather than correcting the system itself.

In the North American context, such maps often confirm the existence of widely reputed "inner cities" popularly blighted for their level of environmental dereliction, poverty, crime, and concentration of minority populations. Indeed, such maps extend a long tradition in geography and urban planning of city mapping that has problematized and attempted to reclaim urban derelict districts through top-down planning focused on urban renewal (Wilson, 1966; Hyra, 2012). Taking the City of Winnipeg as an illustration, numerous maps constructed of the city through the 1980s mobilized census data, including "Native Origin," to depict the concentration of Indigenous Winnipeggers in the central north end of the city – a phenomenon which has had a profound influence on urban and health planning in that city for decades (as will be discussed later in this chapter).

More recently, the map in Figure 7.1 employs the widely used Institut National de Santé Publique du Québec (INSPQ) index (Pampalon et al., 2009). It is noteworthy that this index, a typical census-based deprivation index,

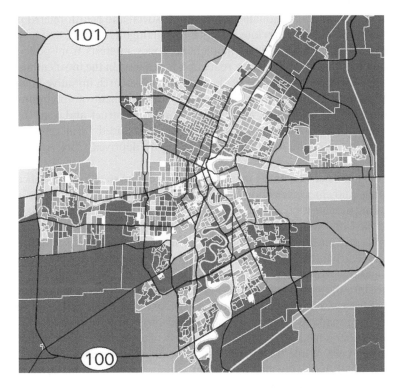

Figure 7.1 Distribution of socioeconomic status in the Winnipeg census metropolitan area (darker shading represents higher combined deprivation)

Note: Combined (material and social) component of the INSPQ Deprivation Index
at the dissemination area level.

Source: Canadian Institutes of Health Information, 2010, reproduced with permission

does not employ variables pertaining to Indigenous ancestry, yet the map
depicts a familiar pattern of deprivation concentrating in the area of the city
just north of the the centre of the map. This juxtaposition merely confirms
the widely known link between Indigenous ancestry and socioeconomic
deprivation, which is particularly localized and severe in the north end of
Winnipeg.

Such maps might appear intuitive to anyone who has had the opportunity to
observe Winnipeg's built environment, revealing a particular "truth" about the
city in a simple and effective representation of its sociospatial gradient. When
visualized in conjunction with outcome measures such as education, crime, or
health, a wide number of population-based inequalities are confirmed.

These visualization techniques have provided important insights for practitioners and policymakers of many stripes (e.g. planning, public health, community development), to build cases and formulate strategies to resolve such

problems. In Winnipeg, the problematization of the urban "Core Area" has been a long-standing rationale for large-scale social and health-related policy interventions, aided in previous instances by analogous analytic and mapping techniques which have served innumerable policy interests from policing to primary health care and poverty reduction in the city. In the most emblematic of these, beginning in the late 1970s, a long-term research initiative known as the Winnipeg Area Characterization Study (Department of Environmental Planning, 1978) undertook a project aiming to construct and map the city according to area-based typologies similarly produced from census data, which resulted in the identification of a highly deprived Core Area in the heart of the city.

In the hands of influential inner-city advocates, the statistical identification, mapping, and characterization of the Core Area would have a major influence in making the case for Canada's largest scale investment in area-based planning, called the Core Area Initiative (CAI). The CAI was the country's first tripartite (federal, provincial, and municipal) agreement aimed squarely at addressing persistent urban decline and its concomitant social problems. Beginning in 1981 and renewed in 1987, the CAI directed a total of C$196 million in public finance into the priority neighborhoods identified in the Area Characterization Study (otherwise known as the Core Area). Over the ensuing decade, investments were made in innumerable social and physical infrastructure projects, all ostensibly aimed at addressing poverty while simultaneously revitalizing the urban core. While the CAI did support many community-based organizations which have provided significant support to burgeoning low-income, immigrant, and Indigenous populations that (mainly at the time) had previously received little to no aid, since then the overall program has been deemed by many to be a failure insofar as achieving its original ambitions. Decades later, numerous legacy infrastructure projects in tourism and retail remain potent symbols of the shortcomings of this massive urban experiment, demonstrating the fallacy of a political imperative that claimed to mitigate social problems, but largely intervened in ways that emphasized municipal economic growth via "bricks and mortar" rehabilitation (Silver and Toews, 2009). Even the CAI's original visionary and lead orchestrator, Lloyd Axworthy (Member of Parliament and Minister of Employment and Immigration at the time that the CAI was launched), was able to "read the tealeaves" halfway through the initiative, noting at the time of its renewal in 1987:

> I think the new phase, where it's really talking about further building development..., is going away from the original idea – which was it had to be a combination of urban redevelopment in a physical sense – but far more important, in terms of getting people training, employment, jobs, better education, a sense of their own individual renewal. And I think it's now reverting back to an old traditional urban renewal idea that if you change bricks and mortars, you'll get something. I think you've got to help change the people. (CKND Eyes West, 1988)

Paradoxically, the same census data that had been deployed to create the Core Area (e.g. poverty rates) as a justification for the CAI, also testifies to the worsening levels of poverty in the inner city during and well after the period of CAI funding.

Therein lies the rub. If these abovementioned deprivation-based approaches lead to intervention measures that potentially worsen the situation for disenfranchised people living in targeted locales (while often enhancing revitalization efforts in these same areas), then what are we doing wrong? Of course, Axworthy was correct to suggest that people are more pertinent objects for intervention in the social determinants of health than "bricks and mortar." Nonetheless, a looming lacuna in the CAI and deprivation-focused interventions more widely may be found in what we tend *not* to scrutinize through indices and maps: we suggest that there are at least three limitations in deprivation mapping which undermine the equity-based goals that they often claim to represent.

First, the transformation of census variables that represent a wide diversity of individual and population characteristics into meta-proxies of deprivation strips away the inherent social complexities (individual life courses, mobilities, experiences) that produce these variables and, in the context of ongoing urban change, put people in their place (both in the social and locational sense). Statistical proxies of deprivation mask the sociospatial heterogeneity of urban life. To reduce social complexity into numbers elides the contextual nature of upstream determinants of health, including important insights into why people live where they do, and how places subsequently affect their health. For example, newer conceptual understandings of the "collective" dimension of health emphasize the relationality between people and the places in which they live (MacIntyre et al., 2002; Cummins et al., 2007). However, reducing multiple variables to aggregated proxies, ostensibly in ways that surface the "social" and "material" dimensions of deprivation, can obscure the intersecting pathways through which structural forces such as racism, classism, or ageism may operate on Indigenous, poor, youth, or elderly bodies and identities to constrain the degrees of freedom in their urban geographies, as well as affect their health (Skinner and Masuda, 2013).

Maps cannot tell us whether aggregated health outcomes of deprived areas are driven independently, additively, or synergistically by the combined sociodemographic profile of its individual inhabitants. Yet we know that being a mother of Indigenous ancestry has little to do with being a single recent immigrant to Canada. While both may live in a highly deprived neighborhood and may have a less than average population health status, each has a unique social explanation. For the former, deprivation is a consequence of 400 years of racializing and oppressing colonialism. Global colonialism has affected many newcomers as well in the form of late twentieth-century neoliberal globalization, transnationalism, and immigration policy, which have pulled people from former European colonies into Canada while pushing them into the margins of Canadian society through racial and religious intolerance. In this sense, deprivation maps are incapable of providing scrutiny of the sources of social mixing and urbanization that have led to overrepresentation or underrepresentation of particular groups or conditions in a given area. Visualization not only avoids historical explanation, it impedes it by reducing complex historical geographies of the city into overly simplistic snapshots of its present demographics.

Second, not only can maps lie (Monmonier, 1996), they also can be fundamentally stigmatizing. When mobilized into the policy and public domain, deprivation maps may be complicit in producing stigmatizing representations of darkly shaded "derelict districts," feeding racializing discourses about the city, and prejudicial attitudes and agendas that place negative labels on inner-city places and people. In this way, deprivation maps continue a long tradition of deficit mapping in both academic and lay contexts that have utilized a wide variety of crude measures of urban decay, such as criminality or social dysfunction, in order to represent probematic areas of the city as blighted and justify interventions. While often useful as the basis for framing issues and justifying interventions, these representations find their way easily into public discourses, particularly when combined with more alarming dependent variables such as crime rates, educational underachievement, and the like.

Invariably, in Winnipeg the specific problem is not just *in* the Core Area, the problem *becomes* the Core Area. In a vicious cycle, complex area-based problems are reduced to statistical proxies by enrolling data from the inhabitants of those areas: these proxies become representations of the problem; these representations come to define particular places as problematic; and the people living in these places become synonymous with the problem. The public sentiment is not so sophisticated that it is capable of discerning the root causes behind such representations. Instead, people are told only to see the pulsing, fear-inducing problem that is the Core Area. Moreover, the people living in these areas become labeled themselves, geographically tainted by their own demographic profile (Woolford, 2001; Skinner and Masuda, 2013). This maneuver provides an easy "out" for racializing discourses about what or who belongs in particular places in the city. It encourages the occasional racist sentiment in Internet commentary about "too many natives Downtown." And in planning discourses, it justifies discourses about "Downtown Revitalization" that focuses on bringing large numbers of more affluent people to the area as a remedy for neighborhood obsolescence (Canadian Urban Institute, 2012).

Third, the typologies that typically depict the city as a social gradient contribute to a localized deficit fix among would-be interveners, by drawing attention to more deprived areas (usually colored darker, redder, or blacker), while giving a free pass to more privileged areas (usually colored lighter, bluer, or whiter). The latter areas nearly always escape explanation; by implication they are "adequate" and in no need of policy attention or resources. Perhaps even worse, low deprivation areas may be presented as intervention benchmarks that appeal to liberal-minded sentiments, offering a "hand up" to disenfranchised groups. The public health and planning impetus becomes equally fixed on the problem of more deprived areas, aiming to correct such deprivations by ameliorating their immediate antecedents. Income support for the poor, educational training for women, and job training programs for Indigenous or criminalized youth are typical social programs that one finds proposed for these areas. Similarly, urban planners develop place-based strategies to reduce poverty, attract investment, improve streetscapes to correct built environment deficiencies in "transitional" communities, often aimed at "mixing" the population, leaving the "complete" communities in the suburbs as conveniently "unmixed" (Wideman and Masuda, 2015). Public health practitioners open breastfeeding clinics for low-income new mothers, and provide needle exchanges for street-involved drug users. Meanwhile, every dollar is counted by commentators perched on the political Right which, when added up, feeds into a frenzy of anti-government and welfare mentality discourses (see Fumano, 2014 for an illustrative example).

What is common among these three limitations is that they fail to take into account the *relational* nature of health inequity. One part of this problem is rooted in the fact that often, studies designs subordinate theory to the methodological expediency of the available data. Relying on census data, rather than real contextual information of actually ill patients and their individual urban experiences and geographies, can obscure the sociospatial determinants of their illness, whether place-based or not. Conversely, the focus on deprivation rather than on privilege limits our ability to examine disproportionate public asset allocation to affluent areas, or to assess prejudicial public attitudes among majority groups that contribute to self-selected, sociospatial segregation from minorities. Rather, we are given a static view that supports endeavors to "fix" deprived people, or worse, to "fix up" deprived places by replacing deprived people with more "creative" ones (Catungal et al., 2009).

If the causes of illness are the denial of basic resources and services to some groups on the basis of racial or class prejudice against them, then simply adding more resources and services misses the point. Instead of just helping those denied, we must think carefully about who is doing the denying, including who benefits from such denial. Health spending, urban planning, social services, and other areas of public governance are not zero-sum games. The affluent, white, and non-disabled are not "naturally" healthier, neither is their good health merely a consequence of their social position. Rather, with privileged social position comes easy access to the resources for basic living (and then some) – many of which are publicly funded, while others accrued through "accumulation by dispossession" (Harvey, 2010). For example, if the best urban assets (e.g. green space, proximity to resources and amenities) are enjoyed disproportionately by the affluent, then this must be a function of governments' unwillingness to intervene in real estate markets that deliver the so-called "commons" to the highest bidders (Banerjee-Guha, 2010). Nonetheless, even if conceding that the right to live in preferred areas of the city is a function of property and class, such rights should not extend to public areas that are adjacent to affluent areas. Yet this is just what happens when urban planning processes overinvest in public spaces which have the same natural or historical value that encourages affluent people to buy into their adjacent properties. Inequities also manifest in social mixing strategies that serve as prescriptions for reducing deprivation. Such plans rarely take place in affluent districts, where they are opposed by NIMBYists ("Not In My Backyard"), but are foisted largely on lower-income districts that are ostensibly in need of "revitalization." Such inequities are often a consequence of the compromises of well-intentioned bureaucrats who respond to the pressure of developers who market an "authentic" or "edgy" urban experience to their well-heeled homebuyers, who end up displacing the very people with whom they are meant to mix (Lees, 2008).

Etymologically, we know that deprivation is not only a *lack* of, but an *act* of depriving something that is essential to life. Deprivation has agency: there is a depriver who withholds something that is wanted or needed. Yet most interventions that are meant to address deprivation focus on the provision of health services and resources to those deprived, rather than tackling the root causes which can be found among those who have benefited from inequality (Pulido, 2015).

Discerning explanatory nuances surrounding the relational dimensions of urban deprivation require much more than a map. Indeed, as Pampalon et al. (2012), the leading proponents of the deprivation index in Canada, readily acknowledge, "the index does not constitute an explanatory framework for social inequalities of health" (p.S21). If this is the case, then what methodologies for social explanation might be available which can account for the relationality of deprivation?

To elaborate a methodology for ascertaining the explanatory dimensions of the social gradient of health, we must go beyond our intuitive readings of deprivation maps. An approach is needed that preserves the inherent diversity of place and respects the complexity of the social, economic, and political *processes* of deprivation, which in turn can offer much-needed interpretive power to the already powerful visualizations offered by mapping methodologies alone. It was just such a challenge – the opportunity for mixed-method participatory research – that we sought to meet in the case study described next.

Investigative Photography for Relational Neighborhood Deprivation Assessment in Winnipeg

Beginning in 2009, a research partnership comprising investigators from the University of Manitoba and several community organizations sought to investigate the relational dimensions of the social determinants of health inequality in Winnipeg. Rather than seeking confirmation of the relationship between social deprivation and health, the partnership study sought an approach that could offer an explanation of area deprivation in health determinants. To do this, we put deprivation maps of Winnipeg into the hands of the inhabitants of deprived neighborhoods to tell us, from their perspective, what deprivation in the city means to them.

Our comparative approach was novel in two ways. First, it intentionally scaled up the assessment of deprivation by comparing low-to-high deprivation neighborhoods, shifting the investigation of health inequity away from the "deficit fix" of individual deprived neighborhoods typically seen in qualitative studies of inner city health. Second, its use of investigative photography departed from conventional photo-mediated methodologies, in that rather than examining lived experience, we engaged inner-city inhabitants as co-researchers to investigate areas of the city that they had not typically experienced (see Masuda et al., 2012).

The rest of this chapter provides an illustration of how our approach addresses the above-cited limitations of deprivation mapping. Drawing from more than two years of empirical work, we will demonstrate how the co-researchers achieved a subaltern and relational revisualization of the social determinants of health inequality in the city that preserved the diversity of urban geographies, and the dignity of inner-city inhabitants.

Method

Procedure

As a first step, we produced the deprivation map shown in Figure 7.2, using a population health index (Odoi et al., 2005) constructed from 18 variables from the 2006 census aggregated at the Enumeration Area level (Table 7.1; see Masuda et al., 2012 for details). This index was derived using a non-hierarchical (K-means) cluster-based technique to construct five demographic typologies. The deprivation score for each typology was calculated as the sum of the variables standardized to a mean of zero. Unlike ordinal approaches (e.g. typically quintiles), this approach preserves the nominal value, or relative degree, of deprivation differences between clusters (noting the admittedly problematic caveat that variables are given equal weight and assumed to be summative).

In contrasting areas of the city falling under clusters 1 (least deprived) and 5 (most deprived), we see proportionally higher levels of those of Indigenous ancestry (7.5 percent vs. 32 percent), more people living alone (6.5 percent vs. 16 percent), and higher numbers of low-income households (5.8 percent vs. 54 percent). Importantly, clusters 2–4 are not necessarily in-between these extremes, but are qualitatively unique. Deprivation in cluster 2, for example, is characterized by a higher immigrant population that is highly mobile and lives alone (both predictors of high deprivation), but also has the highest rate of high school completion of the five clusters by a wide margin (only 26.3 percent have less than high school vs. a 41.9 percent average for all Enumeration Areas).

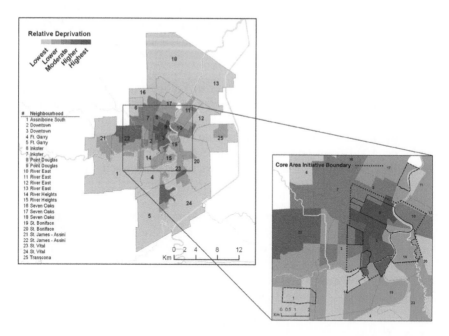

Figure 7.2 Deprivation map of Winnipeg with Core Area Initiative Boundary

Note: A cluster technique of 18 variables from the 2006 census aggregated to Enumeration Area yielded five neighborhood typologies ordered from lowest to highest deprivation (see Table 7.1). Neighborhood names are superimposed on the map in gray lines and neighborhoods visited for assessment are indicated by dotted black lines on the inset map, along with the Core Area Initiative Boundary.

In mapping the index, a picture of Winnipeg emerged that largely resembled the maps shown earlier in this chapter: indeed, highest deprivation does coincide with the Core Area of Winnipeg. On its own, the map is useful. As Odoi et al. (2005) have argued previously, the map can help policymakers and practitioners to focus their efforts on the local population dynamics within each area where population-specific, health-related issues may be more prevalent. Services focused on Indigenous people could focus on the North End (cluster 5), and services for recent immigrants downtown (cluster 4).

However, as with our earlier critique, we have no *prima facie* sense of how Winnipeggers came to sort themselves (or be sorted) in this way, neither what place-based conditions (e.g. health-enhancing or depleting neighborhood characteristics) might coincide with each typology. To answer such questions required that we proceed to the second part of the study, which involved an on-the-ground assessment of each neighborhood typology undertaken by people who have lived a part of all of their lives within the most deprived neighborhoods in the city.

Table 7.1 Average values of census valuables by cluster type

| Cluster | CTAvg | Lowest deprivation | | | | Highest deprivation |
		Cluster 1	Cluster 2	Cluster 3	Cluster 4	Cluster 5
N	167	65	59	24	10	9
COMPOSITIONAL						
%Aboriginal	12.0	7.5	10.6	19.4	13.5	32.3
%Govt$	12.0	6.9	11.9	17.1	14.9	32.3
%Mobility	12.4	10.4	10.8	11.2	31.1	19.3
%HighSchool	41.9	42.0	37.8	50.6	26.3	62.2
%LiveAlone	13.2	6.5	17.9	11.8	29.0	16.0
%LowIncome	15.7	5.8	13.8	27.4	28.8	54.3
%Married	46.7	58.6	42.6	39.8	27.4	26.2
%NewImmigrant	4.1	1.9	3.4	5.3	14.5	10.1
%NonOfficialLang	0.9	0.6	0.6	102	0.9	3.8
%age 65	14.0	11.4	18.5	11.3	12.7	12.4
%SingleParent	19.9	11.5	20.4	29.7	25.5	44.9
%age 20	24.5	26.9	20.4	28.1	18.1	31.3
%Unemployed	5.3	3.7	5.0	6.0	8.4	14.0
%VisibleMinority	14.2	10.4	9.1	26.0	26.5	30.2
CONTEXTUAL						
Dwelling$	C$ 155,853	C$204,204	C$ 142,644	C$ 101,805	C$ 122,764	C$74,139
Median$	C$26,680	C$32,379	C$25,866	C$21,716	C$16,708	C$15,188
%HomeOwner	69.2	89.7	63.9	63.3	16.9	29.3
PopDensity (km²)	2,606	1,377	2,995	3,603	4,386	4,293

Note: CTAvg = City average for all census tracts.

Participants and Data Collection

Starting in June 2010, we recruited a total of 17 community members to participate as co-researchers, each carefully selected with guidance by partners with the
aim of collectively representing as wide as possible cross-section of Winnipeg's
sociodemographic diversity. Roughly equal numbers of co-researchers were
recruited from three neighborhood areas represented by the highest deprivation
cluster, including the Point Douglas, West Broadway, and Centennial neighborhoods. Thus three assessment teams were formed, each consisting of approximately five co-researchers.

To begin, each group of co-researchers was trained together in an investigative photography research method to carry out neighborhood assessments.
Photography was seen to be an appropriate tool, as it afforded an easy and
fast means to capture observed attributes and characteristics of neighborhoods which could be viewed later as the basis for group discussions.

We began the process with a workshop led by a professional photographer
where co-researchers practiced using their digital cameras (which were gifted
to them), learned some key principles of photography, and discussed personal
safety and the ethics of fieldwork. This initial session was meant also to build
rapport within the group, as it was the first time that many had the opportunity
to meet. We followed this session with a preliminary, problem-posing group
discussion about the social determinants of health, and how they link to the
built environment of the city. We encouraged the co-researchers to situate the
social determinants of health within specific places in their neighborhoods, as
well as to think about how past, present, and future conditions have changed
for the worse or better. (As shown already in Chapters 2 through 6, each
geographical location has place-specific social determinants of health, and
Winnipeg is no exception.) Invariably, the co-researchers conveyed an impres-
sive knowledge of the links between the social determinants of health and
places in their neighborhoods. For example, medical clinics illustrated access
to health care, schools and playground conditions represented education and
environment respectively, and so on. These discussions were used to create a
template of place-based social determinants that could be used as a focus for
neighborhood assessments by providing specific topics or objects to look for
and compare. At the completion of the session, the co-researchers collectively
decided upon which neighborhoods to assess in addition to their own. This
decision was informed by the map in conjunction with group preferences, as
well as logistical practicalities. Across the three groups of co-researchers, the
research team ensured that all five of the deprivation typologies would be
represented in the overall analysis.

Scheduling neighborhood assessments with each group in turn over the
next four months, we would set out, usually by bus but sometimes on foot,
to the neighborhoods to be assessed that day. We would find a meeting place
(local coffee shops or picnic tables usually sufficed) to discuss what we knew
about the neighborhood either through direct experience, reputation, or
through brief Internet searches. Then we would plot our routes and review the

priorities that we had identified in our initial discussions on the social determinants of health. The teams ventured out into the neighborhood: sometimes as a full group, other times in smaller teams of two or three individuals. These decisions were left open-ended and usually involved considerations of safety, the size of the neighborhood, or the number of specific places that the team wished to observe.

After the visits, which took between two and four hours, we reconvened at the meeting place for a debriefing session, where photographs were uploaded with interesting insights and experiences informally reviewed and discussed. After all three neighborhood visits were completed, all photos were printed and given to the co-researchers who were asked to reflect on their own photographs and to select, and when possible write a caption for, those photos that they felt most closely or profoundly represented what they wanted to say about their observations during the comparative assessments. One to two weeks later, a research staff member interviewed each co-researcher, where they were given an opportunity to discuss the photographs that they had selected.

Finally, we carried out a group discussion with all the co-researchers in each team. At this meeting, we collected, numbered, and captioned all of the photographs selected from the interviews and laid them out on tables. As a group, we proceeded to organize the photos into themes on the basis of the captions. We then discussed each of the themes, with a particular emphasis on answering this question: "Why are things (e.g. similarities, differences) this way?" All discussions were digitally recorded for follow-up analysis. (In this chapter, all co-researcher participants' names have been pseudonymised to protect their anonymity.)

Data Analysis

From this process, completed independently for each of the three groups, we collected 17 transcripts of individual interviews and three transcripts of the final group discussions. We then subjected the data to a process of coding and thematic integration, which resulted in a voluminous set of data that could be used for purpose-specific interpretation. As our intent in this chapter is illustrative rather than exhaustive, we extracted from this data set a subset of themes that best demonstrate how our participatory method allowed us to interpret the deprivation relationally, in a way that preserves the diversity and dignity of people and places in the city. We address four themes here that illustrate elements of "urban space denied" as a determinant of health inequity.

Findings

Common Spaces Denied

The co-researchers of the West Broadway, Point Douglas, and Centennial neighborhoods felt that the function, meaning, and importance of outdoor urban spaces varied widely across the three neighborhoods. For example, contrasting West Broadway (cluster 5) to Tuxedo (cluster 1) highlighted the dearth of available public space in the former. One co-researcher, Jenna, spoke about her envy of the ample, privately owned green space surrounding an apartment complex in Tuxedo which, perplexingly to her, was signposted with "No Trespassing" signs. She exclaimed, "This is kind of private property ... They have this nice lawn and no one uses it, it's not functional."

For the Point Douglas group, the lack of functional public spaces in their neighborhood did not appear to be as pertinent an issue. Rather than use value, this group's observations of outdoor spaces such as streets, green space, parks, fields, courtyards, and gardens reflected sanitation, cleanliness, hazards, and esthetics, with Trevor and Dominic commenting, "Everyday you see garbage, broken beer bottles" and "It is gross in the North End!" Such dereliction in their neighborhood contrasted with their observations in Seven Oaks (cluster 2) and Crescentwood (cluster 1), which was reflected in Cheryl's comment, "In the North End you don't see those kinds of yards with nice gardens."

The Centennial co-researchers commented on the overall lack of accessibility of urban space for food growing, despite the presence of abundant nearby vacant lots. Their frustration stemmed from a perceived inability to access these vacant lots, which Andrew attributed to "a lack of political will to turn that into usable urban agricultural land." Many of the Centennial co-researchers had originated from rural areas of Asian and African countries, where farming and agriculture were a way of life to provide food for families. Karina spoke about the potential advantage of such skills as a newcomer:

> One of the many skills that newcomers bring is the ability to grow very nutritious food very intensively in very small spaces. So a lot of folks come here, and they have and they already know a sort of economy for growing very simple foods, growing very simply but very well.

Similarly, after viewing photographs of private yards and gardens in the Daniel McIntyre site (cluster 3), Jonathan lamented:

> They managed to plant tomatoes and some vegetables. To me it looks very good because we would be getting fresh tomatoes from his small garden, and vegetables and carrots just on the other side. These are nutritious.

The Centennial co-researchers expressed a desire for garden lots for newcomer and refugee residents to continue applying these skills to produce vegetables and fruit, which are key ingredients in their ethnic diets.

Children and Youth Spaces Denied

Many of the co-researchers are parents and/or carers and expressed concerns related to the diversity of child and youth spaces, facilities, resources, and services across the city. The West Broadway co-researchers praised the availability and quality of child and youth programming offered through community-based organizations in their area. However, Kaila also commented on the number of children and young people that are forced to play in back lanes due to the lack of playgrounds and parks seen to be abundant in other parts of the city. Jennie observed what appeared to be a municipally sanctioned "Children Playing" sign in a Tuxedo alley, wondering whether such a thing could be possible in her own neighborhood:

> They had a sign for children playing, for kids to slow down and Marion had mentioned that she was trying to get something like that in the West Broadway area, and they never did anything with it ... so it just shows that if you have the money, you get what you want.

Point Douglas co-researchers similarly elaborated on traffic safety and signage, but also pointed out other existing dangerous hazards:

> You got kids playing there [next to garbage dumpsters] and they are curious about what is in there. I bet there are thousands of other people that [dispose of dirty needles] – and that is the kids' front lawn. That is all that they have to play in is the streets. (Andrew)

Riel's observation contrasted with the group's perception of the state of the play structures and grounds at schools and community center in Seven Oaks, with Cheryl stating: "It is clean. It is not burned or falling apart and it is not spray painted up. There aren't any alcohol bottles."

Centennial co-researchers shared somewhat different experiences as a result of recent upgrades to Central Park, located in the heart of their neighborhood. Andrew, who lived near Main Street (a strip reputed for open alcohol use, crime, and homelessness), shared his impression that the size of Central Park relative to those in the North End afforded a critical mass that facilitated a more consistent presence of watchful parents:

> Central Park is better there now because the drugs are gone now, and there are more parents with the kids there ... They are with their parents or else some adults are there, but you take these little parks in the North End and there isn't really parents.

Despite this favorable assessment, another Centennial co-researcher, Berniece, pointed out the limits to Central Park as a functional space only during the day and in summer. In the remaining six months of the year, she observed children relying too heavily on indoor spaces and activities offered through neighborhood programs. While such services were seen to be essential, their presence contrasted with the perceived freedom that more affluent families took for granted, via their proximity to green space and higher mobility to access city resources. The need to have constant supervision was seen to be a drain on the already-limited time and resources of parents and service agencies.

Cultural Spaces Denied

Co-researchers across all three groups felt that many visible minorities have been confined to the inner city as a result of the unavailability of subsidized housing and a discriminatory private housing market. All co-researchers in the Point Douglas and West Broadway groups who identified as First Nations or Metis felt that their culture should be reflected in the city, given its high Indigenous population. Visiting St Boniface (cluster 3) and photographing monuments, artifacts, buildings, and memorials celebrating Franco-Manitoban culture in Winnipeg stimulated conversation about the lack of representation of First Nations culture and art in other parts of Winnipeg. One West Broadway co-researcher, Kim, spoke about the distinct differences of her culture:

> As Aboriginal people we do different things differently, like we don't have to go put up a big statue of somebody to honor them. We honor them in different ways: we do ceremonies for them, and just recognize them in different ways.

This form of cultural recognition in the Franco-Manitoban cultures (i.e. public memorialization), which is not as important within the cultures of Manitoba First Nations, was seen to be a form of exclusionary identity validation. The group felt that public spaces in the city to conduct and perform Sundances, pow-wows, drumming circles, and sweat lodges are few and far between. While the entire area of Winnipeg is the traditional territory of Manitoba's First Nations, their representation appears undervalued in most areas. For Carla, the impact of residential schools on Indigenous culture, memory, and displacement equated to a loss of everyday opportunities to connect to the land in the city, noting: "I guess it is hard to kind of get along in this society if you have been colonized."

Co-researchers felt that the city has put the wrong emphasis on investments in Manitoba's First Nations cultures, where centralized commemorative landmarks seemingly located only in tourist destinations were privileged over the provision of lands for cultural practices in neighborhood spaces whose inhabitants are mostly Indigenous.

For example, a Point Douglas co-researcher, Maria, discussed the respect that was given to the limited cultural spaces that had been supported, pointing to the Circle of Life Thunderbird House as emblematic of a sacred space:

> If there were more spaces like sacred traditional spaces, like the Thunderbird House, and stuff like that. You don't see anyone going up there to spray paint it. The drunks are right next to you guys, but they respect it.

Culture was defined differently by the Centennial co-researchers, who emphasized their struggle to adapt to the behavior, values, manners, customs, and norms of Canadians as being crucial to their ability to obtain employment. According to Berniece's reflection on her own experience, "You can work but there are conditions. You don't just get in," – suggesting that employment decisions for newcomers are contingent on their assumed compatibilities with Canadian language and culture.

Grocers also were seen to be important cultural spaces, due to their role in supporting ethnic-cultural diets, particularly for first generation immigrants. One Centennial co-researcher, Brian, stated that it is difficult, "especially for mature people. It is hard to change straight away. Young kids they can fit and they just get used to it very fast, but mature people they take time to change." Berniece, describing an ethnic grocery near her neighborhood, discussed its importance, "because we get much of our food from our culture from our country. I buy spicy [foods], fruit, vegetable[s]."

Culturally appropriate food providers were seen to be important to Indigenous Winnipeggers. Trevor, who lives near Main Street, pointed to the single First Nations-specific grocer located in his neighborhood, which provided traditional food "like bannock, wild mushrooms, wild rice, and wild meat" for Indigenous residents who no longer live on-reserve, but still "crave these foods if we are too busy to cook or if isn't in the budget."

However, while such grocers were deemed essential for both Indigenous and newcomer Winnipeggers, they were of limited utility to those who lived further afield from their locations. In contrast, the vast majority of retail grocers made little to no effort to accommodate non-Western diets. Paradoxically, these community assets were seen to be a geographic barrier for the populations who depended on them, by hindering their mobility. The social geography of food and culture was seen as a significant blind spot to policymakers, who tended to focus their efforts on "fixing" the deficits they saw within traditionally defined "ethnic" areas.

Mobility Denied

The last theme focused on constraints to mobility within and between neighborhoods in the city. West Broadway co-researchers pointed to a river walk that runs adjacent to their neighborhood. The route is a nearly continuous link between the Forks downtown and the city's largest public park in its west end – but it abruptly ends just east of the neighborhood, and picks up again further west. They suspected this gap may have been a consequence of the perceived danger of West Broadway that has been popularly criminalized in public discourse for many years. Kaila contrasted her limited access to the "beautiful trail along the river" adjacent to neighborhoods such as Tuxedo and St Boniface, which in both cases afforded walking and biking access for kilometers in both directions from the neighborhood.

In contrasting their neighborhood to their observations of more affluent areas, Point Douglas co-researchers took note of the remarkable distance to basic amenities and services that they experienced, including grocery stores, physician offices, hospitals, employment opportunities, parks, recreation, and shopping centers. None of these places that they knew about or accessed were seen to be walkable, because the North End is geographically isolated from the rest of the city – hemmed in by the Canadian National railyards to the south and major commuting corridors to the east, west, and north. Many of the interviews and discussions revolved around the difficulty that North End residents had in accessing household amenities, supplies, and sufficient food to support large families. This difficulty was expressed in terms of time constraints:

> It isn't too affordable because if you pay bus fare, the transfer is only good for an hour. So you don't have enough time to go somewhere for an hour. (Dominic)

cost:

> If you have appointments outside of the area, by the time you get back, you have already spent C\$7.50. (Cheryl)

and compromise:

> Even like Safeway, if you want good food, it is way out of the way – and you have so many kids, and you don't have [a] vehicle. So people just go to the corner store, and you just try to pick out what is good and what will last a long time. A big box of Kraft Dinner, or a big box of noodles – stuff like that. (Maria)

These more instrumental mobility constraints were seen to be further exacerbated by the persistent and unalleviated experiences of racism, discrimination, and harassment that they reported when shopping outside of their own neighborhoods.

Discussion and Conclusion

In this chapter, we have illustrated the benefit of mixed-method approaches in overcoming the conceptual and methodological limitations of the widely popular deprivation index used in urban health research. (For another discussion of the value of a mixed-methods approach using GIS, see Chapter 6.) Indeed, deprivation mapping has helped to visualize the social gradient of health, and to confirm the importance of "place effects" on health – both crucial contributions for informing population health interventions. However, with the ease and power of visualization comes the risk of localizing problems and, worse still, perpetuating socially constructed notions of deficit that may exacerbate the stigma that already affects the health and well-being of inhabitants of "deprived areas."

If deprivation mapping as a tool for population health research is here to stay, then it is important that geographers offer our interpretive capacity to investigate place and diversity as determinants of health in order to ensure that the potentially homogenizing effects of such maps are avoided. In most published papers of deprivation and health, accounts of social explanation are at best speculative (see Juhász, 2010 and Kuznetsov, 2011 for good efforts at speculation), and at worst, completely absent. Even with the best of intentions, without the benefit of local expertise, deprivation mapping risks contributing to long-standing and stigmatizing accounts of the neighborhoods identified as "high deprivation." When translated into the public arena, such accounts graft all too easily onto racialized and illness-tainted bodies that become both the analytic objects and popular representations of deprivation, making inner-city inhabitants targets for all kinds of social antipathy. Proponents of deprivation-based research would be wise to insure that their statistics and maps are never presented without an appropriate and rigorous explanatory framework that takes into account the social, cultural, and economic dynamics that contribute to the stratification of urban population diversity at the scale of the city as a whole. It is not enough to concede their lack of explanatory power, because on their own, such maps have a discursive power that can produce socially and politically deleterious effects.

The mixed-method approach illustrated in this chapter provides one way to shift from the deficit fix, which presents homogenized and reductionist images of "high deprivation areas," to a relational view that implicates deprivation at the scale of the city. Our results have provided one method for framing inner-city spaces in a way that preserves their internal sociospatial diversity (no two places are the same), while also juxtaposing the challenges faced in such spaces – in view of the vastly different and highly underscrutinized characteristics of "less deprived" areas of the city. The perspectives provided by the co-researchers in our study have demonstrated amply that these are not two solitudes.

The mixed-method approach to deprivation analysis lends support to an argument that interventions to address health inequities need to pay as much attention to what is happening in the suburbs as in the inner city – and importantly, the interplay between the two. In place of a normative prescription, which would aim to "lift up" the lower end of the social gradient by concentrating services in areas based on measures of statistically derived social deficit, the relational approach would take a whole-city perspective to address the inequities rooted in processes of racialization and social exclusion in housing, vested interests of class and property in the allocation and maintenance of desirable public spaces, and the provision of public resources in garbage and waste collection, to give just a few examples.

Our results suggest that population health interventions should address both the physical manifestations of inequities – for example, in promoting better spatial distribution of public goods such as parks, playgrounds, grocers, clinics, and buses – as well as inequities that arise from the unstated, exclusionary, social consensus that inscribes racialized bodies with markers of illness, criminality, and underachievement. When deprivation maps are accompanied by the deeply contextualized and relational perspectives offered by the very urban inhabitants whose bodies and social position contribute to our ability to construct typologies and visualizations of deprivation, we may not only produce better interventions, but also might contribute to a reversal of the stigmatizing gaze of the map to one that accounts for the complexity of the very diverse and divided city that is Winnipeg, and many other North American cities.

References

Banerjee-Guha, S. ed., 2010. *Accumulation by dispossession: Transformative cities in the new global order*. New Delhi: Sage Publications.

Bell, N. and Hayes, M.V., 2012. The Vancouver Area Neighbourhood Deprivation Index (Vandix): A census-based tool for assessing small-area variations in health status. *Canadian Journal of Public Health*, 103(supp. 2), pp. eS28–32.

Canadian Institutes of Health Information, 2010. Exploring urban environments and inequalities in health. Winnipeg Census Metropolitan Area. Ottawa: Canadian Population Health Initiative.

Canadian Urban Institute, 2012. Winnipeg: Growing in strength and confidence. In: *The Value of Investing in Canadian Downtowns*. Washington, DC, International Downtowns Association, Canadian Issues Task Force, pp. 114–28.

Carstairs, V., 1995. Deprivation indices: Their interpretation and use in relation to health. *Journal of Epidemiology and Community Health*, 49(Supp. 2), pp. S3–8.

Catungal, J.P., Leslie, D. and Hii, Y., 2009. Geographies of displacement in the creative city: The case of Liberty Village, Toronto. *Urban Studies*, 46(5–6), pp. 1095–114.

CKND Eyes West, 1988. CKND EyesWest, a regional newsmagazine, profiles the Core Area Initiative 1 program. Available online at www.youtube.com/watch?v=jVufK2foCfA (accessed February 9, 2015).

Cummins, S., Curtis, S., Diez-Roux, A.V. and Macintyre, S., 2007. Understanding and representing 'place' in health research: A relational approach. *Social Science & Medicine*, 65(9), pp. 1825–38.

Donald, O., 1981. Medical services. In: P.N. Troy, ed. *Equity in the city*. Abingdon: Routledge. pp. 63–84.

Frohlich, N. and Mustard, C., 1996. A regional comparison of socioeconomic and health indices in a Canadian province. *Social Science & Medicine*, 42(9), pp. 1273–81.

Fumano, D., 2014. "Follow the money": Hundreds of millions are spent in the Downtown Eastside every year, but where does it all go? *The Province*, September 30. Available online at www.theprovince.com/news/Follow+money+Hundreds+millions+spent+Downtown+Eastside+every+year+where+does/10247182/story.html (accessed September 30, 2014).

Harvey, D., 2010. The right to the city: From capital surplus to accumulation by dispossession. In: S. Banerjee-Guha, ed. *Accumulation by dispossession: Transformative cities in the new global order*. New Delhi: Sage Publications. pp. 17–32.

Hyra, D.S., 2012. Conceptualizing the new urban renewal: Comparing the past to the present. *Urban Affairs Review*, 48(4), pp. 498–527.

Juhász, A., Nagy, C., Páldy, A. and Beale, L., 2010. Development of a deprivation index and its relation to premature mortality due to diseases of the circulatory system in Hungary, 1998–2004. *Social Science & Medicine*, 70(9), pp. 1342–49.

Kuznetsov, L., Maier, W., Hunger, M., Meyer, M. and Mielck, A., 2011. Associations between regional socioeconomic deprivation and cancer risk: Analysis of population-based cancer registry data from Bavaria, Germany. *Preventive Medicine*, 53(4), pp. 328–30.

Lees, L., 2008. Gentrification and social mixing: Towards an inclusive urban renaissance? *Urban Studies*, 45(12), pp. 2449–70.

Macintyre, S., Ellaway, A. and Cummins, S., 2002. Place effects on health: How can we conceptualise, operationalise and measure them? *Social Science & Medicine*, 55(1), pp. 125–39.

Marmot, M., 2005. Social determinants of health inequalities. *The Lancet*, 365(9464), pp. 1099–104.

Masuda, J.R., Teelucksingh, C., Haber, R., Skinner, E., Zupancic, T., Crabtree, A., Poland, B., Frankish, J. and Fridell, M., 2012. Out of our inner city backyards: Re-scaling urban health inequity assessment. *Social Science & Medicine*, 75(7), pp. 1244–53.

Monmonier, M., 1996. *How to lie with maps*, 2nd ed. Chicago, IL: University of Chicago Press.

Morris, R. and Carstairs, V., 1991. Which deprivation? A comparison of selected deprivation indexes. *Journal of Public Health*, 13(4), pp. 318–26.

Morrison, S., Fordyce, F.M. and Scott, E. M., 2014. An initial assessment of spatial relationships between respiratory cases, soil metal content, air quality and deprivation indicators in Glasgow, Scotland, UK: Relevance to the environmental justice agenda. *Environmental Geochemistry and Health*, 36(2), pp. 319–32.

Odoi, A., Wray, R., Emo. M., Birch, S., Hutchison, B., Eyles, J. and Abernathy, T., 2005. Inequalities in neighbourhood socioeconomic characteristics: Potential evidence-base for neighbourhood health planning. International Journal of Health Geographics, 4(20). Available online at https://ij-healthgeographics. biomedcentral.com/articles/10.1186/1476-072X-4-20 (accessed February 9, 2016).

Padilla, C.M., Deguen, S., Lalloue, B., Blanchard, O., Beaugard, C., Troude, F., Navier, D.Z. and Vieira, V.M., 2013. Cluster analysis of social and environment inequalities of infant mortality: A spatial study in small areas revealed by local disease mapping in France. *Science of the Total Environment*, 454–455, pp. 433–41.

Pampalon, R., Hamel, D., De Koninck, M. and Disant, M.J., 2007. Perception of place and health: Differences between neighbourhoods in the Quebec City region. *Social Science & Medicine*, 65(1), pp. 95–111.

Pampalon, R., Hamel, D., Gamache, P., and Raymond, G., 2009. A deprivation index for health planning in Canada. *Chronic Diseases in Canada*, 29(4), pp. 178–91.

Pampalon, R., Hamel, D., Gamache, P., Philibert, M.D., Raymond, G. and Simpson, A., 2012. An area-based material and social deprivation index for public health in Quebec and Canada. *Canadian Journal of Public Health*, 103(supp. 2), pp. eS17–22.

Pulido, L., 2015. Geographies of race and ethnicity 1: White supremacy vs white privilege in environmental racism research. *Progress in Human Geography*, 39(6), pp. 809–17.

Schuurman, N., Bell, N., Dunn, J.R. and Oliver, L., 2007. Deprivation indices, population health and geography: An evaluation of the spatial effectiveness of indices at multiple scales. *Journal of Urban Health*, 84(4), pp. 591–603.

Skinner, E. and Masuda, J.R., 2013. Right to a healthy city? Examining the relationship between urban space and health inequity by Aboriginal youth artist-activists in Winnipeg. *Social Science & Medicine*, 91, pp. 210–18.

Silver, J. and Toews, O., 2009. Combating poverty in Winnipeg's inner city, 1960s–1990s: Thirty years of hard-earned lessons. *Canadian Journal of Urban Research*, 18(1), 98–122.

Stevens, H., Murdoch, K. and Sale, T., 1980. Human needs and city planning: A study of social conditions in Winnipeg. Report for the Winnipeg Development Plan Review. Winnipeg: Social Planning Council of Winnipeg.

Stewart, M., Reutter, L., Makwarimba, E., Rootman, I., Williamson, D., Raine, K., Wilson, D., Fast, J., Love, R., McFall, S., Shorten, D., Letourneau, N., Hayward, K., Masuda, J. and Rutakumwa, W., 2005. Determinants of health-service use by low-income people. *Canadian Journal of Nursing Research*, 37(3), pp. 104–31.

Townsend, P., Phillimore, P. and Beattle, A., 1988. *Health and deprivation: Inequality and the North*. London: Routledge.

Wideman, T. and Masuda, J.R., 2015. Intensification and neoliberalization: A case study of planning policy in Winnipeg, Canada. *Prairie Perspectives*, 16, pp. 55–67

Wilson, J.Q., ed., 1966. *Urban renewal: The record and the controversy*. Cambridge, MA: MIT Press.

Woolford, A., 2001. Tainted space: Representations of injection drug-users and HIV/ AIDS in Vancouver's Downtown Eastside. *BC Studies: The British Columbian Quarterly*, 129, pp. 27–50.

8 When Is Helping Hurting?

Understanding and Challenging the (Re)production of Dominance in Narratives of Health, Place, and Difference in Hamilton, Ontario

Madelaine C. Cahuas, Mannat Malik, and Sarah Wakefield

On April 10, 2010, the residents of Hamilton, Ontario in Canada, awoke to news of vast health disparities in their city, including a 21-year difference in average age at death between the highest-income and lowest-income neighborhoods (Buist, 2010a). The main regional newspaper, the *Hamilton Spectator*, had just released the first article in its seven-day series, "Code Red," which revealed the results of a study, mapping the connections between health and place. Interviews with top local researchers, health care providers, and political leaders were used to direct attention to various issues raised by the findings. According to the authors, Code Red was intended to highlight growing health disparities in Hamilton in order to raise public awareness of what was seen as an important social problem (DeLuca et al., 2012). The articles stimulated considerable public debate, and ultimately contributed to the development of a municipal strategy that aimed to promote health in the low-income neighborhoods identified in the Code Red articles (City of Hamilton, 2011; Deluca et al., 2012).

Few details about the daily lives of people and communities that call these places home are shared in Code Red. Instead, we see low-income neighborhoods through the gaze of the experts cited: largely professional white men journeying through Hamilton's inner city. We use this silence surrounding the daily experiences of residents living in so-called "Code Red neighborhoods," as a starting point to explore the ways that narratives of health, place, and difference presented in the media – and through research – may have damaging effects on the places and people they intend to help.

In this chapter, we employ Code Red as a case study to show how efforts to uncover spatialized health inequities may work to reinforce dominant notions of particular people and places. Grounded in an intersectionality approach (Crenshaw, 1991; Razack, 1998), we analyze how the narratives mobilized by Code Red (re)produce dominance through:

1) a negative and deeply racialized portrayal of the inner city as a space of deviance and degeneracy inhabited by unhealthy Others;

2)   the suburb as a space of respectability where healthy, responsible (read: white, middle-class) citizens reside (Razack, 2002; Petersen and Lupton, 1996); and

3)   the erasure of resident voices and the privileging of expert (mostly white professional male) voices.

These narratives are reinforced further by an overall failure to account for oppressive power structures (white supremacy, capitalism, patriarchy, colonialism) that embed spatial inequities. Through a detailed content analysis, we identify three specific narratives in the Code Red articles that reproduce dominance: the inner city as a degenerate space; the Code Red woman as irresponsible victim; and the expert as knowing savior. We conclude by presenting the counternarratives of residents and community developers who work closely with residents, to show how dominant narratives are challenged and transformed. Overall, we argue that while it is important and necessary for policymakers and researchers to increase their attention to health inequity, it is also important to address our complicity in reproducing hierarchical power structures through narratives that mark, silence, and materially impact diverse populations. In failing to account for our own complicity, we run the risk of perpetuating inequity, even as we seek to mitigate it.

Placing the Unhealthy Citizen: Innocence, Deviance, Respectability and Resistance

We use intersectionality, a framework that aims to uncover and challenge mutually reinforcing systems of oppression, to ground our analysis (Crenshaw, 1991; Grillo, 1995; see also Chapter 2). Fellows and Razack (1998) draw on Patricia Hill Collins' (1990) notion of "interlocking systems of domination" to argue that power is secured for dominant groups by "marking" subordinated groups as different in relation to an unnamed but assumed norm. In turn, this naturalizes the oppression of non-dominant groups, and obscures how the unmarked norm participates in the domination of others (Fellows and Razack, 1998). Furthermore, subordinated groups are positioned lower in a hierarchy of respectability than dominant groups in relation to this "mythical norm": "white, thin, male, young, heterosexual, Christian, and financially secure" (Lorde, 2007, p. 116). This language of respectability and degeneracy can be traced back to the emergence of liberal democratic societies, wherein respectability signified middle-class membership and having rights over Others (Fellows and Razack, 1998). Respectability and degeneracy were mobilized to validate gender and racial hierarchies, where the pinnacle of respectability was the white, middle-class home (Fellows and Razack, 1998). These hierarchies continue to structure the experiences of people and places in Canadian society.

Razack (2002) argues that our understanding of particular places (and indeed, places themselves) come into existence through systems of domination, and simultaneously uphold these same systems. For example, the national space of Canada is represented as innocent through the nation's origin myth – Europeans peacefully settling empty lands and developing them through their resolute industriousness – which conceals a reality of stolen land, slavery, ongoing Indigenous genocide, and violence against nations of the Global South (Lawrence, 2002; Razack, 2002). This national space of innocence assembles local spaces in hierarchical relations based on how much they belong to this mythical nation; local spaces that do not fit are considered not to belong (Razack, 1998), which justifies further disinvestment and marginalization. In Canada, the production and management of racialized space can be seen in historical analyses of Halifax's "Africville" (Nelson, 2002, 2008), and Vancouver's "Chinatown" (Anderson, 1991). Nelson (2002, 2008) and Anderson (1991) show how racialized, inner-city spaces were constructed as degenerate, making way for slum clearance, eviction, and redevelopment. These cases clearly point to the construction of the inner city in Canada as a racialized space, "the zone in which all that is not respectable is contained" (Razack, 2002, p. 129). They also show how the production of space simultaneously involves the production of "excluded and included bodies" (Razack, 2002, p.10).

Racialized constructions of the slum or inner city are attached to bodies in these spaces, marking them as racialized (Razack, 1998; Teelucksingh, 2006). For example, on the one hand, the bodies of women of color, low-income women, and people who are homeless in the inner city are racialized by positioning them as subordinate in relation to white, middle-class subjects (Razack, 2002). On the other hand, white, middle-class subjects exercise their position of dominance when they travel to spaces of degeneracy for leisure or charity and return to spaces of respectability unscathed and strengthened (for example, when people volunteering in the Global South come to know themselves as good through their efforts to help people (Razack, 2002; Heron, 2007)). That is, they come to know themselves as *experts* and *saviors*, without accounting for how power structures shape these interactions, or their complicity in these structures (Heron, 2007).

Often, these understandings of respectability and degeneracy are overlain with, and supported by, ideas of healthy and unhealthy places that rely on similar tropes. Craddock (1995) described how "the diseased are defined, disempowered and controlled through metaphoric associations of place and affliction, inscriptions of contagious space, and the restructuring of purportedly diseased environments" (p. 958, see also Chapter 7). These associations mark racialized and low-income people residing in the inner city as degenerate and dirty, serving in turn to stigmatize and disenfranchise them further. At the same time, norms of health and respectability become aligned in the ideal of the "healthy citizen," who is understood as "male, European, heterosexual, middle aged and middle class" (Petersen and Lupton, 1996, p. 11). Moreover, ideal healthy citizens seek to protect their own health, as well as the health of others, by engaging in disease prevention (e.g. through diet, immunization, etc.), and leave their bodies open to regulation and intervention (Petersen and Lupton, 1996). Those that do not are understood as unhealthy, without regard for the complex social structures that produce differences in health

(Petersen and Lupton, 1996). Making individuals responsible for their health also can be understood as a part of the development of neoliberal subjectivities more broadly (Jessop, 2002; Staeheli, 2010). This emphasis on individual responsibility further obscures structures of domination, and marks people and places as both deviant and unhealthy.

Although it is incredibly important to interrogate the ways in which dominance is reproduced through space, it is also critical to understand that domination is not a finished project, and that people resist (McKittrick, 2006). Critical "race" scholars (Peake and Kobayashi, 2002; McKittrick, 2006) highlight the importance of telling counter-stories to challenge dominance. Counternarratives and counter-storytelling are long-standing methods that marginalized group members use to voice shared understandings and meanings of their own realities, which often go "suppressed, devalued and abnormalized" (Delgado, 1989, p. 2412). Counternarratives center the knowledge of communities resisting domination, in order to disrupt narratives that reproduce power structures and push for new ways of relating to one another (Nagar and Geiger, 2007).

Feminist geographers such as Rose (1997) and Sundberg (2005) have emphasized the importance of producing non-generalizing, partial, situated knowledge that cannot be understood as universal or objective. In fact, researchers who see themselves as unbiased observers producing objective knowledge may view racialized, low-income communities through a deficiency lens (Solórzano and Delgado Bernal, 2001; Solórzano and Yosso, 2002). Nagar and Geiger (2007) challenge academics to consider how their research can work in the favor of "less privileged communities and places" (p.2). However, asymmetrical relations of power cannot be completely surmounted in the research process, as alliances between academics and marginalized communities remain embedded in these relations (Ahmed, 2000; Nagar and Geiger, 2007). For example, Ahmed (2000) states that scholars' attempts to share power with participants in the research process does not necessarily mean that "the relations of force and authorization that are already implicated in the ethnographic desire to document the lives of strangers" (p.63) have been transcended. For this reason, the power relations that surround the production of texts need to be interrogated, to begin opening up "the possibility of strangers knowing differently to how they are known" (Ahmed, 2000, p. 74). In this chapter, we interrogate the narratives mobilized about "strangers" in Code Red articles, and highlight how low-income residents employ counternarratives to resist and transform dominant constructions of their lives and communities.

Method

Participants and Data Collection

This research combines a content analysis of the Code Red articles and in-depth interviews with key stakeholders. The seven original Code Red articles featured in the *Hamilton Spectator* were published between April 10 and April 18, 2010; we collected 22 pages of text and imagery (including maps) spanning seven days. Our analysis focuses on the original Code Red series, and does not include subsequent Code Red projects such as "Born" (December 2011; Pecoskie and Buist, 2011) or "Barton Street" (May 2013; Buist, 2013). This database was supplemented with a series of in-depth interviews with key architects of Code Red ($n = 2$), residents living in low-income neighborhoods identified in Code Red ($n = 7$), community developers working in those neighborhoods ($n = 5$), and other local stakeholders ($n = 3$). These interviews were not intended to be representative, but rather facilitated in-depth exploration of key issues (Elliott, 1999). To protect the confidentiality of all participants, we use pseudonyms instead of real names when sharing direct quotes from the qualitative interviews.

Procedure

Interviews were conducted between September 2012 and March 2014 and lasted between 30 and 90 minutes. Residents were asked about their personal experiences of their neighborhood and outsider perceptions. Key informants and community developers were asked to reflect on the implications of Code Red, and to describe challenges in implementing a municipal strategy to reduce health disparities. The interviews were recorded and transcribed verbatim for subsequent line-by-line coding (Strauss and Corbin, 1990), and thematic analysis was facilitated by NVivo 9™ software. Content analysis techniques were used to identify key narratives in the Code Red articles, which later were compared to the interviewee responses.

In order to contextualize our observations, the following section provides a brief history of Hamilton, Ontario, focusing on how the spatial arrangements of the city developed over time. We then describe the Code Red series and the lasting effects that it has had on the city, before presenting the insights from our analysis.

Background

Hamilton, Ontario: A History of Spatialized Inequities

The City of Hamilton is located in southwestern Ontario, on traditional Haudenosaunee territory (Firestone et al., 2014). Located on a harbor, and later an important railway junction, Hamilton became a manufacturing hub and eventually was one of the largest steel-making hubs in North America (Buzzelli and Jerrett, 2004). Yet the history of Hamilton is a contested one, where Black, Indigenous, immigrant and working-class peoples have struggled against spatialized inequities by fostering Black institutions, protesting slavery and racism, asserting treaty rights, and challenging exclusionary development practices (Cruickshank and Bouchier, 2004; Orkin and Klippenstein, 2003; Shadd, 2010).

By the early twentieth century, Hamilton's industries attracted many working-class and immigrant families to the city, who were stigmatized for residing in poor-quality housing adjacent to industry (Freeman, 2001). At the same time, growth in the city's suburbs was facilitated by the annexation of neighboring farmland and building of new roads (Freeman, 2001). For example, Black farmers residing on the Hamilton Mountain in a community called "Little Africa" faced intense racism and increasing challenges to staying on the land, pushing some to move to the lower city for work (City of Hamilton, 2010; Shadd, 2010). Later, the introduction of master planning in the postwar period served to harden perceptions about "declining" areas, limit the scope for residential renewal, and drive residents out of the urban core. For example, town planner E.G. Faludi created zoning regulations to designate neighborhoods located beside industry as "declining," "blighted," and "slum," which marked them for removal and dismissed the need for affordable housing for working-class families (Cruikshank and Bouchier, 2004, p. 464).

Like many cities across North America, the manufacturing sector in Hamilton declined due to changes in the global economy after the 1960s (Beauregard, 2009). This led to the closure of many companies, and left surrounding communities exposed to environmental hazards (Wakefield et al., 2001; Wakefield and McMullan, 2005; Beauregard, 2009). Additionally, poor planning decisions by local elites have had lasting negative effects on the image of Hamilton's downtown (Cruikshank and Bouchier, 2004). In particular, a major city-led redevelopment of the downtown core in the 1960s led to the demolition of 44 acres of the city's original commercial district, replacing it with an indoor, privately managed commercial space (Slote, 2011). The process of commissioning the redevelopment raised concerns that key business interests in the city had driven the process without much regard for the views of local residents (Freeman, 2001).

More recently, the city's handling of the Red Hill Valley expressway drew criticism from the general public and members of the Haudenosaunee Confederacy (Orkin and Klippenstein, 2003; Salter, 2013). Local First Nation peoples challenged this development, as it would cut through and negatively impact Haudenosaunee territory and violate the Albany Treaty of 1701 (Orkin and Klippenstein, 2003; Salter, 2013). Local residents also rallied against this development, as the environmental impact would deteriorate already poor air quality for east end communities (Craggs, 2013). Yet proponents of the expressway successfully pushed through their plans for increased development in 2007, calling the highway, "a gift that will keep on giving" in terms of establishing businesses and jobs (Craggs, 2013). As the descriptions above demonstrate, the history of Hamilton is replete with seemingly well-meaning efforts to transform the inner city, but which have taken place without engaging the voices of the low-income, racialized residents, and Indigenous peoples already active in their communities. It is against this backdrop that the Code Red series of newspaper articles emerged. While these articles were written with positive social change in mind (a point we elaborate below), they serve as a window into how particular places become marked (Fellows and Razack, 1998) as deviant, without sufficient recognition of how these narratives reproduce dominance and inequity.

Situating Code Red

Code Red emerged as a collaborative project between the *Hamilton Spectator* and researchers at McMaster University (a major Canadian university located in Hamilton). According to the key authors of Code Red, its main purpose was to demonstrate significant differences in the social determinants of health and health outcomes between Hamilton's neighborhoods (e.g. income, hospitalization rates), in a way that would be accessible to a lay audience and spur public debate (DeLuca et al., 2012). In order to meet their objectives, the authors accessed almost 400,000 hospital records for Hamilton residents, which included the patients' demographic information, type of services used, and a geographic marker identifying the census tract in which they lived (DeLuca et al., 2012). This data was used to develop 26 maps showing how different neighborhoods ranked in terms of health and socioeconomic variables (Buist, 2010a; DeLuca, 2012). These maps, presented in the Code Red articles, documented many significant disparities in health, health care utilization, and socioeconomic status (Buist, 2010a). In addition, they were color-coded: "green was used to indicate better parts of the city," followed by lighter shades of green, and finally red to signify the areas that fared worst on each indicator (DeLuca, 2012, p. 321).

The text accompanying the maps provided a variety of so-called expert opinions and reflections, but few personal accounts of people living in the neighborhoods identified in Code Red. Four relatively short stories of people sharing their experiences of prostitution, teen pregnancy, homelessness, and inefficient long-term care for older adults appeared in the series. When asked how he identified stories to include, a lead Code Red reporter stated that it was having a sense of a good story:

> I've had a lot of experience obviously in the business for many years and so you just sort of get a sense of who's going to make for a good story [...] I can remember just sitting at the table and my jaw was probably on the table just listening to her tell me this horrifying story about how she got on to the wrong path in life and the types of things that had happened to her. You know ... for someone like me who lives a comfortable life, it's beyond belief.

This statement points to how the audience of Code Red is not necessarily the people living in low-income neighborhoods, but white, middle-class readers who may be *shocked into helping* people living in poverty. The main authors have stated publicly that they were concerned about the possible stigmatization of neighborhoods identified in the report, but "felt that the positive outcomes for the community outweighed the potential stigma that might be attached to these neighborhoods" (DeLuca et al., 2012, p. 326). In an interview we conducted, one of the lead reporters reiterated this:

> I'm very sensitive to the whole issue of stigmatization, which is something I've been asked about and something I really struggled with ... []
> But what would the alternative be? [...] You can't just bury your head in the sand.

Indeed, the series significantly influenced public debate and municipal politics to the extent that six months after the release of Code Red, a mayoral election was won by the only candidate who embraced Code Red as a campaign issue (Deluca et al., 2012). Code Red also garnered attention from provincial and federal levels of government and continues to grab the attention of the public, as more than 184 articles have been published in the *Hamilton Spectator* referencing the series (Deluca et al., 2012).

One of the most visible changes spurred by Code Red was the establishment of a citywide initiative called the Neighbourhood Action Strategy (City of Hamilton, 2011, 2016). The strategy uses a community development approach in tandem with a municipal planning process to engage low-income residents in developing plans to improve neighborhood health (City of Hamilton, 2011). Since the initiative began in 2011, residents in ten neighborhoods – with the support of community developers, service providers and city staff – have developed neighborhood action plans that articulate a vision for the neighborhood and describe specific projects to reach that vision, ranging from reducing traffic congestion, to improving food security through urban agriculture (City of Hamilton, 2013).

Why, then, have we chosen to write about the damaging effects of this media series and research study when it appears to have done so much good? In the next section, we show how research and media reports on health and place are embedded in relations of power, histories, and contexts. We argue that research examining health differences across places – whether reported in the media, or in more traditional academic forums – may work to reproduce relations of domination and subordination, even when motivated by a desire for positive social change.

In the following section we present three narratives in Code Red that serve to mark the places and bodies in Hamilton's inner city as deviant and unhealthy in relation to the unmarked "spaces of innocence" in the suburbs (Razack, 2002). We also show how these narratives position particular (i.e. white, male, professional) bodies as knowledgeable about how to define and solve the problem of the inner city, while low-income residents are scripted as passive victims.

Findings

Uncovering Narratives of the Unhealthy City

The Inner City as a Space of Deviance

The first article of the Code Red series, provocatively entitled "Worlds Apart," describes the vast differences between Hamilton's neighborhoods in terms of wealth and health. In this article, six maps are presented that illustrate statistics on a number of health and socioeconomic variables (Buist, 2010a). From these maps, the viewer can see how the red areas coalesce in the downtown, north, and east end areas of the city, whereas the green areas can be found on the outer suburbs of the city. The text beside each map shows statistics on how the top and lowest ranking census tracts fared. One map in the series showed the percentage of families headed by a female lone parent, indicating that this was understood as a problem in the same way as poverty and ill-health (Buist, 2010a, p. WR6).

These maps were accompanied by narratives intended to contextualize the maps, including this passage, where the author describes what he sees in his journey to the lowest-ranking census tract in Hamilton:

> On a brisk winter morning, kids in pyjama bottoms are pushing babies in strollers along Wentworth Street North. Three blocks over, a scruffy young man walks a menacing-looking pit bull, the dog's muzzle absent. Bits of garbage kicked up by a stiff wind dance and spin in front of the grimy stores on King Street East. (Buist, 2010a, p.WR5)

In this description, the esthetics of the place – and the people in it – are emphasized and found deficient in ways that reinforce dominant constructs of respectable dress and conduct, without explicitly naming them as such. Through the author's lens, the reader comes to see this place as full of chaos and disrepute. In addition, the reader is introduced to the figure of the deficient mother: a narrative we problematize later.

The city is presented as a place of deep socioeconomic and health divides, with inner-city neighborhoods represented as places of poverty, decay, and illness. The article emphasizes that some neighborhoods in Hamilton appear more similar to countries in the Global South in terms of life expectancy and health outcomes. The term "Third World" (Buist, 2010a, p. WR1) was invoked four times, followed by the author's or interviewees' sentiments of "shock," "outrage," or "horror." For example, one north end neighborhood's ranking in life expectancy is pegged as being equal to "Nepal, just ahead of Pakistan and worse than India, Mongolia and Turkmenistan" (Buist, 2010a, p. WR1). Another seven inner-city neighborhoods were said to have greater percentages of low birthweight babies than sub-Saharan Africa. Conversely, suburban areas are described as healthy neighborhoods where people use fewer health care resources, and thereby cost taxpayers less money. In fact, the geography of Hamilton is described in the first article as a "healthy ring with a rotten hole centered on the lower inner city" (p.WR2).

What is the purpose of these comparisons, and what narratives do they mobilize? We argue here that the inner city is understood as a space of deviance and degeneracy *because* of its closeness to racialized "Third World" spaces (Buist, 2010a, p. WR1). The "unhealthy" inner city is understood as an aberration, while the "healthy" suburb is normalized. As one Code Red interviewee stated:

> I think the extent of the poverty and the disparities are more gaping than any of us would have known going into this ... It would have been reminiscent of what you might anticipate in Detroit or the south side of Chicago or some Third World countries, certainly not what you expect in southern Ontario. (Buist, 2010a, p. WR2)

This statement points to well-known racialized places as locations where it seems it would be normal or reasonable to encounter poverty. Here, places are understood as naturally occurring instead of produced through social, political, and economic processes that reproduce dominance and are resisted (McKittrick, 2006). The invocation of the "Third World" Other also works to reify problematic notions of "Third World" (Buist, 2010a, p. WR1) degeneracy and the superiority of the "First World" (Mohanty, 2003), and more specifically, Canada as an innocent nation.

Further, the articles outline the multiple costs associated with providing health care, particularly in inner-city neighborhoods:

> The differences are astounding. In one inner-city neighbourhood ... the total cost for hospital bed, emergency room and ambulance use was [C]$9.15 million for the two years of data collected. More importantly, it means there's a difference of [C]$8.63 million in hospital, ER [emergency room] and ambulance costs between the top and bottom neighbourhoods in Hamilton. (Buist, 2010c, p.Go4)

This emphasis on health care costs works to reinforce dominant notions of the inner city as a burden, inhabited by unhealthy citizens; and conversely, the suburb as a space of respectability where healthy citizens reside.

The Code Red Woman

As noted earlier, the marking of inner city spaces as deviant is not only "raced" and classed, but also gendered. Of the fairly limited portrayals of residents in the articles, many of the longest and most memorable described the experiences of women. Consider the following description of coming to downtown Hamilton, narrated by a health care worker interviewed for the Code Red series:

> "One of the first things that shocked me was driving down the street, maybe 2 o'clock in the morning, and seeing parents and kids running across the street," she said. "What are kids doing up so late at night? Or moms pushing their babies in strollers down the street that late at night. Totally shocked." (Buist, 2010a, p.WR1)

As this is the first description of the area in the series that does not draw on the health data analysis, its placement is telling. The health care worker goes on to describe a couple of encounters she had with local women while on the job:

> "Her mascara is running, she's got one shoe on, it's cold out but she has no real clothes on for winter or the weather, her purse is half strewn all over the sidewalk," Bartley recalled. "She says that she's running from somebody and she doesn't need any help. She was a street person, so she works on the street for money. Eventually, she said that she's addicted to cocaine and she doesn't know how she got there, so we just took her to the hospital." (Buist, 2010a, p.WR2)

> "There was a girl slumped over on the toilet," Bartley said. "Her boyfriend was there and they had pulled a baby out from the toilet. She didn't even know she was pregnant, she says, and her boyfriend is screaming in the background, wanting to have a paternity test to see if the baby was his [...] And I'm thinking, as they're yelling in the background, this is like a Jerry Springer Show." (Buist, 2010a, p.WR4)

In each of these cases, the women portrayed are seen as lacking control and respectability, both because of their behaviors (not only prostitution and substance use), and their lack of self-care. The women are described as disheveled and pitiable, almost to the point of absurdity; ultimately they are scripted as irresponsible women. Similarly, the very last story of the first Code Red article introduces the reader to Karen De Silva, who is called a "broken person" – her story is told in the following way:

> Raised in the Jane–Finch area of Toronto by her alcoholic grandmother, because that was the better choice than being raised by her drug-addicted mother. Sexually abused at a young age by a family member. In and out of foster homes, a constant runaway. Then other problems kicked in. Exotic dancer at age 16, heavy crack cocaine user by age 18, a baby removed from her care at age 21, prostitute by 22 ... She needed the cash because she'd already spent the rent money on drugs. (Buist, 2010a, p.WR7)

In these few sentences, again the reader is introduced to the figure of the absent or deficient mother and woman who has failed to care properly for her children. De Silva herself is scripted first as a vulnerable child, then as an irresponsible mother for turning to prostitution. Women continue to be presented as both victims of, but partially culpable for, their circumstances in the remainder of the series – particularly in a later article where descriptions of teen mothers suggest their choices are predetermined by their own parenting (Pecoskie and Buist, 2011).

Ultimately, this works to propagate notions of inner-city degeneracy and victimhood, erasing the complexity of these neighborhoods and the agency of racialized women such as De Silva, who have navigated and survived extremely oppressive conditions. Instead, the judge, counselor, nurse, and psychiatrist in the story are scripted as heroes. This pattern also can be seen in a story about a local doctor who runs a maternity clinic:

> He recalls the case of a young woman who showed up in the 15th week of pregnancy, addicted to crack cocaine and vomiting all the time. "She required an awful lot of resources," said Price … "But in combination with my nurse practitioner, with the social worker in the clinic, with the public health nurse and the dietitian, we were able to get her off the crack cocaine." (Buist, 2010b, p.Go5)

These stories are told to demonstrate how priority areas in Hamilton use up a greater share of hospital resources than affluent neighborhoods. Noticeably absent from the portrayals of these women is any discussion of how hierarchical power structures form conditions for violence against low-income, racialized women. In the next section, we explore how the Code Red series positions (usually white, middle-class male) professionals as experts and saviors, and in ways that reproduce gendered, racialized, and classed bodies as deficient and unhealthy subjects.

Experts, Saviors, and Victims

In the first article of the Code Red series, the reader is introduced to nine people identified as experts in health and poverty in Hamilton (several more experts are introduced in later articles) (Buist, 2010a). Throughout the series the reader is pointed to their personal accounts of working in Hamilton's inner city, or their thoughts on the Code Red data.

The first article also contained nine photographs: four are portraits of the cited experts (two of which can be seen in Figure 8.1), and two are small images of the primary author Steve Buist and photographer Gary Yokoyama. There was also a relatively small photo of Karen De Silva. The remaining two pictures presented images of the neighborhoods with the lowest health outcomes according to Code Red. One photo focuses on a building with broken windows and graffiti and a lone cyclist in the background (see Figure 8.2).

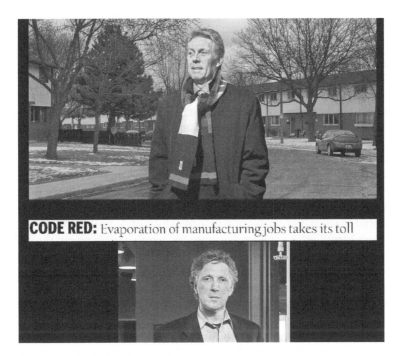

Figure 8.1 Two professionals featured as experts: Fred Eisenberger, Mayor of Hamilton (above), and Mark Chamberlain, President and CEO of Trivaris Ltd and Chair of the Hamilton Roundtable for Poverty Reduction (below), in the Code Red series

Source: Buist, 2010a, p.WR4; reprinted with permission from the *Hamilton Spectator*

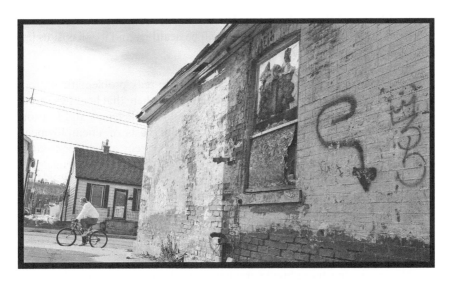

Figure 8.2 CT0050, the lowest rated of Hamilton's 130 census tracts, according to Code Red. The image highlights a dilapidated space

Source: Buist, 2010a, p.WR7; reprinted with permission from the *Hamilton Spectator*

The other shows a young man and two women, with one holding a small child; none of them are named, and none are looking at the camera. The caption under the image reads "neighbours on Roxborough Street in the east end enjoy the warmth of early March. This neighbourhood, or census tract, has the highest rate of cardiovascular ER visits in Hamilton" (Buist, 2010a, p. WR5). It is not known whether the people in the image are family or friends, what they think about where they live, their struggles and hopes, or what their ideas are in terms of neighborhood change.

Conversely, many of the experts identified in the article series are quoted to define the problem or as providing thoughts about solutions. In the final article, six people provide their opinions on how to solve the problems raised by Code Red in short editorials – all of them white, male professionals. Overall, men were identified in expert roles more frequently than women: throughout the series, 12 out of a total of 15 experts were male, and all appeared to be white. Also, the two key female professionals featured in the series largely spoke about their own experiences of providing services to people, rather than being given space to discuss solutions to health disparities, or provide policy advice.

None of the expert editorials in the final Code Red article were written by residents from any of the neighborhoods identified as having poor health outcomes in Code Red; and in many cases, the quotations from experts exhibited a clear sense of division from residents: for example, in terms of the use of "us" and "they":

> "If I can help this person get a job, they'll be healthier and it will cost us less money. If I can help a person through a mental illness, they'll be healthier and they will cost us less money. If we can help a person go from homelessness to a home, they will be healthier and it will cost us less money." (Buist, 2010a, p.WR2)

This division between "us" and "them" appears to reify problematic notions of who is a healthy or an unhealthy citizen. It is clear here that healthy citizens are understood as largely white, middle-class subjects (Petersen and Lupton, 1996). There is also a reference to the economic costs of unemployment, mental illness, and homelessness, which healthy citizens are understood to bear the burden of, without accounting for the contributions and struggles of low-income communities.

In the Code Red narratives, professionals are scripted as knowledgeable saviors whose heroism is laudable, and residents are positioned as passive victims. For example, a doctor highlights his compassion in helping people who are so different from him:

> "Every single person breaks my heart," said Guenter. ... "From the day that they were conceived through to the time I meet them, they have been up against some circumstances that are completely foreign to me,

circumstances that I cannot imagine growing up in. But I have to say there are many joys around this work, and the joy is to see when people can actually surmount that set of circumstances." (Buist, 2010a, p.WR5)

While this sense of commitment to those in need is laudable, it can serve to reify relations of dominance and obscure the complex power hierarchies that create inequities. Instead of asking what power hierarchies sustain these differences and inequalities, healthy citizens are positioned to help unhealthy Others. However, our interviews with residents in these neighborhoods tell a different story, which we turn to below.

Contesting Code Red and Imagining New Possibilities through Counternarratives

In this section we draw on semi-structured interviews with residents and community developers working in the low-income neighborhoods identified by Code Red. The interviews highlight how residents and community developers working closely with residents interpret and contest the dominant narratives mobilized in Code Red. It is clear from the interviews that there is a strong consensus among participants that outsiders view where they live as a "ghetto" or "slum," but that insiders have a deep sense of pride in their neighborhood. It is also clear that while residents may view themselves as stigmatized subjects, they also see themselves as agents with the capacity to resist, contest, and transform dominant narratives of their neighborhood by creating counternarratives.

The residents interviewed reported great dissatisfaction with Code Red's portrayal of their neighborhoods. They noted how there was significant silence around residents' perspectives and experiences, and that the authors did not address their concerns and grievances. For example, Anna said:

> This neighborhood is actually – it's kind of funny that we don't tend to sit back and say "poor us, poor us, poor us." When the Keith neighborhood was named in the Code Red articles, the first thing we did was say, well how dare you, Steve Buist! And we challenged him to come see what it's like. [...] and then we finally just decided that it doesn't really matter what Steve Buist says about the neighborhood – we're gonna make it the way that we want it. Some of the things he said are here, but what he didn't talk about was the great people – and what he didn't talk about is what we do have. All he wanted to do is talk about what we don't have.

Participants felt that their neighbors were viewed as lazy and blamed for their poverty. They contested this understanding of low-income residents by pointing to how their neighbors were "hardworking people," and emphasized the need for a living wage and the ways that changes in the global economy negatively impacted working-class communities. This can be seen in the following quote, where Anna challenges the poverty tropes propagated in Code Red:

> Anyone who is poor is seen to be lazy. Well, you're just not working hard enough. If you don't have enough, it's because you're not putting in the work necessary – and I think that is strongly reflected in Hamiltonian attitudes towards poverty. You know, maybe it goes back to the years of Hamilton being a manufacturing boomtown, when there was no want for work – no matter how uneducated you were. That's probably a strong factor in it, but nowadays, when we've watched the manufacturing sector collapse in upon itself … that concept is carrying through, despite the fact that there's just not enough work here. The press has also got a big thumb in that. They like to report numbers.

It is clear that resident participants had a clear understanding of the historical context that has produced social, economic, and spatial inequities. However, the negative tropes, dominant narratives, and stigmatizing language that Code Red employed are also understood as constructed by media for profit. For example, during a qualitative interview, Ben explained:

> The Hamilton Spectator invented Code Red … They invented it. It could've been any title, but we've grabbed it and we've accepted it as an actual official designation or an official label – and it is not – [but] we bought into it and we keep using that language. I avoid that language because it's a corporation – it is a for-profit corporation. The same way that Coca-Cola reinvented Christmas, the *Spectator* has reinvented Hamilton, the lower city of Hamilton – and I won't perpetuate it.

There is a concerted effort on the part of neighborhood residents to be mindful of the language used to characterize their communities and neighbors. The residents are working to actively change the way people talk about poverty, and instead frame neighborhood challenges around social and economic inequity. For example, Doug shared:

> It [poverty] just kept getting put in for everything – like in the paper. It just made it look like everybody in the area was lazy, no good, didn't give a damn about nothing. Sure you're always going to have some people that may be just like that but not everybody's like that. There are a lot of people that work long hours and are good decent people but because they don't make C$17 or C$18 an hour, it doesn't make them any less of a person.

> We often use "financial inequity" [as our term]. We have a different average household income in this neighborhood than, say, they do in Ancaster [an affluent suburb]. That doesn't mean that Ancaster is any better, it just means that it's a little unequal.

The residents are also developing their own media forums where they can tell their stories from their points of view, and share them directly with other community members. Residents are aiming to focus on community strengths, assets, and communicating collective successes in their media.

While the residents contested the dominant narratives propagated in Code Red, many also pointed to the ways in which multiple changes occurred in the city because of the media series. The most prominent example is the Neighborhood Action Strategy. Residents and community developers working within the Strategy have said that it has helped to connect resources to communities in order to support residents in developing and implementing asset-based action plans aimed at improving health in their neighborhoods. Overall, residents and community developers have indicated that despite the gains of the Strategy, the dominant narratives and language of Code Red that cast residents as victims and professional people as so-called experts still persist. For example, there have been times when residents have felt disempowered and excluded by these experts. During the interviews with community developers, Sophie described neighborhood meetings "overrun with service providers," with "people in authority coming in and saying this is what we're going to do." These outside actors include city staff and service providers, as well as researchers and students from the local universities and colleges who want to learn about efforts to combat poverty and disparities in health, but whose commitment to the neighborhoods tends to be transient. Another community developer, Mary, noted that these outsiders can fail to see residents as knowledgeable equals:

> At heart, I think the service providers ... don't want to sit there and listen to people ... possibly people complaining. [...] Maybe they think "I didn't go to years of school to sit here and listen to you ..." There's still that power difference, we are the professionals and you are the client.

Again, this points to the importance of listening and engaging residents as equal, knowing partners on their own terms. Overall, while residents are cautiously optimistic about the effect that the Strategy might have on their neighborhood, they are concerned about the extent to which those attempting to partner with them are willing to see them as equals in the process.

Discussion and Conclusion

This chapter has used the Code Red series of newspaper articles to explore how efforts to document geographic disparities in health can work to further marginalize and stigmatize particular people and places. In particular, it has highlighted how the reproduction of particular narratives – namely, the inner city as degenerate space; women as irresponsible victims; and the expert as knowing savior – all continue to position the inner city as a racialized space of deviance and degeneracy inhabited by unhealthy Others (Razack,

2002; Petersen and Lupton, 1996), and to silence residents in lieu of expert (read: white professional male) voices. These narratives re-embed spatial inequities, even as the Code Red authors and other social actors are seeking to reduce them. More specifically, they reproduce norms of respectability that privilege white, male, affluent actors: these actors describe the problem and solutions, and are the implicit standard against which others are judged. In contrast, women, low-income and racialized people are portrayed as out of control: they are seen as passive victims, but also the cause of their own afflictions through irresponsible behavior, and thus are constructed as at least partially to blame for the oppression, exclusion, and violence that they endure. This is reinforced further by an overall failure to pay serious attention to the power structures (patriarchy, white supremacy, colonialism and capitalism) that shape peoples' lives.

These findings resonate with literature on space and subjectivity, where the production of places also produces included or excluded bodies (Razack, 1998, 2002). The observed mobilization of health and disease in ways that align with existing conceptions of the degenerate inner city echoes other, mostly historical, work in health geography, which has shown how describing places as "diseased" serves to legitimate elite strategies to reshape the inner city and disempower residents (Craddock, 1995; see also Shah, 2001; Craddock, 2004). In our case, the narrative of contagion (Craddock, 1995) has been replaced by a neoliberal ideal of healthy citizenship that the degenerate, inner-city subject fails to achieve. In both cases, the deviancy of the inner city – and the people who live in it – is both validated and reproduced by invoking health as an issue of concern.

The role of research here – and in particular, the mapping of neighborhoods by sociodemographic and health indicators – is important to consider. While the maps presented in Code Red might be seen to speak for themselves in terms of the data that they present, the maps also serve to homogenize the diversity of people living in neighborhoods. When numbers are mapped to entire areas, the experiences of the diverse and multifaceted individuals residing in these areas are lost (see also Chapter 7). While the Code Red authors did recognize the potential for stigma when developing the series, they saw their options as either reporting the data, or doing nothing. We would instead argue that choices about the selection, (re)presentation, and interpretation of data are not neutral, but can serve as powerful – if not always conscious – tools of domination (see Ahmed, 2000).

In addition, while there is no question that many of the solutions proposed in Code Red would go a long way towards improving the health of residents in Hamilton's inner city, our point here is to draw attention to how rarely the voices of those most affected by intersecting systems of oppression are actually present, particularly in terms of framing the problem and identifying solutions. At most there were personal stories, and even then only selective ones, emphasizing challenges rather than the full scope of their lives. Those most affected were not asked how the data from the Code Red study should be interpreted, or about solutions to the inequities documented. Instead, it was the experts who described their experiences and talked about solutions, and this reinforced their taken-for-granted power.

In opposition to these narratives, we have presented the perspectives and concerns of residents to show how dominant narratives can be challenged and transformed. In this section we demonstrated how residents contested the dominant narratives circulated in Code Red and voiced their own counternarratives of their neighborhoods. They identified ways to begin imagining new forms of relating to one another by discarding stigmatizing language, developing new media outlets, and understanding residents as knowing, resilient, and active. They also highlighted potential difficulties in working in partnership with the people and organizations who fail to treat them as equal.

It is important to note that we are *not* arguing that the author and publishers of Code Red are bad actors who single-handedly created and propagated the narratives described here. Rather, we aim to demonstrate that Code Red is an example of how underlying narratives of dominance are (re)produced in and through the media and reports on health inequities. It is also not our intention to position ourselves – or this reading of the evidence – as somehow outside or above the social relations and oppressive power structures that shape academic work (see Ahmed, 2000; Nagar and Geiger, 2007). Like all research, our interpretation is admittedly partial, and also incompletely (re)presents residents of Hamilton's inner city. Finally, our intention is not to foreclose the possibility that individuals and institutions can learn and change: for example, a recent follow-up series in the *Hamilton Spectator* attempted to foreground the voices of residents and highlight their positive work in the Strategy (see Pecoskie, 2014).

Overall, in highlighting the narratives and impacts of Code Red as well as resident responses to the series, we seek to emphasize how the good intentions of dominant actors – including researchers – cannot always be assumed to lead to positive consequences. Therefore, it is important for researchers and others to be reflexive and examine their complicity in reproducing oppressive relations, in order to begin seriously addressing the interlocking structures of power in which we are all implicated.

References

Ahmed, S., 2000. *Strange encounters: Embodied others in postcoloniality*. London: Routledge.

Anderson, K., 1991. *Vancouver's Chinatown: Racial discourse in Canada, 1875–1980*. Montreal: McGill-Queen's University Press.

Beauregard, R.A., 2009. Urban population loss in historical perspective: United States, 1820–2000, *Environment and Planning A*, 41(3), pp. 514–28.

Buist, S., 2010a. Worlds apart: Glaring disparities in wealth and health have taken a shocking toll on a huge number of Hamilton's people. *The Hamilton Spectator*, April 10, p. WR1.

Buist, S., 2010b. Band-aid fixes getting us nowhere. *The Hamilton Spectator*, April 12, p. Go4.

Buist, S., 2010c. Starting life on 'the right trajectory'. *The Hamilton Spectator*, April 13, p.Go4.

Buist, S., 2013. Barton Street: A Code Red project. *The Hamilton Spectator*, May 18, p.BA1.

Buzzelli, M. and Jerrett, M., 2004. Racial gradients of ambient air pollution exposure in Hamilton, Canada. *Environment and Planning*, 36, 1855–76.

City of Hamilton. 2010. Little Africa Plaque (Early Black community on Hamilton Mountain) (CS10032). Hamilton: City of Hamilton. Available online at www.hamilton.ca/NR/rdonlyres/C724DF1F-1C9E-4A38-820F-EA97C31AAB05/0/Apr07EDRMS_n85765_v1_5_6__CS10032__Little_Africa_Plaque.pdf (accessed September 30, 2014).

City of Hamilton, 2011. Neighbourhood development strategy (CM11007). Hamilton: City of Hamilton. Available online at www.hamilton.ca/NR/rdonlyres/FC73E139-6402-4CE6-BF38-7B92F782A129/0/May09EDRMS_n167008_v1_7_3__CM11007.pdf (accessed July 12, 2014).

City of Hamilton, 2013. Neighbourhood action strategy annual report (V1). Hamilton: City of Hamilton. Available online at www.hamilton.ca/NR/rdonlyres/88A4B4C4-2251-4ED7-B6DF-1C27CB64399B/0/NeighbourhoodInitiatives AnnualReport_FINAL.pdf (accessed July 12, 2014).

City of Hamilton, 2016. Neighbourhood action strategy. Available online at www.hamilton.ca/city-initiatives/strategies-actions/neighbourhood-action-strategy (accessed February 2, 2016).

Craddock, S., 1995. Sewers and scapegoats: Spatial metaphors of smallpox in the nineteeth-century San Francisco. *Social Science & Medicine*, 41, pp. 957–68.

Craddock, S., 2004. Beyond epidemiology: Locating AIDS in Africa. In: E. Kalipeni, S. Craddock, J.R. Oppong, and J. Ghosh, eds. *HIV and AIDS in Africa: Beyond epidemiology*. Malden, MA: Blackwell, pp. 1–10.

Craggs, S., 2013. 5 years later, was the Red Hill Valley Parkway worth it? CBC News, January 2. Available online at www.cbc.ca/news/canada/hamilton/news/5-years-later-was-the-red-hill-valley-parkway-worth-it-1.1275560 (accessed September 30, 2014).

Crenshaw, K., 1991. Mapping the margins: Intersectionality, identity politics, and violence against women of color. *Stanford Law Review*, 43(6), pp. 1241–99.

Cruikshank, K. and Bouchier, B.B., 2004. Blighted area and obnoxious industries: Constructing environmental inequality on an industrial waterfront, Hamilton, Ontario, 1890–1960. *Environmental History*, 9(3), pp. 464–96.

Delgado, R., 1989. Storytelling for oppositionists and others: A plea for narrative. *Michigan Law Review*, 87(8), pp. 2411–41.

Deluca, F., Buist, S. and Johnston, N., 2012. The Code Red project: Engaging communities in health system change in Hamilton, Canada. *Social Indicators Research*, 108(2), pp. 317–27.

Elliott, S.J., 1999. Qualitative approaches in health geography: Introduction. *Professional Geographer*, 51(2), pp. 230–2.

Fellows, M.L. and Razack, S., 1998. The race to innocence: Confronting hierarchical relations among women. *Journal of Gender, Race and Justice*, 1, pp. 335–52.

Firestone, M., Smylie, J., Maracle, S., Spiller, M. and O'Campo, P., 2014. Unmasking health determinants and health outcomes for urban First Nations using respondent-driven sampling. *BMJ Open*, 4(7), pp. 1–8.

Freeman, B., 2001. *Hamilton: A people's history*. Toronto: James Lorrimer & Co.

Grillo, T., 1995. Anti-essentialism and intersectionality: Tools to dismantle the master's house. *Berkeley Women's Law Journal*, 10(1), pp. 16–30.

Heron, B., 2007. *Desire for development: Whiteness, gender, and the helping imperative*. Waterloo: Wilfred Laurier University Press.

Jessop, B., 2002. Liberalism, neoliberalism, and urban governance: A state-theoretical perspective. *Antipode*, 34(3), pp. 452–71.

Lawrence, B., 2002. Rewriting histories of the land: Colonization and indigenous resistance in eastern Canada. In: S. Razack, ed. *Race, space, and the law: Unmapping a white settler society*. Toronto: Between the Lines, pp. 21–46.

Lorde, A., 2007. Age, race, class, and sex: Women redefining difference. In: A. Lorde, ed. *Sister outsider*. New York: Crossing Press. pp. 114–23.

McKittrick, K., 2006. *Demonic grounds: Black women and the cartographies of struggle*. Minneapolis, MN: University of Minnesota Press.

Mohanty, C.T., 2003. Under western eyes: Feminist scholarship and colonial discourses. In: C.T. Mohanty, ed. *Feminism without borders: Decolonizing theory, practicing Solidarity*. Durham, NC: Duke University Press. pp. 16–42.

Nagar, R. and Geiger, S., 2007. Reflexivity and positionality in feminist fieldwork revisited. In: A. Tickell, E. Sheppard, J. Peck and T. Barnes, eds. *Politics and practice in economic geography*. London: Sage Publications, pp. 267–78.

Nelson, J.J., 2002. The space of Africville: Creating, regulating, and remembering the urban "slum." In: S. Razack, ed. *Race, space, and the law: Unmapping a white settler society*. Toronto: Between the Lines, pp. 211–32.

Nelson, J.J., 2008. *Razing Africville: A geography of racism*. Toronto: University of Toronto Press.

Orkin, A. and Klippenstein, M., 2003. Sacred promise: Hamilton's Red Hill Valley expressway project violates important 1701 Crown–Iroquois treaty rights. *The Hamilton Spectator*, December 13, p.F8.

Peake, L. and Kobayashi, A., 2002. Policies and practices for an antiracist geography at the millennium. *The Professional Geographer*, 54(1), pp. 50–61.

Pecoskie, T., 2014. High hopes, ambitious plan. *The Hamilton Spectator*, September 15. Available online at www.thespec.com/news-story/4858916-high-hopes-ambitious-plan/ (accessed October 1, 2014).

Pecoskie, T. and Buist, S., 2011. Born: A Code Red project. *The Hamilton Spectator*, November 19, p.WR1.

Petersen, A.R. and Lupton, D., 1996. *The new public health: Health and self in the age of risk*. Thousand Oaks, CA: Sage Publications.

Razack, S., 1998. *Looking white people in the eye: Gender, race and culture in courtrooms and classrooms*. Toronto: University of Toronto Press.

Razack, S., 2002. *Race, space, and the law: Unmapping a white settler society*. Toronto: Between the Lines.

Rose, G., 1997. Situating knowledges: Positionality, reflexivities and other tactics. *Progress in Human Geography*, 21, pp. 305–20.

Salter, C., 2013. *Whiteness and social change: Remnant colonialisms and white civility in Australia and Canada*. Newcastle-upon-Tyne: Cambridge Scholars Publishing.

Shadd, A., 2010. *The journey from tollgate to parkway: African Canadians in Hamilton*. Toronto: Dundurn.

Shah, N., 2001. *Contagious divides: Epidemics and race in San Francisco's Chinatown*. Berkley, CA: University of California Press.

Slote, K.D., 2011. *The transformative city: Creating meaningful and creative public space in Downtown Hamilton*. Unpublished MA thesis, University of Waterloo.

Solórzano, D. and Delgado Bernal, D., 2001. Critical race theory, transformational resistance and social justice: Chicana and Chicano students in an urban context. *Urban Education*, 36(3), pp. 308–42.

Solórzano, D. and Yosso, T., 2002. Critical race methodology: Counter-storytelling as an analytical framework for education research. *Qualitative Inquiry*, 8(10), pp. 23–44.

Staeheli, L.A., 2010. Political geography: Where's citizenship?. *Progress in Human Geography*, 34(3), pp. 393–400.

Strauss, A., and Corbin, J., 1990. *Basics of qualitative research: Grounded theory procedures and techniques*. Newbury Park, CA: Sage.

Sundberg, J., 2005. Looking for the critical geographer, or why bodies and geographies matter to the emergence of critical geographies of Latin America. *Geoforum*, 36(1), pp. 17–28.

Teelucksingh, C., 2006. *Claiming space: Racialization in Canadian cities*. Waterloo: Wilfred Laurier University Press.

Wakefield, S. and McMullan, C., 2005. Healing in places of decline: (Re)imagining everyday landscapes in Hamilton, Ontario. *Health and Place*, 11(4), pp. 299–312.

Wakefield, S.E.L., Elliott, S.J., Cole, D.C. and Eyles, J.D., 2001. Environmental risk and (re)action: Air quality, health and civic involvement in an urban industrial neighbourhood, *Health & Place*, 7(3), pp. 163–77.

9 Constructing the Liberal Health Care Consumer Online

A Content Analysis of Canadian Medical Tourism and Harm Reduction Service Provider Websites

Cristina Temenos and Rory Johnston

This chapter analyzes the websites of two kinds of Canadian health service providers that target very different populations: people who use illicit drugs and seek harm reduction services; and people who go abroad for private medical care (i.e. medical tourists). Illicit drug users who access harm reduction services tend to be socially and economically marginalized, experience high levels of comorbidity, and often have needs that are difficult to meet in traditional health care settings (Marlatt, 2002; Hunt et al., 2010). In contrast, medical tourists have the social and economic capital to pursue medical care outside of the Canadian system, when the services offered domestically do not meet their desires or needs (Ramirez de Arellano, 2007; Connell, 2013). In their accessing contested services (i.e. forms of care that are stigmatized by some groups) at the margins of existing networks of care, these distinct groups share common ground in the contemporary landscape of Canadian health care. Because of the enormous differences in the typical socioeconomic position of these services' intended users, harm reduction care providers and medical tourism facilitators inherently capture a diverse range of Canadians whose care-seeking does not fit the existing norm. Therefore, examining the practices of these providers and facilitators provides a unique opportunity to compare and contrast the language and rhetoric used by emerging contested care services when marketing themselves to these "atypical" Canadian patient groups.

We present the findings of a content analysis of the websites of Canadian medical tourism facilitators and harm reduction service providers in order to meet the challenge of broadening, as stated in Chapter 1, "The focus of diversity [to be] not solely on differences or difference, but also on recognizing and identifying those commonalities shared among particular population groups, places, and contexts." Doing so provides a deeper understanding of the kinds of shared discursive tactics which simultaneously identify and legitimize the increasingly diverse health care needs of contemporary Canadians, and the responses of emerging Canadian care providers. We argue that the ideological framework that works to validate these contested services is drawn from broader liberal values which typically emphasize the importance of individual needs or desires, choice, and responsibility over collective social norms and economic priorities (Bondi, 2005). This same liberalized logic that works to make these new forms of care acceptable are those that also currently underpin much of the political-economic decision-making processes and public discussion in Canada.

The content analysis presented in this chapter draws on the self-care deficit nursing theory (Orem, 1980) – a theory of care used in both clinical nursing practice and social sciences research (Denyes et al., 2001; Chaboyer et al., 2013; Fullagar and O'Brien, 2014). In analysing care practices, this theory fixes patients as rational managers of their own regimes of care. This fundamentally liberal approach to theorizing care uptake and delivery is helpful in understanding how medical tourism facilitators and harm reduction service providers construct their very different users as having legitimate needs, using liberal concepts and language that emphasize individual choice, personal responsibility, and pragmatic rationality. In the next section we provide a brief introduction to medical tourism, harm reduction, and the self-care deficit nursing theory, in order to orient the reader further to the rationale and contribution of our analysis.

Medical Tourism

By definition, medical tourism involves the private purchase of health services. As such it is a significant departure from the core, publicly funded structure of the Canadian health system that has developed into a critical component of national identity (Forget, 2002; Snyder et al., 2011). The traditional (although never constitutionally formalized) rights-based conceptualization of health services has provided a strong ideological foundation for a health care system that is, in theory, publicly financed and accessible to all Canadians, regardless of income or location (Forget, 2002). In practice, there is varying access to publicly funded services across the country's provinces and territories, depending on what services are deemed necessary, and where physicians and facilities are located (Romanow, 2002). This variance serves as a driving factor behind Canadians traveling internationally for care, but more broadly as a key site for ongoing ideological struggle in Canadian society. This struggle contests traditional collectivist ideals that underpin the existing health system against a liberal political-economic outlook that frames health care as a commodity (e.g. Angell, 2008; Martin and Dhalla, 2010; Humphreys, 2013). Proponents of this latter conceptualization of care aim to liberalize Canadian health care by privatizing various components of the health system: primarily, the public financing monopoly that serves to control costs and universalize access to health care for citizens (Steinbrook, 2006; Esmail, 2014). This perspective argues that individual Canadians are unjustly denied the freedom to address their own health care needs by using their own resources to meet them. With few exceptions, Canadians seeking to access private medical care that is covered through public insurance must exit the Canadian health care system and travel to purchase their treatments privately outside of the country, engaging in the practice of medical tourism (Snyder et al., 2011).

The global medical tourism industry is reported repeatedly to be growing (Lautier, 2008). Medical tourists assume a great deal of responsibility over their trajectory of care, often identifying their care provider, assessing the quality of care, and financing treatment themselves. The degree of responsibility that medical tourists assume distinguishes them from those that engage in cross-border care, where the formal components of a domestic health system support patients accessing international care by providing referrals and reimbursement (Johnston et al., 2012). Due to varying definitions and poor surveillance, little is definitively known about who medical tourists are, both globally and within Canada (Crooks et al., 2010). However, qualitative work examining the experiences of Canadian medical tourists and facilitators demonstrate that these patients travel for many reasons, including the affordability of uninsured care, through access to care not approved or offered in Canada, to avoiding waitlists for care (Johnston et al., 2012). This research also indicates that there is no typical medical tourist with regard to gender, socioeconomic status, or medical condition, suggesting diversity among and within medical tourist patient groups. Rather, the strongest single influence on the likelihood to travel for care is familiarity with the destination country or with international travel more broadly, with many Canadian medical tourists reporting familial or personal ties abroad that set their trip in motion (Johnston et al., 2012). Thus, Canadian medical tourists are likely to be as diverse as the general population, with as many intersecting axes of difference as Canadian patients domestically.

Because of the many responsibilities that they assume, medical tourists represent prototypical liberal consumers of health services, portrayed by proponents as rational actors choosing the highest-quality care at the lowest price on the global market (Horowitz et al., 2007; Lunt et al., 2010). However, this portrayal of medical tourists as empowered consumers is at odds with studies which have found many of these patients at the margins of their home systems, and thereby driven abroad for care that they would prefer to access locally (Crooks et al., 2010; Kangas, 2011; Johnston et al., 2012). Additionally, as a break from established norms of care delivery, medical tourism is contested by physicians and scholars sometimes as unsafe, unethical, or both (Birch et al., 2010; Connell, 2013).

Canadian medical tourism facilitators (MTFs) are one of the two service provider groups that we examine in this chapter. MTFs are usually former medical tourists, travel agents, and/or people who have preexisting personal ties to countries with active medical tourism sectors. For a fee paid either directly by the patient, or embedded into the fees charged by the clinic abroad, they arrange for patients' medical care abroad, often within their own network of physicians and medical facilities, serving as agents who specialize in booking medical services for a fee (Dalstrom, 2013). They often advertise their services online, and also attract new clients through word-of-mouth. As such, they are one of the most visible fixtures relating to medical tourism available for analysis. We employ their websites in this chapter in order to explore how this contested practice is communicated as safe and legitimate by those involved in providing its services.

Harm Reduction

In a similar vein to the debate around the privatization of health care in Canada, currently there is an ongoing debate in the country regarding how to increase access to health services for people who use drugs, including addiction treatment services. The traditional view of psychoactive substance misuse (including illegal drugs, regulated pharmaceutical drugs, alcohol, and tobacco) has been structured around collectivist moral and legal conceptions of this behavior as a criminal matter that negatively impacts society (Marlatt, 2002). This long-dominant conception has been losing traction among policymakers and the public in recent years in the face of growing evidence in support of public health approaches to substance misuse, including harm reduction (Percival, 2009; Marlatt and Witkitewitz, 2010). Harm reduction is a pragmatic public health approach to people who use drugs that centers on risk reduction, individual risk management, and providing low threshold access to health services and behavioral interventions for people who wish to alter or stop drug misuse (Marlatt, 2002). There are many forms of harm reduction that exist along a continuum of care. Further, harm reduction is aimed at risk reduction strategies in other areas of health and social service provision, such as sex work, housing, and mental health treatment. For the purposes of this chapter we discuss harm reduction specifically for people who use drugs.

In the domain of drug use, the goals of harm reduction are to offer a judgment-free approach to providing health services for people who use drugs, reduce the risks of drug misuse to the user, and mitigate and alleviate the social and biomedical risks of drug misuse to society (Marlatt, 2002). Harm reduction services are committed to meeting a drug user "where they are at," rather than requiring abstinence from psychoactive substances before general health or addictions treatment services can be accessed. This individualistic, risk-management view has grown in popularity due to its effectiveness with reaching populations which face high barriers to accessing health services, a general acknowledgment from health service professionals that traditional abstinence-based addictions treatment has a low success rate, and in part to the heavy collective economic burden of a law-and-order approach to managing the negative impacts of substance use in society (Marlatt, 2002; Strathdee et al., 2010; Stöver, 2013).

Despite a large, global body of evidence that harm reduction health services have high rates of success in providing access to care for marginalized populations, and in reducing the negative health outcomes associated with drug use (e.g. spread of infectious diseases, deaths from overdose), provision and access to such services remain geographically uneven and highly contested in Canada and elsewhere (McCann, 2008; McCann and Temenos, 2015). Like the debates surrounding the role of medical tourism role in a collectivized health care system, the contested terrain of harm reduction lies in ethical arguments about the value of individuals (Rhodes, 2009; Strathdee et al., 2010). Opponents of harm reduction proffer arguments that frame the drug user as someone who chooses to break the law, and therefore is undeserving of limited publicly funded resources for health services. However, the mandates of public health policy lay in providing equitable access to health services and reducing population-level morbidity and mortality rates, which harm reduction health services have a record of achieving.

Generally, the people accessing harm reduction services are highly marginalized in mainstream Canadian society. As noted above, often they are characterized as "problematic" or "chaotic" drug users, meaning that their drug use affects other goals, ambitions, and ways of living. As such, typically they are precariously housed, and often do not work in the formal economy. Those accessing harm reduction services tend to be male, of ethnic minorities, and have an average age between 35 and 65. There are high levels of comorbidity and decreased life expectancy among this group. Through entrenchment in poverty and the ongoing marginalization of people who use drugs, this population experiences high barriers to accessing traditional health care systems and services, and is constructed as apart from Canadian society. Importantly, it has been noted that harm reduction service provision has the dual effect of empowering marginalized individuals seeking care, while also surveilling and disciplining them into responsible and rational citizens or consumers (Fischer et al., 2000, 2004).

Providing a content analysis of Canadian harm reduction service provider website, together with Canadian medical tourism services, enables us simultaneously to consider the strategies employed by two alternative care options that operate within and outside of Canada's public health care system, thereby adding depth to our understanding of the diversity of care options available to Canadians. Second, this analysis highlights the importance of a key point of access – service website – for two patient groups that represent two very different areas contested in the landscape of the Canadian health care system. Finally, it exhibits commonalities among the diverse user groups, enabling us to talk across the differences between harm reduction and medical tourism to consider how contested practices arise in the light of patients whose needs are unmet in the mainstream Canadian health care system.

Overview of Self-care Deficit Nursing Theory

Self-care deficit nursing theory articulates the provider–patient relationship as one of managing a "self-care deficit" in the patient. This model advances a view of patients as individuals who are temporarily unable to care for themselves, but who universally desire and seek to manage their own health needs. As summarized by Denyes et al.:

> Both the concept and the theory of self-care (Orem, 1995) express the view of human beings as attending to and dealing with themselves. This view is important and complex because the individual, the self, is both the agent of action (the one acting) and the object of action (the one acted upon). (2001, p.48)

In Orem's framework, providers exist in relation to patients as temporary carers and educators, working to support patients in their own journey to recovery and ultimately, self-management of their condition. Five basic components comprise the theoretical framework (Denyes et al., 2001), which we describe later. While this framework has been critiqued for a narrow and normative conception of patienthood that hinges on all people being (or desiring to be) rational, non-disabled actors (Browne, 2001; Wilkinson and Whitehead, 2009; Fullagar and O'Brien, 2014), we identified it as an excellent fit for structuring our analysis of how contested health services construct and mobilize liberal ideals in care delivery because of its overlap with liberal political-economic conceptions of the individual.

The self-care deficit nursing theory framework highlights commonality among diverse groups of care providers and diverse patient groups. Further, it highlights a scaled geographic focus of each patient group and provider: those accessing harm reduction service providers as hyperlocalized individuals, in contrast with medical tourism facilitators and medical tourists engaging in long-range travel to access treatments outside of Canada. In addition to its relevance to this analysis, it is an established clinical theory currently used by care providers in Canada and elsewhere (Wilkinson and Whitehead, 2009; Fredericks, 2012).

Rationale

At first glance, medical tourism and harm reduction do not share very much in common. However, on further inspection, both of these relatively novel health care practices emerge from the persistent political, cultural, and economic shift towards liberalism that Canadian society has undergone in the past few decades. Larner (2000, p. 13, as quoted in Bondi (2005, p. 500) states: "Neo-liberal strategies ... encourage people to see themselves as individualized and active subjects responsible for enhancing their own well being." Often, online health resources such as websites are now a first point of contact between service providers and the public, as well as a venue in which knowledge exchange is mobilized (Bennett and Glasgow, 2009; Lunt et al., 2010). While there has been much work examining how an individual is constructed subjectively under liberalized forms of governmentality (for examples, see Larner, 2000; Bondi, 2005), there has been less research on the mechanisms and technologies through which this happens. This chapter seeks to understand better the way in which service providers unique to these two very different health practices, and these two very different patient groups, each mobilize liberal concepts in online promotional materials in order to represent themselves as relevant and legitimate options to their potential users. In so doing, common practices and ideas that work to manage and discipline the evolving health-seeking behaviors and attitudes of diverse populations such those in as Canada present themselves for constructive critique and, potentially, modification.

Method

Data Collection

Prior to beginning data collection, we prospectively decided that online resources by Canadian MTFs and Canadian harm reduction service providers (HRSPs) would serve as the source materials for a content analysis. An exhaustive online search of active MTFs was conducted using the search terms "Canada," "medical tourism," "medical tourism facilitator," "medical tourism broker," "medical travel," "medical travel facilitator," and "medical travel broker." The websites identified were supplemented by an existing private database of active MTFs maintained by the SFU Medical Tourism Research Group. An exhaustive online search for Canadian HRSP websites was conducted over the same period, using the terms "Canada," "harm reduction," "SEP" (syringe exchange program), "needle exchange," "HIV/AIDS," and "drug treatment." These searches were performed in December 2012, with the websites downloaded to our hard drives so that the materials would remain a stable point of reference, regardless of future changes made to the websites.

In total, 23 websites were identified for inclusion: 11 MTFs and 12 HRSPs. As websites often consist of numerous pages with a broad range of categories, it was decided that only the content of the "home," "frequently asked questions," and "about us" pages would be reviewed, as they were found on the sites of both MTFs and HRSPs. Following this, we reviewed the websites of both HRSPs and MTFs, copying and pasting all relevant text into a shared spreadsheet. Relevance was predetermined, as all statements referring to the providers, their services, and service users as this would illustrate how each factor was articulated by the providers themselves.

Analysis

A content analysis of the websites' text was performed using a thematic framework derived using five of the self-care deficit nursing theory domains identified by Denyes et al. (2001):

1) self-care;
2) self-care agency;
3) self-care requisites;
4) therapeutic self-care demand; and
5) self-care practices and systems.

Table 9.1 The five domains of self-care deficit nursing theory

Self-care domain	Description
Self-care	The core drive to maintain or recover one's health and well-being
Self-care agency	The capacity to learn and enact self-care practices
Self-care requisites	The technologies and resources necessary to engage in and sustain self-care practices
Therapeutic self-care demand	A desire and ability to seek effective self-care measures, and the ability to distinguish harm from therapy
Self-care practices and systems	The professional or expert knowledge and networks that enable and support self-caring

The self-care deficit nursing theory framework is used to break down self-care routines, in order to identify points of intervention where caregivers can facilitate establishing and maintaining individual patients' self-care practices. Adapting these analytic domains to structure our content analysis is useful in breaking down and understanding how liberalized subjectivities within biomedical health care systems are composed across different services, meeting the needs of a diverse range of patients.

During the data collection process we copied text from each website into a shared spreadsheet organized into the five analytic domains of self-care deficit nursing theory described above. Thus, these categories served as qualitative coding categories. If statements touched on multiple self-care domains, copies of the statement were included within all relevant categories. A meeting was held following this first stage of data collection and analysis, wherein discrepancies in interpretation were identified, discussed, and resolved by reorganizing outlier statements.

Findings

Our analysis of the 23 service provider websites found that the statements describing the nature of the services, providers, and users in the online materials of MTFs and HRSPs fell into all five of the domains of the self-care deficit nursing theory framework. As expected, the content of MTF and HRSP websites diverged, given their diverse roles and audiences; but the language used by the two provider groups converged thematically around a number of shared concepts and values. What emerged from the analysis was a normative understanding of how patients should act for successful service uptake and outcomes. This section outlines the most common of these concepts present in each of the five self-care domains within the websites analysed.

Self-care: A Drive to Achieve Health

Statements articulating the core concept of self-care were found on many of the HRSP websites, framing harm reduction measures as simple, pragmatic approaches to meeting an existing need for safer drug use practices. For example, one websites noted:

> It was pretty clear that the people coming to the program were asking for lots of different kinds of services and had lots of health needs. The program keeps on growing and working with the community to meet these needs. (Streetworks, n.d.)

Many of these websites actively work to distance themselves from the normative and moral frameworks with which their patients might conflict, instead articulating their users as having unmet needs that HRSPs seek to address. A website noted: "We offer services in a non judgmental way that recognizes that people will use drugs, and we try to minimize the harm associated with their drug use" (City of Toronto, 2012). These kinds of messages demonstrate how the underlying demand for HRSPs is presented as existing inevitably, consequently rendering the necessity of the services as self-evident.

Self-care messaging was usually located in definitions of medical tourism or company mission statements on the websites of MTFs. Here, medical tourism was presented as a natural response to financial or temporal barriers to care. The desire to achieve and remain in good health through medical interventions was presented as basic and universal. Some websites appealed to historical examples of medical travel that reinforce this framing. For example:

> Health Tourism has been in existence for centuries. Even in ancient times, people would travel to far off lands looking for better and more effective cures that were not available in their own country. Today the catalysts for traveling to seek medical procedures in other countries include lengthy wait times and escalating healthcare costs. (Choice Medical Services, 2007)

Two websites specifically sought to counsel their Canadian audience on the acceptability and ease of privately purchasing care abroad despite their inability to do so domestically, in effect naturalizing the desire for self-care. One such example states:

> These patients are extremely unlikely to forgo the wait times that everyone they know is dutifully embracing if they are not comfortable with the process ... I pay enormous attention to getting my clients to feel comfortable with and embrace an undertaking that asks them to step into the unknown. (International Health Care Providers, 2001)

This mirrors the same basic frame employed by HRSPs, presenting the under-lying demand as long-standing and natural, justifying the need for the service being offered.

Self-care Agency: The Capacity to Care for Oneself

Statements on the HRSPs' websites relating to self-care agency were struc-tured around the notion of empowering drug users both as individuals and as a group. Often, the goal of empowering drug users to improve their own health was stated explicitly, with the means to personal empowerment most commonly being tied closely to education, particularly regarding risk awareness. For example: "We are committed to supporting drug users to focus on their health and well-being through: raising awareness, education and empowerment," (Mainline, n.d.), and "To encourage self-esteem in sub-stance users and other clients and an awareness of health issues" (Ottawa Site Needle & Syringe Program, 2012). Alternatively, the means to empowerment was articulated more broadly in issues of advocacy, esteem-building, and strong, respectful relationships with health care providers. Thus, agency was constructed by HRSPs primarily as a matter of capacity-building in order to support empowered (i.e. informed, self-directed) choices.

As the intermediary role of MTFs complicates the notion of self-care agency in terms of purely self-managed care, many websites sought to con-struct their role as assistants for their already competent clients, educating and directing them to the best care in a stress-free manner. This is captured in one facilitator's statement:

> While many of our clients are capable of coordinating their own health care in the fee-for-service sector, due to our expertise in facilitating and managing our clients' health care, and our extensive research of facilities across the country, we are able to reduce the amount of time and steps involved in order to move from diagnosis to medical treatment. (Timely Medical Alternatives, n.d, a)

Self-care agency among the websites of MTFs was articulated most often in an expansion of options for frustrated health care consumers. Individual empowerment was not explicitly mentioned, but the implicit concept was prevalent across the majority of the websites reviewed. For example, state-ments such as "Since 2003, Timely Medical Alternatives has helped thousands of Canadians leave the increasingly long public waiting lists, and take matters into their own hands" (Timely Medical Alternatives, n.d. b), and "Fast and efficient medical solutions – Take your own health in hand" (Service Sante, 2012), employ the concept of empowering disenfranchised patients. These sites thereby portray medical tourism as a means for individuals to reclaim their individual agency by allowing them to choose their preferred course of medical care.

Self-care Requisites: Resources Required for Self-care

The self-care requisites articulated in HRSP websites focused on specific outreach, services, and education approaches. For example: "We use a multi-faceted approach to service delivery that includes: fixed site, street outreach [and] mobile component" (City of Toronto, 2012). While medical supplies and procedures were highlighted as important resources and technologies, knowledge translation was a key focus of capacity-building found on many HRSP websites. One such example states: "Here is some information about drugs that can be helpful to take care of yourself and your friends or family" (Streetworks, n.d.). In some cases, the value of integrated resource utilization and knowledge translation capacity was explicitly attested to: "support and education is very important for people engaging in and affected by risky behaviours" (Mainline, n.d.). This last example also points to an underlying emphasis on responsibility within HRSP websites. The technological and resource focus for HRSP websites in this sense provide information to be taken up by the person accessing the information. Further, the sites' focus on "multi-faceted approaches" also highlights an acknowledgment on the part of service providers that they are dealing with individual and diverse patients, and that they are not trying to offer a "one-size-fits-all" model of care.

In contrast, self-care requisites within MTF websites focused primarily on the financial resources to achieve travel for medical purposes and the cost of care. Affordability of services was commonly highlighted, with statements such as: "Are you aware that private healthcare in Canada & the U.S. is not as expensive as you may think?" (Timely Medical Alternatives, n.d. b), and "Our packages cost significantly less than all other similar offshore packages" (Surgical Tourism Canada, 2012a). While the cost of care was the dominant message in this domain for MTF websites, biomedical and technological advancement also was highlighted. For example: "The medical tourism industry has matured substantially ... through improvements in technology, internationally trained specialists, concierge services and the introduction of internationally recognized accreditation processes" (Angels Global Healthcare, 2010). The messages in this domain thereby present medical tourists as being alienated from the Canadian health care system, yet still desiring Canadian standards of care – a frustrated desire that medical tourism can address (affordably).

Therapeutic Self-care Demand: Seeking Effective Treatment

For HRSPs, issues relating to therapeutic self-care demand were found in an emphasis on the quality of outcomes, and appeals to evidence-based health practices. Statements about risk reduction were common within HRSP websites: "to reduce the risks associated with those practices while improving their quality of life" (Cactus Montréal, 2005); or: "The Ministry of Health acknowledged the urgent need to implement harm reduction strategies to control the epidemic [of HIV and Hepatitis C]" (Ottawa Site Needle & Syringe Program, 2012 SEP). Pragmatic solutions also were present under this domain: "We provide practical support ... to help improve the quality of [users'] lives" (AIDS Calgary, 2009). Harm reduction health services are provided in most circumstances as a public health intervention, and often focus on reaching custom solutions for individuals who both face barriers accessing health services, and have an elevated risk of contracting blood-borne disease. Pragmatism about therapeutic health service provision, supported by evidence in order to effectively manage risk, was prevalent across this domain.

Hospital accreditation, quality of care, and experience stood out as dominant themes under the domain of therapeutic self-care demand on the websites of MTFs. The international accreditation of hospitals affiliated with MTFs was found regularly to be prominently displayed or discussed on one page of a websites. This accreditation chiefly serves to legitimate care providers beyond the Canadian health care system, and usually was explained as in the following example:

> Clients can now be assured of the quality of care they receive because there is an international standard of care accreditation, or Joint Commission International (JCI). This is an international benchmark of care for hospitals abroad that also regulate US hospitals. There are over 500 JCI accredited hospitals in the world. (Gateway Health International, 2012)

Often, the concepts of quality of care and risk management were emphasized through personal experience and company philosophy. One facilitator's vision, for example, is: "To be a trusted avenue into the global healthcare market by creating a safe and successful experience for the Medical Tourist through the reduction of unnecessary risks" (Angels Global Healthcare, 2012) – highlighting the role of the facilitator in creating a "successful" personal experience for the individual patient. In its mission statement, another facilitator similarly highlights the role of quality: "To provide access to clients looking for medical care at world class healthcare facilities that offer safe, state of the art technologies and procedures and personalized one on one medical consultations and follow up care" (Gateway Health International, 2012) – simultaneously acknowledging and marketing many different elements that compose high-quality care. Together, the themes of risk management and expertise were most prevalent in the messages of therapeutic demand.

Self-care Practices and Systems: Enabling Knowledge and Networks

Ongoing social and community support was the predominant issue that emerged under the domain of self-care practices and systems among the HRSP websites. Readily available and continued treatment for medical issues such as addiction, HIV/AIDS, Hepatitis C, and mental health needs, as well as medical support systems, were highlighted. One service provider succinctly sums up these three features in the following statement, where it "offers counseling and support in addition to methadone provision" (City of Toronto, 2012 SEP). Another service provider states that "we contribute to meaningful and trusting relationships" (Mainline, n.d.). The social services such as counseling offered by HRSPs deepen and extend the scope of care provided beyond material resource provision, which was detailed above. Comprehensive social, well-being, and care systems were also present in the HRSP websites, "from primary care to treat disease and infection, to addiction counseling and treatment, to housing and community supports" (Vancouver Coastal Health, n.d. a). While sometimes professional networks were invoked to indicate the quality and range of systems available, for example in saying: "Clients are supported by a team of nurses, counsellors and support staff" (Vancouver Coastal Health, n.d. b), it was just as common for peer and volunteer networks to be emphasized as sources of expertise. Thus, a very wide range of practices and providers were invoked by HRSPs in situating themselves for potential users.

The websites of MTFs predominantly focused on their facilitation of practices that support continuity of care and their stable relationships with existing care networks, working to establish themselves as one professional among a network of professionals. For example:

> We do not cut corners, we do not advertise cheap packages, we offer a complete, comprehensive TOP QUALITY service from start to finish ONLY AT OUR JCI ACCREDITED PARTNER FACILITIES. We are healthcare professionals! On returning to Canada after treatment we arrange regular follow ups with local physicians. [sic] (Surgical Tourism Canada, 2012b)

Similarly, numerous providers prominently employed testimonials from former clients, drawing on their personal experiences to communicate the care offered as safe and familiar. In contrast with HRSPs, a much less diverse range of providers and indicators of quality were referred to by MTFs, limited to accounting for recognizable accreditation, medical training, and the personal experiences of facilitators and former clients, in order to communicate messages of expertise and professionalism.

Discussion

Unlike other chapters, this analysis does not seek to examine axes of diversity within the users of HRSPs and MTFs. Instead, it allows for a more nuanced understanding of how diverse populations, and the multiplicity of their care needs and/or desires, are affirmed as they arise within a health care landscape – itself situated within, and informed by, wider political-economic trends and values. As such, our discussion aims to generate a better understanding of the common ideological intersection that informs the provision of care targeting Canadian drug users and medical tourists, and likely extending to other forms of (contested) care provision in Canada. We do so by exploring the shared discursive tactics across the websites of two different contested Canadian health care services. We discuss the findings presented above in the context of three cross-cutting themes that emerged from our content analysis: expertise, agency-as-choice, and risk management.

Expertise

Claims of expertise are important for legitimizing health care services and rendering ethically contested practices neutral, thereby freeing potential users from concerns which otherwise might discourage them from accessing care. Both Canadian HRSPs and MTFs utilize expertise as a way of sanctioning entry into the particular service, thereby reducing one barrier to access. In the case of MTFs, expertise claims are grounded in hospital accreditation regimes, the training of affiliated physicians, and the personal experience and professionalism of facilitators. This focus on expertise serves to legitimize the patients, the facilitator, and health services outside of Canada. Similarly, HRSP websites mobilize expertise through appeals to scientific evidence and to the experience of professionals and those in the community. Appealing to evidence-based success is unsurprising, because the philosophy of harm reduction is based on biomedical and positivist scientific paradigms. Yet because it is still in an ongoing process of integration into the Canadian health care system, education around harm reduction remains focused on outlining and validating its basic principles to both people to whom the services are targeted, and the general population (McCann, 2008, McCann and Temenos 2015). Thus, scientific, value-free neutrality is employed by both MTFs and HRSPs via expertise to facilitate the use of their services.

In order to legitimize their services, MTFs frame medical tourism as a practical, ethically neutral, and rational mode of care delivery that is focused on individual patients' needs. At the same time, these claims build trust in MTFs' expertise in the practice of medical tourism, and its associated procedures and services. Coupling this approach with a focus on accreditation practices allays moral and technical concerns around users' mobility between systems, thereby sanctioning traveling for care. This expertise-as-legitimacy is, in part, further "borrowed" from the constellation of established service providers identified by both HRSPs and MTFs as being part of their therapeutic networks.

Finally, HRSP websites presented expertise as direct experience. Leveraging the personal experiences of the service providers, and the involvement of "peers" (active or former illicit drug users) in the programs as either employees or volunteers, legitimacy was further established through a focus on experiential expertise in the field. Highlighting peer involvement in HRSPs contributes to understanding harm reduction as a low-threshold service, and implicitly invites the potential client into a community of equals while explicitly showcasing both the efficacy of the service and the value that former clients have placed in it. MTFs' utilization of client testimonials operate in much the same way. While a minority of MTF websites highlighted the personal experiences of facilitators in vetting foreign facilities and care providers, appeals to direct experience with care abroad were less common among this group. Instead, expertise was constructed more often as a part of a reliable and pleasant consumer experience via the personal professionalism of the facilitators, and the number of times that they had arranged for care abroad. The common utilization of experience-as-expertise across the two groups is important for understanding how this component of legitimacy is mobilized. It demonstrates that personal experience – even differently constructed as relatable knowledge or commodifiable service – is highlighted regularly as a signifier of quality in a liberalized health services market. If novel care demands continue to emerge and diversify, the ways in which "expertise" is constructed successfully may be critical in anticipating which services become firmly established and ultimately accepted.

Agency-as-Choice in Accessing Health Services

Agency-as-personal choice was a prevalent frame throughout the websites of both MTFs and HRSPs. This is in contrast with conceptions of personal agency-as-capacity, or as deriving from structural factors that facilitate or inhibit personal options and ability. In the case of MTF websites, personal choice was constructed around choice and control over decisions of whether and when to access private health services – many of which, inevitably, are found outside of the Canadian health care system. It is important to note that MTF websites are offering commercial services related to accessing a wider variety of health care services, not health care itself. Therefore, the position of MTFs within the system of care frames them as enablers within a decision-making process, rather than an agent of change in and of themselves.

In addition, choice was valorized in harm reduction websites, but emerged from empowering their users through education. By engaging in active language, providers indicate to website users that personal control and choices in regard to drug use are valid and possible, while at the same time directing readers how to achieve them – actively, through "awareness." These examples demonstrate *how* personal choice and empowerment align with the self-care deficit nursing theory's assessment of self-care agency, exhibiting the hallmarks of empowerment, knowledge acquisition, and self-sufficiency. They also resonate with Bondi's examination of decision-making as a form of empowerment: constructing the client as an agent of change and in control of their health outcomes, and functioning as "a technology of subjectivity that recruits people into active self-management and fosters neoliberal forms of (individual) freedom" (2005, p. 504).

The common view of users of both MTFs and HRSPs as active agents engaged in rational decision-making functions in a complementary role to that of "expertise" as outlined above. By constructing their users as rational agents best suited to assess and select their own care routines, the particular visions of agency-as-choice advanced by MTFs and HRSPs work to legitimize further their users' desires for particular modes of care and care delivery. This co-construction of legitimacy through informed agency among users, and expertise among providers, suggests one key tactic that contested health services, however diverse, use to carve out their own space in a liberalizing health service environment. Similarly, the historical or "inevitable" frame adopted by both HRSPs and MTFs in outlining the rationale for their services indicates the common values from which these two different services emerge. The outlook that drug use and traveling for medical care have always, and will always, occur justifies the providers that address this naturally existing demand. A liberal outlook justifies such supply-side responses to these natural existing demands, especially those which then align themselves with values of risk management and professionalism in meeting them. Within this framework then, valid choices are preceded by natural demands, which require appropriately tailored responses that the providers step in to fill. Given the potential for an ever-increasing range of services emerging to meet the needs of a diverse population in a liberal society, those which are able to mobilize narratives of the "natural" or "inevitable" may have a greater likelihood of uptake or long-term acceptance.

Risk Management

The theme of risk and risk management was found across the websites of both MTFs and HRSPs, but was mobilized in very different ways across these two groups. For HRSPs, risk is understood as implicit in drug use, and serves as a key justification for the care provider to exist. By utilizing harm reduction services, ultimately people can reduce their risk of poor health in the immediate and far future. Risk management is framed as an end goal and basic rationale for harm reduction, highlighted within statements found in the categories of self-care and self-care agency that indicate desires and actions associated with health practices. In contrast, MTFs invoked the language of risk and risk management in order to emphasize the safety of medical treatments abroad, and the systems in place to ameliorate potential harm. The language of risk, harm, and success all fell within the five domains of the self-care deficit nursing theory framework, closely tied to service quality, comprehensiveness, and the associated issue of hospital and facilitator accreditation. Acknowledging risk in this way served only to emphasize safety, working to position risk management as a means to recruiting potential patients rather than an end of the service itself.

The differences outlined above demonstrate how the concept of risk can play a shifting discursive role in constructing liberalized health service consumers, serving as a modifiable variable under an individual's control, or as a signal of quality within the health care market that a rational actor can interpret competently. The variable but central role that the concept of risk plays across such different providers is consistent with arguments by scholars who have situated the concept of risk and risk management as central to neoliberal rationality, rhetoric, and management techniques (e.g. O'Malley, 2000; Gray, 2009). The coding scheme derived from the self-care deficit nursing theoretical framework assisted in identifying the presence of messages about risk, while also highlighting the different ways that it is used by each service provider.

While never referred to as risk management among the MTF websites, this theme emerged through the above-mentioned focus on service quality, comprehensiveness, and accreditation of health care facilities. The predominate focus of MTF websites on the high quality of services abroad, and managing the risks of medical travel, makes it clear that these are significant in informing decisions to engage in medical tourism – no doubt dictated by a lack of familiarity with the quality of health services outside of the Canadian health care system. This foregrounded acknowledgment of the importance of good care vis-à-vis managed risk is an additional means through which MTFs work to legitimize their services, as in so doing they present themselves as responsible health care players. HRSP websites were focused more directly on risk management and risk reduction through encouraging the individual to utilize the services offered, a focus on need-specific service acquisition, and choice about when and where to access services. MTF websites articulate the notion of risk as ever-present but effectively managed through quality measures, rather than engaging with risk management as a means of patient agency. Thus, both services situate themselves within an existing landscape of risk which, in turn, they work to modify. This acknowledgment of ever-present risk justifies the necessity for the providers, while their efforts to reduce it for their clients legitimize their roles.

Conclusion

Cultivating and Disciplining Diversity

To engage in self-care, there is an assumption that the individual is, or should be, empowered to make decisions about if and how to care for oneself. Further, there is a more foundational belief that the individual will desire to make rational decisions focused on risk management and improving their health outcomes. This analysis shows some of the ways that contested service providers in a liberal political-economic climate such as Canada's position themselves as facilitating latent desires and the exercise of personal choice.

This content analysis' inclusion of a diverse overall user population via the use of two very different patient groups (see Chapter 2) allows us to explore some of the similarities and differences in the use of language and ideological concepts between the providers of care to both groups. The target audiences of both HRSPs and MTFs are people whose needs or desires have not been met by the Canadian health care system. By positioning themselves as providing personal choice in care, service providers are providing a *radical sense of choice* for the Canadian health care user by adopting a consumer language and outlook from the wider economic and social spheres. This radicalism positions them on the periphery of established networks of care and governance in the Canadian health care system, requiring both providers to work actively at constructing a legitimate place for themselves and their users or clients in a constellation of existing care providers. The messages that emerged through our content analysis were surprising in their similarities between HRSP and MTF websites, considering that the patient groups (while diverse within themselves) neither overlapped in their care needs, nor in their characteristics.

Evaluating the websites of Canadian MTFs and Canadian HRSPs using a self-care framework facilitates an understanding of whether and how health services interpret and construct their users as liberal subjects driven by choice and self-interest. In a self-reinforcing fashion, this liberal political-economic frame encourages the identification of diversity by valorizing individual desires and choices, then provides the broad validation criteria for the means to meet them. The very different kinds of service provision examined in this analysis allow us to identify and understand some of the common discursive tactics and themes informing how contested health service providers interpret themselves and their users. With differing degrees of success, both medical tourism and harm reduction are in the process of integrating themselves into the existing Canadian health care landscape. How they are understood, accessed, and affect people's notions of legitimacy are important considerations, as the Canadian health care landscape continues to evolve in response to the shifting health needs of its diverse population.

References

Angell, M., 2008. Privatizing health care is not the answer: Lessons from the United States. *Canadian Medical Association Journal*, 179(9), pp. 916–19.

Bennett, G.G. and Glasgow, E.G. 2009. The delivery of public health interventions via the internet: Actualizing their potential. *Annual Review of Public Health*, 30(1), pp. 273–92.

Birch, D.W., Lan, V., Karmali, S., Stoklossa, C.J. and Sharma, A.M., 2010. Medical tourism in bariatric surgery. *American Journal of Surgery*, 199(5), pp. 604–8.

Bondi, L., 2005. Making connections and thinking through emotions: Between geography and psychotherapy. *Transactions of the Institute of British Geographers*, 30(4), pp. 433–48.

Browne, A.J., 2001. The Influence of liberal political ideology on nursing science. *Nursing Inquiry*, 8(2), pp. 118–29.

Chaboyer, W., Ringdal, M., Aitken, L. and Kendall, E., 2013. Self-care after traumatic injury and the use of the therapeutic self-care scale in trauma populations. *Journal of Advanced Nursing*, 69(2), pp. 286–94.

Connell, J., 2013. Contemporary medical tourism: Conceptualisation, culture and commodification. *Tourism Management*, 34, pp. 1–13.

Crooks, V.A., Kingsbury, P., Snyder, J. and Johnston, R., 2010. What is known about the patient's experience of medical tourism? A scoping review. *BMC Health Services Research*, 10(266). Available online at http://bmchealthservres.biomedcentral.com/articles/10.1186/1472-6963-10-266 (accessed February 12, 2016.

Dalstrom, M., 2013. Medical travel facilitators: Connecting patients and providers in a globalized world. *Anthropology & Medicine*, 20(1), pp. 24–35.

Denyes, M.J., Orem, D.E. and Bekel, G., 2001. Self-care: A foundational science. *Nursing Science Quarterly*, 14(1), pp. 48–54.

Esmail, N., 2014. *The private cost of public queues for medically necessary care: 2014 edition*. Vancouver: Fraser Institute. Available online at https://web.archive.org/web/20130810015508/http://www.fraserinstitute.org/uploadedFiles/fraser-ca/Content/research-news/research/publications/private-cost-of-public-queues-for-medically-necessary-care-2013.pdf (accessed January 29, 2016).

Fischer, B., Rehm, J. and Blitz-Miller, T., 2000. Injection drug use and preventive measures: A comparison of Canadian and Western European jurisdictions over time. *Canadian Medical Association Journal*, 162(12), pp. 1709–13.

Fischer, B., Turnbull, S., Poland, B. and Haydon, E., 2004. Drug use, risk and urban order: Examining supervised injection sites (SISs) as "governmentality." *International Journal of Drug Policy*, 15(5–6), pp. 357–65.

Forget, E.L., 2002. National identity and the challenge of health reform in Canada. *Review of Social Economy*, 60(3), pp. 359–75.

Fredericks, S., 2012. The influence of country of origin on engagement in self-care behaviours following heart surgery: A descriptive correlational study. *Journal of Clinical Nursing*, 21(15–16), pp. 2202–8.

Fullagar, S. and O'Brien, W., 2014. Social recovery and the move beyond deficit models of depression: A feminist analysis of mid-life women's self-care practices. *Social Science & Medicine*, 117, pp. 116–24.

Gray, G.C., 2009. The responsibilization strategy of health and safety: Neo-liberalism and the reconfiguration of individual responsibility for risk. *British Journal of Criminology*, 49(3), pp. 326–42.

Horowitz, M.D., Rosensweig, J.A. and Jones, C.A., 2007. Medical tourism: Globalization of the healthcare marketplace. *Medscape General Medicine*, 9(4), pp. 33. Available online at www.ncbi.nlm.nih.gov/pmc/articles/PMC2234298/ (accessed February 12, 2016).

Humphreys, A., 2013. Canada must offer private options along with universal health-care to combat long wait times: Report. *National Post*, October 28. Available online at http://news.nationalpost.com/2013/10/28/canada-must-offer-private-options-along-with-universal-health-care-to-combat-long-wait-times-report/#__federated=1 (accessed November 18, 2014).

Hunt, N., Albers E. and Montanes-Sanchez, V., 2010. User involvement and user organizing in harm reduction. In: T. Rhodes and D. Hendrich, eds. *Harm reduction: Evidence, impacts, and challenges*. Luxembourg: Office of the European Union, pp. 369–92.

Johnston, R., Crooks, V.A. and Snyder, J., 2012. "I didn't even know what I was looking for": A qualitative study of the decision-making processes of Canadian medical tourists. *Globalization and Health*, 8(23). Available online at www.ncbi.nlm.nih.gov/pubmed/22769723 (accessed February 12, 2016).

Kangas, B., 2011. Complicating common ideas about medical tourism: Gender, class, and globality in Yemenis' international medical travel. *Signs*, 36(2), pp. 327–32.

Larner, W., 2000. Neo-liberalism: Policy, ideology, governmentality. *Studies in Political Economy*, 63, pp. 5–25.

Lautier, M., 2008. Export of health services from developing countries: The case of Tunisia. *Social Science & Medicine*, 67(1), pp. 101–10.

Lunt, N., Hardey, M. and Mannion, R., 2010. Nip, tuck and click: Medical tourism and the emergence of web-based health information. *Open Medical Informatics Journal*, 4 pp. 1–11.

McCann, E.J., 2008. Expertise, truth, and urban policy mobilities: Global circuits of knowledge in the development of Vancouver, Canada's "four pillar" drug strategy. *Environment and planning A*, 40(4), pp. 885–904.

McCann, E. and Temenos, C., 2015. Mobilizing drug consumption rooms: Inter-place networks and harm reduction drug policy. *Health and Place*, 31, pp. 216–23.

Marlatt, A., 2002. *Harm reduction: Pragmatic strategies for managing high-risk behaviors*. New York: Guilford Press.

Marlatt, G.A. and Witkiewitz, K., 2010. Update on harm-reduction policy and intervention research. *Annual Review of Clinical Psychology*, 6, pp. 591–606.

Martin, D. and Dhalla, I., 2010. Privatizing health care is risky for all of us. *The Globe and Mail*, November 11. Available online at www.theglobeandmail.com/news/national/time-to-lead/privatizing-health-care-is-risky-for-all-of-us/article1395420/ (accessed November 18, 2014).

O'Malley, P., 2000. Uncertain subjects: Risks, liberalism and contract. *Economy and Society*, 29(4), pp. 460–84.

Orem, D., 1980. *Nursing: Concepts of practice*, 3rd ed. New York: McGraw Hill.

Percival, G.L., 2009. Exploring the influence of local policy networks on the implementation of drug policy reform: The case of California's substance abuse and crime prevention act. *Journal of Public Administration Research and Theory*, 19(4), pp. 795–815.

Ramirez de Arellano, A., 2007. Patients without borders: The emergence of medical tourism. *International Journal of Health Services*, 37(1), pp. 193–8.

Rhodes, T., 2009. Risk environments and drug harms: A social science for harm reduction approach. *International Journal of Drug Policy*, 20(3), pp. 193–201.

Romanow, R.J., 2002. *Building on values: The future of health care in Canada*. Ottawa: Commission on the Future of Healthcare in Canada. Available online at http://publications.gc.ca/collections/Collection/CP32-85-2002E.pdf (accessed November 18, 2014).

Snyder, J., Crooks, A., Johnston, R. and Kingsbury, P., 2011. What do we know about Canadian Involvement in medical tourism? A scoping review. *Open Medicine*, 5(3), pp. e139–48. Available online at www.ncbi.nlm.nih.gov/pmc/articles/PMC3205829/ (accessed February 12, 2016).

Steinbrook, R., 2006. Private health care in Canada. *New England Journal of Medicine*, 354(16), pp. 1661–4.

Stöver, H., 2013. Multi-agency approach to drug policy on a local level: "The Frankfurt Way." Briefing paper for 2013 International Conference on Drug Policy and Policing, Open Society Foundation, Frankfurt, November 14. Available online at www.opensocietyfoundations.org/sites/default/files/The_Frankfurt_Way.pdf (accessed November 18, 2014).

Strathdee, S.A., Hallett, T.B., Bobrova, N., Rhodes, T., Booth, R., Abdool, R. and Hankins, C.A., 2010. HIV and risk environment for injecting drug users: The past, present, and future. *The Lancet*, 376(9737), pp. 268–84.

Wilkinson, A. and Whitehead, L., 2009. Evolution of the concept of self-care and implications for nurses: A literature review. *International Journal of Nursing Studies*, 46(8), pp. 1143–7.

10 Lived Experience in Context

The Diverse Interplay between Women Living with Fibromyalgia and Canada's Health Care System

Valorie A. Crooks

According to Gesler and Kearns (2002), health geographers are interested in connecting the macro (e.g. social systems) and micro (e.g. individual lived experiences) through considerations of "structure and agency, society and individual, hegemony and self-expression, cultural norm and personal biographies, [and/or] social systems and everyday practice" (p.64). They argue that geographic investigations of such seeming opposites are important and useful, as such interactions – those between the micro and macro – happen in and over space and time. In the context of this chapter, it can be understood that there are constraints inherent in the organization and delivery of health care services in Canada that shape chronically-ill women's negotiations of this institution, and that such women are able to engage in decision-making, thereby exercising agency, that also directs such negotiations, all of which happen over and in space and time. For example, such negotiations can take place in the health care clinic, where the institution and the individual simultaneously are brought in place. The decision-making that informs chronically-ill women's negotiations of such institutions can be informed by activities and interactions undertaken in a variety of places, ultimately generating diverse experiences of this single institution.

In this chapter, I examine chronically-ill women's negotiations of health care. I specifically examine those experiences reported by a group of 55 women managing fibromyalgia syndrome (FMS), living in three communities in the Canadian province of Ontario. FMS most commonly occurs in women, and is characterized by lasting fatigue and bodily pain in multiple points. FMS has no known cause or cure, and it is also difficult to diagnose, as there is no measurable approach to determining its presence or ruling out its absence. As a result, FMS is one of a handful of diagnoses known as "contested chronic illnesses," in that there are some who believe it is psychosomatic in nature. An outcome is that there is a minority of doctors who are reluctant to diagnose and/or treat it, leaving patients on their own to figure out how to best manage the chronic pain and fatigue. In this chapter I qualitatively explore how women managing this contested chronic illness navigate some of the structural issues and challenges inherent in health care, and conversely, the decisions and actions that they take which shape how they experience this same institution. In so doing I draw out how diversity in access to care (e.g. affordability, physical distance, physician availability, perceptions of care quality), social location (e.g. income, access to transportation, geographic location, access to health information), and bodily experience (e.g. symptom management, coping with pain and fatigue, desire to seek medical intervention) shape these women's journeys as patients. (These axes of diversity are among the social determinants of health introduced in Chapter 2.) In the two sections that follow, I provide some background context prior to introducing the study and sharing the findings of the interviews conducted.

Structural and Organizational Challenges in Canadian Health Care

It is no secret that Western-style systems of health care, which are organized around allopathic medical traditions, are better suited to address the needs of people affected by acute or even fatal illness than those living with chronic conditions such as FMS (Armstrong and Armstrong, 1996; Rothman and Wagner, 2003; Epping-Jordan et al., 2004). Despite the fact that the numbers of people (and particularly women) reporting living with chronic illnesses are increasing due to myriad factors such as population aging, advances in modern medicine, and clearer diagnostic processes, these Western-style health care systems – Canada's included – have difficulties meeting the needs of this large patient group. The complexity involved in managing chronic illnesses, along with the frequent involvement of more than one service provider, has created a situation where "even knowledgeable [primary] practice teams have difficulty consistently providing optimal care to all of their patients" (Rothman and Wagner, 2003, p. 258). Further, the focus on curative practice and intervention often leads to patients' psychosocial needs being unmet (Armstrong and Armstrong, 1996).

The allopathic underpinnings of Canada's public health care system have resulted in the costs of non-Western treatments such as homeopathy and acupuncture, and allied health care such as chiropractic treatment and massage therapy – regardless of their anticipated or proven benefits – not being covered. Meanwhile, people living with chronic illnesses such as FMS are becoming increasingly interested in using non-Western and allied health approaches to symptom management (Caspi et al., 2004). Furthermore, the focus on allopathic medicine during practitioners' training has left some Canadian family doctors and specialists unwilling to treat patients who are pursuing such treatments, or even unwilling to discuss such options during appointments (see for example, Crooks and Chouinard, 2006).

There are organizational aspects to the delivery of health services in Canada that exacerbate the difficulties found in meeting some patients' needs, including those living with chronic illness in certain areas. Canada is a geographically large country, and physical access to health care services varies greatly between places. For example, people living outside of major cities and metropolitan centers frequently lack close physical access to most specialist services, allied health, and non-Western practitioners, even to family doctors (Schuurman et al., 2010; Crooks and Schuurman 2012). One outcome of this particular situation is that family doctors practicing in communities where there are no specialists on-site often take on the role of managing chronic illnesses themselves (Canadian Institute for Health Information, 2003), even though they may lack this training (Rothman and Wagner, 2003). Another outcome of this situation for patients is that the expense of traveling to and from non-local practitioners, with few exceptions, is paid out-of-pocket. Thus, while the costs of specialist appointments are covered by Canada's public Medicare system, material resources play a role in people's abilities to access them.

Family doctors are the cornerstone of Canada's health care system: not only do they provide essential primary care and preventative care, and ongoing symptom monitoring for people managing chronic illnesses such as FMS, but they also serve as gatekeepers to secondary and tertiary care (Donald Watt, 1987). Meanwhile, family doctor shortages are reported frequently in Canada in communities of all sizes (Talbot et al., 2001). For example, in 2001, 12 percent of Canadians reported not having a family doctor (Canadian Institute for Health Information, 2003). In urban centers, often people in such a situation are left to manage their health – and sometimes complex chronic illnesses like FMS – in walk-in clinics (Crooks et al., 2012). Other communities are becoming increasingly reliant on locum practice where there is no steady, on-site family doctor. The causes of people managing their health or a chronic illness outside the practice of a family doctor are wide-ranging, and can include choosing to leave a family doctor for one reason or another, only to find that other medical practices are not any taking on new patients, or having a family doctor retire and not automatically being included in a new practice (Crooks et al., 2012).

One significant outcome of not having a family doctor – and the increasing amounts of physician turnover – is that many people lack interpersonal and informational continuity of care in their journeys through Canada's health care system (Saultz and Albedaiwi, 2004; Stewart, 2004; Crooks et al., 2012). Continuity is one of the pillars of care, particularly primary health care, in Western health systems such as Canada's (Crooks et al., 2012). When it is lacking, one's ability to access appropriate care is compromised (Rothman and Wagner, 2003), particularly negatively affecting those managing chronic illness that require ongoing symptom monitoring. Moreover, because often there is no one set way to manage chronic illnesses such as FMS, being switched between family doctors may result in management programs being changed due to the transition and the new doctor's beliefs as to how best to treat symptoms, ultimately resulting in a lack of continuity of care.

Patient Agency in Navigating the Health Care System

While it can be seen from the above discussion that the structure and organization of the system of health care services in Canada certainly impacts on the journeys of the chronically-ill patients through it, patients are not exclusively passive participants. Instead, the desire to increase concordance and partnership in doctor–patient relationships is resulting in patients becoming increasingly active decision-makers. The decision-making they engage in, in turn, also shapes their journeys through Canada's system of health services and interactions with specific practitioners. Caspi et al. state that "for medical decisions with more than one reasonable option, patient participation in decision-making is often necessary to optimally match management decisions with patient preferences" (2004, p. 64). The change in paradigm within the allopathic medical tradition to seeking out shared decision-making in the doctor–patient relationship or partnership is slowly resulting in a shift away from the traditional, paternalistic-style of decision-making, whereby doctors exclusively made decisions for patients (Roter, 2000).

While shared decision-making is being embraced by many Canadian practitioners, and is even being supported through health policy initiatives (Holmes-Rover, 2005), there are still decisions that patients make outside of this realm which shape their journeys through the health care system, and even possibly their health. For example, while the decision to pursue a particular treatment might be made in consultation with a family doctor, the decision to discontinue seeing a particular family doctor or specialist, or to not continue with a particular treatment option, may be made by an informed patient alone (Crooks et al., 2012). In addition, the increasing amount of health information available online is allowing patients to become better informed about the conditions with which they are living, including FMS. While patients' use of such information can lead to a more even distribution of power, shared decision-making, or even partnership between doctor and patient, another outcome is that such knowledge may empower patients to make decisions on their own (Crooks, 2006; Lee et al., 2014). However, it is important to recognize that the validity and accuracy of some of this online information has been brought into question by health experts, in that misinformation sometimes is used to inform decision-making which can have negative implications for health and navigating health care (Car et al., 2011).

Most broadly, Holmes-Rover (2005) suggests that patients sometimes engage in "rational agency," whereby they will do whatever they feel is necessary in order to maintain their health. They may end up making decisions based on what they feel is best for themselves and their health, regardless of whether or not other sources or people are consulted. Decisions made by patients, sometimes alone and at other times in consultation with others, can result in actions being taken that negatively or positively affect both their relationships with doctors, and/or their journeys through health care systems such as Canada's. Such decisions may be made by patients out of a desire to exercise more control over their health and/or health care by engaging in what is sometimes referred to as "patient agency" (Schneider et al., 2010; Thomas et al., 2010).

The brief discussions presented in this section and the one above illustrate some important aspects of the diverse interplay between patients and the larger system of health care services. The system determines which services are available locally and for which treatments costs are covered, while shared or independent decision-making by the patient determines which ones will be pursued. Such decisions are affected by one's access to information and material resources, in that a patient may decide to pursue chiropractic treatment, only to find that he/she is unable to afford to do so. As mentioned previously, current challenges within Canada's system of health care have resulted in some patients not having regular family doctors and/or lacking interpersonal continuity in care; while for some of them, deciding to search for a more supportive family doctor who will discuss the use of non-Western treatments, or who will acknowledge the legitimacy of FMS as a diagnosis, is what will expose them to such problems in the first place. While we can understand that this complex interplay exists, it is rarely discussed beyond the conceptual level. Existing studies tend to focus either on decision-making (e.g. Caspi et al., 2004), or on the system of health services (e.g. Rothman and Wagner, 2003), rather than on both. This leaves us wondering how exactly patients' lives are shaped by the larger system of health services and how, in turn, they make decisions that affect or mediate this impact and their journeys through this social institution.

I believe that this interplay is simultaneous, and thus warrants exploration from both sides. In the remainder of the chapter I do exactly this, by examining how the structure and organization of Canada's health care system shapes the experiences of chronically-ill patients with FMS, and how the decisions that such women make guide their journeys through it. Through this examination I show how factors as diverse as access to care, social location, and the body shape, mediate, and guide this interplay. In the section that follows I provide some background details on the study, before going into depth about the results.

Method

Research Design

Women who had developed FMS and were living in one of three communities in the province of Ontario, Canada – the cities of Hamilton (a large city in a populous area of the province), North Bay (a small-sized city in a northern area of the province), and Sudbury (a medium-sized industrial city located in a northern area of the province) – were sought out in this study. The study purpose was to document and explain the life-changing and simultaneous processes of negotiating a changing, sociospatial life after developing a chronic illness, and of becoming a chronically-ill patient and negotiating the health care system. More specifically, the ways in which women's bodily experiences, roles, and routines of everyday life, relationships with others, and negotiations of social institutions were affected by, and sometimes changed as a result of, their lives with FMS were examined. A snowball sampling strategy (Miles and Huberman, 1994) was used to identify participants, with the first contacts having been made through local support groups and the Arthritis Society offices in each city. The data were collected between August 2003 and January 2004, after first receiving approval from McMaster University's research ethics board.

Participants and Data Collection

In-depth semi-structured interviews were conducted with a total of 55 women throughout the data collection period. Their ages ranged from 35 to 88, with the average being 58 years. On average, they had lived with the symptoms of FMS for 14 years, with the shortest period being less than a year and the longest being 54 years. The average length of time since diagnosis was just under nine years (ranging from less than a year to 23 years). Finally, most women lived with at least one other chronic illness in addition to FMS, with one woman managing as many as five chronic illnesses simultaneously. The women's dwelling types were quite varied. Twenty-seven owned family homes and lived with other family members; five widowed women owned family homes in which they lived alone; and five single women lived alone in owned homes. Five women rented family homes, four rented subsidized family housing, and nine lived alone in rented housing.

Each of the interviews took place at a location of the interviewee's choosing. Of the 55 interviews, 49 were conducted either in the women's houses or in a public place, one was conducted at a woman's place of employment, and five were conducted over the telephone. The five telephone interviews were conducted when face-to-face conversations were not possible because the interviewee and I were in different cities at the time of interview. At the start of the interview, each woman was informed of her rights as a participant, including the right to refuse to answer a question and the right to withdraw from the project at any time. Every woman who booked an interview agreed to participate after having been informed of these rights and signing a consent form, and no participants withdrew from the study after completing the interview. In order to maintain anonymity, pseudonyms chosen by the participants are referred to in the remainder of this chapter.

Data Analysis

The questions asked of participants during the interviews were structured using a guide organized under six subheadings:

1) background information;
2) experiences within spaces of health care;

3) experiences outside spaces of health care;
4) everyday life;
5) identity; and
6) demographics.

The interview data were transcribed verbatim after all the interviews had been completed. These transcripts were then entered into NVivo ™, which is a qualitative data management program. A coding scheme consisting of 10 free and 152 tree nodes (organized by 12 parent categories) provided a means by which to organize the data. This scheme was created in three main stages. First, a preliminary scheme was generated after the interviews had been completed and before the transcripts had been reviewed, based primarily on the structure of the interview guide. Second, after the transcripts had been reviewed, the preliminary scheme was revised to include nodes that emerged from the dataset. Finally, the scheme was revised during the coding process, which included the elimination of redundant nodes. The constant comparative technique (Boeije, 2002) was employed in data analysis. The primary form of comparison was at the "between nodes" level, particularly between conceptual and experiential nodes.

Throughout the processes of data collection and analysis it became clear that the women shaped their experiences of the health care system and their experiences as patients, which in turn was shaped by the structure and organization of this same system. In other words, an interplay between structure and agency emerged from their discussions of accessing health care, interacting with physicians, and managing FMS. In the sections that follow I examine this interplay, and in so doing show the significance of factors such as geographic location, physician availability, care quality, access to transportation, income, ability to exercise patient agency, symptom management, and the wider embodiment of FMS in guiding this interplay.

Findings

How System Structure and Organization Shaped Patient Experiences

Physical access to, and the affordability of, local or even regional health care and alternative health treatments shaped the women's journeys through the health care system. As discussed above, the burden of paying for the services provided by some allied health professionals including rehabilitation therapists, and most non-Western practitioners such as chiropractors and naturopaths, falls on individuals' shoulders. For people who are chronically ill, the expenses incurred as a result of using such treatment can be burdensome, given that such conditions typically require management for an extended period of time. For many such costs are prohibitive, particularly for those who are unable to work full time or who do not have private health insurance cover – despite the health benefits they anticipate from such treatments.

During the interviews, 26 of the women commented specifically on the unaffordability of health treatments and services not covered by the public system. For example, Gisele was unable to continue seeing a naturopath practicing close to her house in North Bay because the cost had exceeded what she could afford on her limited income through Canada Pension Plan disability benefit (a contributory benefits program). Tracey could no longer afford to pay for naturopathic treatments despite experiencing the "best care [she had] ever received" under the care of a naturopath in Hamilton. After finding chiropractic treatment and massage therapy to be of help in managing her FMS, Marilyn decided that the benefits outweighed the costs of such treatment:

> Conventional medicine is fantastic as far as they go, but alternative medicine that I have … [has] helped me in what I've had to do myself – and last year it cost me C$5,600 of my own money to do what was good for me … I can't, you know [afford to spend that money]. Drugs are okay, but I try to [avoid them], because of reactions to them. I try to stay away from it as much as possible and do what's more natural to the body, because the body recognizes more natural things.

For Arlene, a lack of private medical insurance had left her in a position where she felt she could no longer allow herself to even ask or read about new treatments for FMS, in order to avoid feeling disappointed when cost was a barrier. As she said: "I don't check into a lot of stuff because there's not a lot of stuff I can really afford." The reality for many of these 26 women was that despite the observed or anticipated benefits of treatments such as chiropractic, massage therapy, and naturopathy, the costs were too high for regular use which, in turn, restricted their use of them and their abilities to manage the symptoms of FMS at times.

Women receiving income assistance or pensions who once worked found out-of-pocket health care costs to be particularly prohibitive given their limited income, which often fell far short of what they had grown accustomed to when performing paid labour. Ann's family doctor had encouraged her to seek the advice of a naturopath to guide her use of herbal remedies; however, she was unable to afford both the cost of seeing a naturopath regularly and cost of the herbs and supplements. As she explained:

> I'm on really good terms with the people at the health food store. I spend a hundred dollars a month there, and take all the, you know, I had changed my diet … I take the things that I think I need to. My doctor [in theory] really does not want me to spend three hundred dollars on a naturopath because he knows I can't afford it. So I've made the appointment to see one twice, but it's just expensive. All these things are really expensive – and you get to the point, like my income has become more limited. I'm an educated person, I have a university education – but my income is so limited that I can't afford all these things that they're recommending.

Ann's comment conveys the struggle faced by many of the women with restrictive incomes, whereby managing the symptoms of FMS with limited access to material resources meant having to choose one treatment over another – if any at all – due to the lack of affordability of non-Western treatments in particular.

Access to health services cannot be defined solely in economic terms. The physical accessibility of local or even regional health care services and other interventions such as non-Western treatments, along the with lengthy wait times associated with a dearth of service, also negatively affected some of the women's abilities to manage FMS. Twenty-five of the interviewees talked specifically about perceiving a lack of local services and treatments: four of whom lived in Hamilton, nine in Sudbury, and the remaining 12 in North Bay. In Hamilton and Sudbury the women's concerns reflected the fact that they felt there simply were not enough family doctors and specialists to allow everyone to receive care locally, even though the services were there. In Sudbury and North Bay there was also a perception shared by several of the participants that their local care was not as good as that which would be received in Toronto (a major metropolitan center in the province's south), and that they had inadequate local care. While it is difficult to assess the accuracy of such perceptions, given that there are multiple ways in which they can be interpreted, having such concerns raised during the interviews is not surprising in view of the increasing lack of confidence in the health care system reported by Canadians (e.g. Wilson and Rosenberg, 2004). These women's perception, that health care services elsewhere were better than those available locally, may have been informed by such a lack or loss of confidence. The most frequently cited challenge in North Bay with respect to the issue of physical access to services was the lack of rheumatological care in the city. For example, despite Janice's desire to see a rheumatologist to help manage her FMS, the lack of a practice in North Bay, and physical impairments that restricted her from driving and traveling long distances (to Sudbury), had prevented her from accessing such specialist care elsewhere.

Many of the women decided to change family doctor in order to find a more supportive physician (discussed later on in this chapter). Yet such change also occurred as a result of physician retirement or turnover, making it an event beyond the women's control which, for some, diminished their abilities to manage the symptoms of FMS. Ten of the participants experienced this type of change in the receipt of health care: four of whom had family doctors retire while they were under their care, and six of whom lost family doctors due to the practitioner leaving for another clinic or downsizing his/her patient load. Cecile, Lynn, and Caroline had yet to find a new family physician after losing their previous one to retirement or turnover. Caroline shared this about her experience:

> The last doctor that finally sent me to the rheumatologist, she left town –
> and Sudbury's really bad for that. There's like, 30,000 people that don't

have doctors at the moment. So I've been going to emergency walk-in clinics, and through them … I've been sent to see a rheumatologist or to see other … specialty doctors. That's the only way I can do it. So I've been pretty unlucky. Yes, I did leave certain doctors because they couldn't help me.

The retirement or departure of a physician who is thought of as being particularly helpful, knowledgeable, and/or supportive can be a challenge to those managing chronic illnesses, as it means having to learn how to interact with a new family doctor – one who may have a different view of how to manage FMS, or even of the legitimacy of the illness itself. Maria still did not feel as comfortable with her "new" family doctor of six years, whom she had been consulting since the passing of her previous family doctor. For Maria, the loss of her family doctor was like the loss of a family member. That type of comfort and closeness with a practitioner was something that took time to build, and which perhaps she may never experience again. Gayle had also yet to find a family doctor as supportive as the one she had seen for 14 years before she went into semi-retirement. Since then, Gayle decided to leave a family doctor whom she felt did not address her mental and spiritual health; and since then, based on the recommendation of a friend, had started to see a doctor infrequently in Kitchener – just over 460 km from Sudbury.

Decision-making and Participants' Patient Journeys through the System

It is important to remember that the decision to seek treatment, or to follow up on a treatment regimen, is one that ultimately rests with an individual. The pursuit of non-Western and allied health treatments discussed above played a big role in the women's decisions regarding managing FMS and their lives with the illness. Twenty-one of the participants had tried chiropractic treatment, four had tried acupuncture, seven had visited naturopaths or homeopaths, two had seen nutritionists, 28 had seen massage therapists, and 18 women had tried physiotherapy. Many had tried combinations and permutations of these interventions in order to assist them with managing FMS, as Maggs said: "And, oh, just try everything!" Thirteen were still actively using such services at the time of interview. while many others had discontinued some or all of them completely, primarily due to cost or effectiveness, or even both. All but one of the women also were seeing a family doctor and/or specialist at the time of the interview (her situation is discussed in greater detail below).

Thus, seeing allied health professionals or using non-Western therapies was done in addition to choosing to pursue treatment through conventional means such as family doctors, rheumatologists, neurologists, pain psychiatrists, and others. The women's decisions to pursue such treatments were likely informed by a multitude of factors, including a desire to have relief from symptoms, hearing from others about the success of a particular treatment, and dissatisfaction with the limited allopathic treatments available. While for the most part the participants did not discuss the rationale for such decisions in the interviews, Caspi et al. (2004) tell us that decisions to pursue alternative treatments are informed most often by combinations of personal experience, information found online, and testimonials from others.

For Freda, the decision that had the most significant impact on her ability to manage FMS and its impact on her life was to no longer pursue discussion of treatments for her FMS, including requesting referrals, with her family doctor. She talked about the experiences that led to this decision:

> I've kind of given up on care here, and I've, in a way, given up on what care I would get out of town too because it's harder to get places, you know? ... You need to find the right specialist to see. You know, and the doctors here [North Bay] have pooh-poohed it [FMS] ... I had an abusive practitioner here for three years or so, and I finally found another woman doctor who is very nice, very good – but ... the first thing she said was, "I know little about fibromyalgia." I didn't say, "Well, do you plan to learn something?", because I knew it wouldn't happen. She happens to be extremely busy ... and so, I don't even expect to bring up anything or have her search for anything.

While Freda still had a family doctor, she considered herself to have "given up" on accessing health care for her FMS, and had decided not to bring it up during doctor–patient interactions. Her decision was informed by experiences such as having discouraging interactions with former doctors, having seen doctors who discounted the legitimacy of FMS as a diagnosis, and the illness-related difficulties that she had with traveling outside of North Bay to access specialist care.

Dee made a similar decision in response to ineffective treatments, but also continued to see a family doctor:

> I no longer use any of the health care services, because they were so, they're not only non-existent, they make you feel worse. I found that the best thing I did was get out of the health care system – because all they could do was make me feel worse. They never, ever made me feel better.

Although Freda and Dee's experiences were not common among the women, they do raise another important issue with regard to the role of decisions in the use of health care services: people can decide to discontinue treatments or services, just as they decided to use them in the first place. While these two women's situations reflect an extreme, many of the women opted to discontinue everything from drug therapies through seeing specialists to using acupuncture for a variety of reasons, including their effectiveness, recommendations from others and self-help sources, as well as the costs associated with accessing those treatments not covered by the public system.

Choosing to try new interventions and discontinue others seemed to be one of the constants that the women talked about in terms of managing FMS. In other words, change was a constant for those who managed this chronic illness using health care services or other interventions. This was due at least in part to the fact that managing a chronic illness for which there is no known cause, cure, or set course of treatment involved trial and error when attempting to identify a regimen of care that worked well. Frances had been living with FMS for close to 20 years at the time of her interview. She had become tired of this type of constant change in treatments and therapies:

> You know, everyone claims to have a cure for fibromyalgia, and I have tried so many things – and have spent so much money on it – and you know what? None of those made an iota of difference.

Although Frances still saw a family doctor and rheumatologist, the constant state of change in things such as medicines and exercise regimens that came about from trying new therapies, interventions, and treatments was no longer part of her life, as these did not produce the desired outcomes of reduced pain and fatigue or increased energy. Just like Freda and Dee, discussed above, she found that the best decision to make in the face of ineffective, and sometimes costly, treatments was to discontinue pursuing new treatments and services altogether.

Another type of decision made by many of the women regarding health-related services was to change family doctors and specialists. Seventeen women talked about making such a change out of the desire to find a practitioner who was thought of as being more supportive of their needs, meaning the he/she would consider a range of possible treatments and/or act in partnership with patients, or was simply willing to acknowledge the existence of their FMS. The experiences shared by Arlene and Pat during their interviews are telling:

> I found a doctor that doesn't tell me it's all in my head. You know, she's not an expert on fibromyalgia, but between her and my chiropractor, like I manage better than I did with my family doctor. He was … "old school" is being kind. (Arlene)

> Plain and simple, he was treating me like a whiny, menopausal woman … So you think I … like, do you think it's fun being sick? Like, if you're looking for attention or pity, you're not going to get it … and I wasn't. I was just looking for understanding – and I wanted him to acknowledge that there was something wrong with me. (Pat)

Their decision to change family doctors was done out of necessity in order to try to find a practitioner who was willing to acknowledge their symptoms and assist with making a diagnosis. In Arlene's case, she wanted to find a doctor who believed the cause of FMS to be more than psychological, while

Pat sought out a family doctor who was willing to support her application for disability income support and recognized disability to be an outcome of FMS. Marilyn and Gloria changed family doctors as a result of conducting research into FMS and their desires to be managed by practitioners who were willing to discuss alternative treatments. For many of the 17 women who had decided to switch doctors, the search for a new practitioner was difficult, due to the shortage of local family doctors taking on new patients. Such decisions, then, did not always lead to the desired outcome of finding a practitioner who was more supportive of their needs – such as the desire to develop a working partnership – or receptive to treating women with FMS.

Discussion and Conclusion

The findings shared above revealed that many of the participants I spoke with came face-to-face with some of the institutional limitations in the delivery of health care services reported by people living with chronic illnesses. Such problems were outlined at the beginning of this chapter, and include:

- a lack of funding for non-Western and allied health treatments, despite their increasing use;
- a lack of physical access to specialists and sometimes even family doctors for those living in certain communities;
- family doctor shortages in communities of all sizes; and
- a lack of interpersonal continuity of care.

Some of these realities were experienced by the women as a result of their own decisions, such as interpersonal discontinuity in care due to going through several family doctors in order to find one they regarded as supportive. Others were a result of organization and structure of the system, such as no new family doctor available to take over the practice of a retiring practitioner, which resulted in the women having no family doctor at all.

The findings draw a distinction between changes in care and the use of health care services over which the women had some degree of control, despite the constraints placed on their decision-making; and those over which they had little or no control. The experiences shared in the interviews, for example, showed that the women's decision-making mediated the impact that the health care system had on their lives and their journeys through it, doing so in diverse ways depending on their access to care, social locations, and bodily experiences. The perceived need for such decision-making on the women's part, particularly that informed by a desire to find a doctor viewed as being more supportive of their needs, reflects the reality that the time and preparation put into appointments and nurturing a supportive working relationship with doctors did not always yield the desired outcome. The experiential evidence also revealed that constraints such as access to material resources, and variations in how supportive of the illness experience doctors treating FMS were, shaped the women's decision-making and/or their abilities to act on the decisions they had made regarding their health and use of health care services. The women's bodies also constrained their decisions, as some women chose not to travel to distant specialists because this was too physically and mentally taxing. Their bodily experiences, and doctors' readings of their embodied performances as patients, also informed their decision-making, in that women chose to leave practitioners who did not seem to address their physical symptoms. The women also chose to discontinue treatments that did not achieve the desired relief from symptoms. Thus, it is the chronically-ill body, a chronically-ill woman's positioning in society and space, as well as social relations of power, that will constrain her negotiations of this institutional system (a system that was introduced in brief in Chapter 1).

These findings help to connect the micro and the macro in understanding the forces that shape the lives of women living with FMS. We can see how small actions or negotiations undertaken by the women at the micro-scale were done in response to this macro-scale institutional system. In addition we can see how the ways in which the system impacts either negatively or positively on the individual depends in part on his/her responses to its organization and service delivery. Although not discussed explicitly above, the institution focused on in this chapter (i.e. the public health care system) is informed by larger processes such as state restructuring and the global neoliberalization of the state, which involve changes such as privatizing public services and increasing individual responsibility for ensuring his/her own personal well-being (Armstrong and Armstrong, 1996; James, 1999; Chouinard and Crooks, 2005). The women's engagement in these systems thereby also connects them to global processes of change, which allows us to understand that their individual experiences in and of the space of care provision are not only intersectional and relational, but also translocal. Their individual experiences in place shape, and are shaped by, these larger social institutions, which are informed by even larger national and global processes.

Other geographers have highlighted connections between the macro and micro in the context of relationships between individuals and state-run institutions. For example, Chouinard (1999, 2001), argues that there has been an erosion of basic human rights for people with disabilities in the province of Ontario, and that this is an outcome of neoliberal influences on the economy and governance – as reflected in cuts to Human Rights Commission funds. One outcome of these specific funding cuts is that people with disabilities – especially disabled women who are even further marginalized by the state and in society in general – have become "shadow citizens," in that in principle they have rights, such as the right to not be discriminated against, but in reality the funding does not exist in Ontario or Canada to enforce these rights through federal or provincial human rights commissions. James's (1999) research into the closure of hospitals in the province of Saskatchewan has illustrated how the restructuring of the health care system has had a great impact on local citizens. For example, James found that the people who reported difficulties in physically accessing more distant health care services as a result of local hospital closure – such as elderly and disabled populations – used such services less often than the general population, while also reporting poorer health status. Furthermore, the shift to community care facilities has meant more work for private citizens, in that family and friends are now increasingly expected to assist in service delivery, such as feeding and administering medication. Much of this work has fallen on women, as they are the ones most frequently responsible for meeting family health care needs (see Roberts and Faulk, 2002). The present study and those conducted by Chouinard (1999, 2001) and James (1999) lend support to Dyck et al.'s (2001) argument that the global neoliberal shift, and the institutional policies and practices that it guides, have direct implications for the daily lives of Canadian citizens. As Dyck and colleagues state:

> [W]hatever the geographical scale, the simultaneity of local and global relations plays out in women's lives, shaping their health experiences, their access to resources for promoting a healthy life or managing disease or trauma, and their ability to use quality health care services. (2001, p.14)

The findings shared here echo this, while also pointing to the complex ways in which access to care, social location, and the body interact with one another to shape a diverse range of outcomes for women managing FMS.

Acknowledgments

This research was funded by a grant awarded from the Arthritis Health Professions Association. The author is also funded by a Scholar Award from the Michael Smith Foundation for Health Research.

References

Armstrong, P. and Armstrong H., 1996. *Wasting away: The undermining of Canadian health care*. Toronto: Oxford University Press.

Boeije, H., 2002. A purposeful approach to the constant comparative method in the analysis of qualitative interviews. *Quality & Quantity*, 36(4), pp. 391–409.

Canadian Institute for Health Information, 2003. *Health care in Canada*. Ottawa: Canadian Institute for Health Information.

Car, J., Lang, B., Colledge, A., Ung, C. and Majeed, A., 2011. Interventions for enhancing consumers' online health literacy. *Cochrane Database of Systematic Reviews*, 15(6), CD007092. Available online at http://onlinelibrary.wiley.com/doi/10.1002/14651858. CD007092.pub2/pdf (accessed February 12, 2016).

Caspi, O., Koithan, M. and Criddle, M.W., 2004. Alternative medicine or "alternative" patients: A qualitative study of patient-oriented decision-making processes with respect to complementary and alternative medicine. *Medical Decision Making*, 24, pp. 64–79.

Chouinard, V., 1999. Body politics: Disabled women's activism in Canada and beyond. In: R. Butler and H. Parr, eds. *Mind and body spaces: Geographies of illness, impairment and disability*. New York: Routledge. pp. 269–94.

Chouinard, V., 2001. Legal peripheries: Struggles over disabled Canadian's places in law, society and space. *The Canadian Geographer*, 45(1), pp. 187–92.

Chouinard, V. and Crooks, V.A., 2005. "Because they have all the power and I have none": State restructuring of income and employment supports and disabled women's lives in Ontario, Canada. *Disability & Society*, 20(1), pp. 19–32.

Crooks, V.A., 2006. "I go on the Internet; I always, you know, check to see what's new": Chronically ill women's use of online health information to shape and inform doctor–patient interactions in the space of care provision. *ACME: An International E-Journal for Critical Geographies*, 5(1), pp. 50–69. Available online at http://ojs. unbc.ca/index.php/acme/article/view/748 (accessed June 1, 2015).

Crooks, V.A. and Chouinard, V., 2006. An embodied geography of disablement: Chronically ill women's struggles for enabling places in spaces of health care and daily life. *Health & Place*, 12(3), pp. 345–52.

Crooks, V.A. and Schuurman, N., 2012. Interpreting the results of a modified gravity model: Examining access to primary health care physicians in five Canadian provinces and territories. *BMC Health Services Research*, 12(230). Available online at http://bmchealthservres.biomedcentral.com/articles/10.1186/1472-6963-12-230 (accessed February 12, 2016).

Crooks, V.A., Agarwal, G. and Harrison, A., 2012. Chronically ill Canadians' experiences of being unattached to a family doctor: A qualitative study of marginalized patients in British Columbia. *BMC Family Practice*, 13(69). Available online at: http://bmcfampract.biomedcentral.com/articles/10.1186/1471-2296-13-69 (accessed February 12, 2016).

Donald Watt, W., 1987. The family physician: Gatekeeper to the health-care system. *Canadian Family Physician*, 33, pp. 1101–2.

Dyck, I., Davis Lewis, N. and McLafferty, S., 2001. Why geographies of women's health? In: I. Dyck, N. Davis Lewis and S. McLafferty, eds. *Geographies of women's health*. London: Routledge, pp. 1–20.

Epping-Jordan, J.E., Pruitt, S.D., Bengoa, R. and Wagner, E.H., 2004. Improving the quality of health care for chronic conditions. *Quality and Safety in Health Care*, 13, pp. 299–305.

Gesler, W.M. and Kearns R.A., 2002. *Culture/place/health*. London: Routledge.

Holmes-Rover, M., 2005. Likely consequences of increased patient choice. *Health Expectations*, 8(1), pp. 1–3.

James, A., 1999. Closing rural hospitals in Saskatchewan: On the road to wellness? *Social Science and Medicine*, 49(8), pp. 1021–34.

Lee, K., Hoti, K., David Hughes, J. and Emmerton, L., 2014. Dr Google and the consumer: A qualitative study exploring the navigational needs and online health information-seeking behaviours of consumers with chronic health conditions. *Journal of Medical Internet Research*, 16(12), pp. e262. Available online at www. jmir.org/2014/12/e262 (accessed February 12, 2016).

Miles, M.B. and Huberman, A.M., 1994. *Qualitative data analysis*. Thousand Oaks, CA: Sage Publications.

Roberts, J. and Faulk, M., 2002. *Women and health: Experiences in a rural regional health authority*. Winnipeg: Prairie Women's Health Centre of Excellence.

Roter, D., 2000. The enduring and evolving nature of the patient–physician relationship. *Patient Education Counseling*, 39(1), pp. 5–15.

Rothman, A.A. and Wagner, E.H., 2003. Chronic illness management: What is the role of primary care? *Annals of Internal Medicine*, 138(3), pp. 256–60.

Saultz, J.W. and Albedaiwi W., 2004. Interpersonal continuity of care and patient satisfaction: A critical review. *Annals of Family Medicine*, 2(5), pp. 445–51.

Schneider, H., Le Marcis, F., Grard, J., Penn-Kekana, L., Blaauw, D and Fassin, D., 2010. Negotiating care: Patient tactics at an urban South African hospital. *Journal of Health Services Research & Policy*, 15(3), pp. 137–42.

Schuurman, N., Berube, M. and Crooks, V.A., 2010. Measuring potential spatial access to primary health care physicians using a modified gravity model. *The Canadian Geographer*, 54(1), pp. 29–45.

Stewart, M., 2004. Continuity, care, and commitment: The course of patient–clinician relationships. *Annals of Family Medicine*, 2(5), pp. 388–90.

Talbot, Y., Fuller-Thomson, E., Tudiver, F., Habib, Y. and McIsaac, W., 2001. Canadians without regular medical doctors: Who are they? *Canadian Family Physician*, 47, pp. 58–64.

Thomas, F., Aggleton, P and Anderson, J., 2010. "Experts", "partners" and "fools": Exploring agency in HIV treatment seeking among African migrants in London. *Social Science & Medicine*, 70(5), pp. 736–43.

Wilson, K. and Rosenberg, M.W., 2004. Accessibility and the Canadian health care system: Squaring perceptions and realities. *Health Policy*, 67(2), pp. 137–48.

11 Aging, Gender, and "Triple Jeopardy" Through the Life Course

Rachel V. Herron and Mark W. Rosenberg

In this chapter, we explore the intersections of gender and age with a particular focus on older Canadian women and the challenges they face as providers and recipients of care. Feminist scholars have a long-standing interest in the gendered dimensions of care and the ways in which women are constructed as the caregivers *of* choice, even if they are not the caregivers *by* choice. As the Canadian population ages, these debates about who cares are intersecting increasingly with issues of aging. Indeed, many older women face a "triple jeopardy" of declining health, declining social support, and declining resources. We draw on recent research and secondary data from the Canadian Community Health Survey (CCHS) to explore these intersections.

Introduction

As health researchers, we imagine that the work we do ultimately will enhance the health, well-being, and care that people experience. Thirty years after its writing, Margaret Atwood's *The Handmaid's Tale* cautions us that "better never means better for everyone ... It always means worse, for some" (Atwood, 1985, p. 245). She reminds us that the better future we seek will draw on the contexts, identities, and structures that we have around us today. We begin with reference to Atwood's novel because of its focus on gender and inequity in a future world. In her dystopia, women are reduced to a functional status as childbearers, older women are disposable, and a group of elite, mostly men, control the rights of others. The societal structure is upheld by the notion that it is improving the conditions of life, at least for some.

As Chapters 1 and 2 in this volume have shown, understanding the diversity of health experiences today is central to improving health equity across multiple forms of difference, both now and in the future. In this chapter, we explore the diversity and health of older women in contemporary Canada, and attempt to make a few careful projections about the future. We draw on intersectionality as a framework for exploring diversity, particularly the many social and physical roles that intersect in older women's lives, shaping their opportunities over time and across space. In spite of the many improvements that Canadian women experience in their lives compared to past generations, they face declining health, declining social support, and declining resources, while they are simultaneously expected to be caregivers in the home. However, in keeping with our interest in the future, we suggest that the social positions that disadvantage the majority of older women today will intersect differently in the future and, at some point in time, may allow a greater majority of older women to reposition themselves outside of caregiving.

The chapter begins by looking at how women have been traditionally characterized as caregivers. Drawing on these constructions of gender, we discuss the difference between, and meaning of, gender and women as well as the strength of intersectionality as a framework for exploring difference and diversity among older women. The remainder of the chapter focuses on recent studies and secondary data analyses to illustrate the complex and changing conditions of older women in Canada. The chapter concludes with a summary of the limitations of our approach, and future directions for research that ultimately seeks to enhance the lives of older women in Canada.

Women, Aging and Caregiving in the Canadian Context

Experiences of health and ill-health are linked intrinsically to the places where we live, and the ways in which care is constructed in these places. Care involves a complex web of relationships, responsibilities, roles, and rights, all of which play out at different scales and in different settings (Atkinson et al., 2011). In the last half of the twentieth century, the care of older people in Western countries has shifted largely away from institutional settings to community settings (Milligan and Power, 2010). Successive rounds of health care restructuring from the late twentieth century to the present day have placed additional pressure on communities and families to provide more complex care for longer periods of time. Under this neoliberal agenda, family-based care is viewed as the primary and most appropriate form of care. However, the responsibility of care is not borne evenly within families, communities, and institutions. As care has moved back into the domestic sphere, gendered assumptions about who cares best have been reinforced.

Feminist scholars have long pointed out that interpretations of care are based on sociocultural constructions of gender that ascribe particular responsibilities, qualities, and rights, to women (Aronson, 1991; Dyck et al., 2001; Giesbrecht et al., 2012). In spite of advances in women's rights across the Western world, health care systems and policies in many of the most developed countries are based on constraining assumptions about women, aging, and caregiving. For example, women tend to be viewed as heterosexual and married with children (Grigorovich, 2013). As they age they are thought, by and large, to have spent at least some portion of their lives in caregiving roles as a daughter, wife, mother, and/or grandmother (Armstrong and Armstrong, 2004). Outside of the home, women often are expected to perform caregiving roles in their communities, including childcare, meal preparation, and generally providing social support to neighbors and community groups in need (Herron and Skinner, 2011; Seaman, 2012). In health care settings, there are significantly more women in caring professions such as nursing, personal support work, and other ancillary work such as housekeeping and food services that contribute to the overall health of an individual. Taken together, it is estimated that women provide approximately 80 percent of formal and informal care (Armstrong et al., 2008).

Although women tend to provide more hours of more intimate care over their lives than men, they are more likely than their male counterparts to experience declining social and material resources which can affect their health and access to care in later life. Women tend to experience more interruptions in their work, take on more flexible employment, and receive less pay throughout their lives; this affects their financial resources to put towards health promotion, prevention, and treatment in their earlier years and in later life. Generally, women are more prone to developing chronic diseases, more likely to be institutionalized in old age, have longer lengths of stay in institutional settings, and fill a greater number of long-term care beds (Bird and Rieker, 2008). This is due in part to their longer life expectancy: in Canada, women live approximately four years longer than men (Statistics Canada, 2013). As heterosexual married women tend to outlive their partners, who are often older and experience poor health before they do, they are more reliant on home and institutional care to provide for their daily needs when they can no longer for themselves. Furthermore, if their partner is healthy, men may not have experience or confidence in performing traditionally gendered activities of daily living such as bathing, dressing, grooming, and homemaking (Robinson et al., 2014).

Although there are many factors that may disadvantage older women, they face additional disadvantages in the form of ageism and sexism. The widespread discourse of population aging as a *problem* constructs older people, in general, as a homogenous group defined by their needs, passivity, and inability to contribute to their own care and communities (Waldbrook et al., 2013). While older people are expected to be passive, older women face particular pressure to look and act younger rather than show their age (Clarke and Korotchenko, 2011). In the context of health care, there has been a tendency to view declines in older women's health as normal aspects of aging, and to characterize those women who persistently advocate for themselves as "too demanding" (Aronson, 1991; Angus et al., 2012). Moreover, assumptions about the "nature" of gender, caregiving, and ageing place pressure on women to perform to specific norms, disadvantaging those who do not fit into this framework.

Understanding Women and Gender

Understanding normative pressures around care and the diversity of older women's experiences of health and health care requires us to engage with ongoing discussions about the differences between, and meanings of, sex and gender (Kazanjian and Hankivsky, 2008). There are no singular definitions for sex and gender (Springer et al., 2012). In general, biological sex is used to refer to aspects of the body (commonly thought of in terms of reproductive organs, hormones, and chromosomal differences), while gender is used to refer to sociocultural roles associated with masculinity and femininity. Both categories are broad and, to some extent, socially and politically constructed (Sothern and Dyck, 2010). Traditionally, women have been the driving force behind gender equity politics and policies because women's health is affected disproportionally by gendered practices (Hankivsky, 2012). However, gender does not apply exclusively to women, and there are great differences in gender and sex experiences among women. Furthermore, gender and sex are exclusionary categories for people who do not identify with one specific sex (e.g. intersex) or gender (e.g. transgender).

In this chapter, we focus on women because of their gendered role in providing care and the specific challenges they share in negotiating care. We draw on intersectionality to explore the diversity within these experiences, with attention to the complex social construction of women's identities and place within the Canadian context.

Health, Diversity, and Intersectionality

Many scholars have identified intersectionality (introduced in Chapter 2) as a useful framework for exploring the relationship between gender and sex, and their interaction with other factors such as class, "race," sexuality, and age (Hankivsky, 2012; Bauer, 2014). Conceptually, intersectionality has a rich history in the social sciences. African American legal scholar Kimberlé Crenshaw (1989) coined the term "intersectionality" as a means of understanding the multiple marginalizations of black women. She posited that gender/sex and "race" were neither separate nor additive in producing experiences of marginalization, but instead that they should be understood as having intersecting and multiplicative effects on the experiences of black women. While feminist scholars have built on intersectionality theory over the last 30 years, geography has adopted it only relatively recently (Valentine, 2007; Giesbrecht et al., 2012). One of the strengths of intersectional analysis is that it allows us to view the complex dimensions of inequality with particular attention to context and history (Hankivsky, 2012). As such, health geographers have much to contribute to, and learn from, intersectional analysis, with their focus on the social and physical positioning of people across space and in place.

Although initially much of the theoretical development and application of intersectionality stemmed from qualitative research, there has been a burgeoning interest in modeling intersectionality quantitatively (Bauer, 2014). For example, Seng et al. (2012) examined the relationship between marginalized identities (e.g. education, income, "race" and/or ethnicity, and gender) and mental health outcomes across three levels: structural, contextual, and interpersonal. Their work not only contributed to debates about how to undertake quantitative intersectional analysis, but also demonstrated the multiple ways and scales in which the effects of intersectionality can impact on the individual. Indeed, the weight and significance of particular identities and social positions may change in relation to the setting or scale. Using similar quantitative approaches, Veenstra (2013) explored self-reported hypertension in association with "race," class, gender, and sexual orientation. He found that these social identities had mitigating and aggravating effects on health status. Wealthier black men, wealthier bisexual respondents, and wealthier South-Asian women were all more likely than expected to report hypertension. What these two studies hold in common is that they each use intersectionality theory and quantitative methods to demonstrate the complex and often contradictory relations between different social positionings. However, they have controlled for, rather than investigated, the intersection of age with other variables.

In her introduction to a special issue on intersectionality and health in *Social Science & Medicine*, Hankivsky (2012) suggested that the trinity of gender, class, and "race" have predominated intersectional studies, while age has been relatively underexplored. A handful of studies have used intersectionality theory to look specifically at health in older adults (Koehn et al., 2013). For example, Mair (2010) used an intersectional framework to explore the relationship between social ties, depression, "race," and gender in older adults, illustrating the shared benefit of marriage across "race" and gender, differences between black women's and white women's social ties, and the potential vulnerability of black men who tend to have fewer social ties. Warner and Brown (2011) modeled trajectories of functional limitation across racial and/or ethnic and gender differences in older adults, demonstrating that women of all racial and/or ethnic groups have higher levels of functional limitation than white men and men of the same "race" or ethnicity. Most recently, Hinze et al. (2012) examined gender, "race," and education and their intersecting effects on the social relationships, health behaviors, health conditions, and depressive symptoms of older black women. All three studies compared the outcomes of men to those of women, using white men as the baseline for better outcomes and accounting for diversity among older women, in terms of "race" and socioeconomic status. There is still a need to consider diversity among older women in greater depth.

Qualitative approaches are well suited to exploring the range and value of different social and physical positions in older women's lives. Giesbrecht et al. (2012) provide a critical diversity analysis of female caregivers using the Compassionate Care Benefit program, offering a foundation for future intersectional analyses. They demonstrated that the negative consequences of caregiving are not experienced uniformly across women. Culture, gender, geography, life stage, and material resources affect both the opportunities of caregivers and the person for whom they cared during end-of-life care. Although this study draws on interviews with front-line workers rather than the informal caregivers and care recipients themselves, it points to the value of examining axes of difference as they are experienced in relation to health care. The study also offers a more contextually specific view of the meaning of different axes: for example, Giesbrecht and colleagues identified access to material resources rather than socioeconomic status as an axis of difference, and in so doing, they were able to offer concrete examples of the ways in which female caregivers' socioeconomic position impinges on opportunities of care (i.e. in accessing equipment, medication, transportation, and respite).

Both quantitative and qualitative studies have begun to show the strength of intersectional approaches in examining the complexity of aging as an accumulation of histories, contexts, and social and physical positions. Still, there is a need for more research on the diversity of older women's circumstances. Older women may share experiences of sexism and ageism, but the experiences of women at 45, 65, and 75 years of age are not likely to be the same. Although "race," class, gender, sexual orientation and so on form significant intersections in the lives of people at all ages, their significance is rooted in particular histories and contexts.

As geographers, we hope to identify some of the changing contexts of older women's lives. We have chosen six variables to frame our discussion: education, labor force participation, income, immigration, marital status, and living arrangements. This is by no means an exhaustive list; our selection reflects some of the most significant changes for women in Canada as we see them. We discuss each of these variables in the following section, looking carefully at how they intersect across older age cohorts, and with regard to women's involvement in caregiving and care receiving. We acknowledge that the phrase "care receiving" implies dependency. Our aim is not to reinforce the passive view of older women as "care recipients;" instead, we hope to demonstrate the multidirectionality and contingency of older women's needs and contributions to care.

Intersections in the Lives of Older Women in Canada

Education

One of the greatest disadvantages that today's older women face is their significantly lower levels of education, in comparison to their male counterparts and younger women. Low levels of education are associated with mortality rates, but also health-related quality of life long before death (Ross et al., 2011). In general, women with low levels of education are more likely to be positioned in health-damaging life circumstances throughout their life course, be distanced from places of power and decision-making, and experience more oppression and discrimination. Intersectional analyses have shown that higher levels of education seem to ameliorate the health of people experiencing other multiple forms of marginalization, and that highly educated people benefit more from having a close network of friends than those with less education (Hinze et al., 2012; Veenstra, 2013).

Following current trends, older women of the future will have higher levels of education than the current cohort of older women in Canada. In general, this trend is likely to contribute to the health of older women. In the USA, higher levels of education have been shown to have the greatest impact on health for women in racialized minority groups (Hinze et al., 2012). Still, Ross et al. (2011) indicate that more highly educated and more affluent women in Canada experience a decline in their health-related quality of life that is slightly more accelerated than poorer women, rather than experiencing a delayed decline like their male counterparts. They suggest that this may be linked to survivorship, further emphasizing the need to explore age, sex, and health in relation to marital status and gendered expectations surrounding caregiving.

Labor Force Participation

In the past, women were typically homemakers: they were seen as ideal caregivers for children and older adults because, presumably, they were available and their flexible schedules enabled them to provide care when needed. However, in the last half of the twentieth century, women's participation in paid labor outside the home increased significantly. In 1973, 45 percent of women aged 25–44 participated in the labor force; by 2013, women's participation (aged 25–44) in the labor force had increased to 83 percent (Statistics Canada, 2014). Women with more education and involvement in the labor force are more likely to have experience of negotiating and advocating for particular needs for themselves, as well as others. In addition, they may benefit from social support networks built through their work. Moreover, labor force participation not only improves the financial resources that women have available to them in later life, it also enhances their decision-making power as care recipients and caregivers. Contemporary women may be less likely than ever to see themselves as caregivers. Joseph and Joseph (2013) indicate that instead of taking leave from work to become full-time caregivers for a spouse or parent, some women are choosing to go to work as relief from caregiving. Increasingly, it would seem that some (advantaged) women might have the choice to provide tangible support or not.

In contrast, labor force participation may increase work overload, self-reported stress, and work-related injuries and illnesses among particular groups of women, in Canada and elsewhere. Middle-aged women and younger old women may face demands to balance paid work with providing care for children, grandchildren, and aging parents at the same time (i.e. the "sandwich generation"), which can impact negatively on their overall health (Pillemer and Suitor, 2013). Often, these potential negative consequences of labor force participation for some women are exacerbated by low income and racial inequities (Do et al., 2014).

Income

Undeniably, economic resources underpin many of the assumptions that we have about healthy aging and care. The overall health of low-income, older women is shaped by the economic conditions in which they live, and have lived, throughout their lives. Limited economic resources may impinge on their opportunities for social engagement (Rozanova et al., 2012), housing (Waldbrook, 2013), nutrition (Matheson and McIntyre, 2014), and decision-making. As a key social determinant of health, income shapes the care that older women need, are able to receive, and often are obligated to provide informally.

Just as education and labor force participation are increasing among women, compared to older women in the past, more women report having a personal income; however, their income generally declines as they age. In spite of the publicly funded universal health care system across Canada, older women's abilities to access and make the best use of health and social support services are affected by economic resources – particularly in relation to such things as transportation, medication, respite, and equipment (Giesbrecht et al., 2012). Lower-income families tend to depend on informal family care to make resources spread further, placing lower-income older women in a precarious position of poorer health as well as preferred caregiver. This precarious position is particularly common among immigrant women in Canada.

Immigration

The pattern of immigration has changed significantly over the last century, contributing to the diversity of the Canadian population as a whole, as well as the diversity of older women's health and care needs. Traditionally, the majority of immigrants came to Canada from Europe, the UK, and the USA, whereas today the majority of immigrants to Canada come from India and China (Singh Setia et al., 2011). A number of factors may contribute to the disadvantages experienced by immigrants in relation to health, including migration-related stress, issues associated with recognizing credentials obtained in their country of origin, language or cultural differences, lack of experience and knowledge of the Canadian health care system, and discrimination and racism at the individual and structural levels. Immigrant women in particular enter Canada as family-sponsored immigrants or dependent immigrants, relegating them to dependent positions within the family and Canadian society (Stewart et al., 2006). Many of the women are not fluent in either official language (i.e. French or English), and childcare responsibilities may present barriers to their taking federally funded language courses while they are eligible. Even if they were active in the labor force in their country of origin, they are more likely to be at the lower end of the labor market or unable to work in Canada, which may exacerbate their isolation within Canadian society. Although they may benefit from family social support and support from a broader ethnic community, they are likely to have more limited independence.

The bulk of studies on immigrant health in Canada have focused on issues of health equity between Canadian-born and foreign-born Canadians. Much of this work centers on whether, and under what circumstances, there may be a healthy immigrant effect – whereby immigrants to Canada generally have fewer chronic conditions and better health compared to the average Canadian (McDonald and Kennedy, 2004). Subsequent studies have indicated that immigrant health may converge with that of the wider Canadian population, or decline over time in Canada (Newbold, 2005; Dean and Wilson, 2010). Disputes about the existence of a healthy immigrant effect increasingly have explored the intersectionality and social determinants of immigrant health, in order to shed light on its complex time path. Using data from the CCHS, Kobayashi and Prus (2012) found that middle-aged women immigrants were much more likely to report poor health compared to Canadian-born women, regardless of visible minority status, age, income, and health behavior. Furthermore, Singh Setia et al.'s (2011) analysis of the Longitudinal Survey of Immigrants to Canada demonstrated that women from countries lower on the development index were at greater risk of poor self-reported health. In the absence of targeted policies and programming towards immigrant women experiencing poorer health in their younger years, their poorer health status is likely to continue into later life. Conversely, Kobayashi and Prus (2012) found that non-white elderly (65+) female immigrants who had been in Canada for fewer than 10 years were less likely to rate their health negatively compared to Canadian-born females. This finding was explained by differences in demo-graphic, economic, and lifestyle factors. Overall, recent research illustrates the importance of considering the intersections of age, gender, "race," and ethnicity in older women's health. There are still relatively few studies that examine diversity within the immigrant population and in later life. Newbold (2005) notes that black people are more likely to transition from healthy to less healthy, while Chow (2010) indicates that Chinese immigrants are more likely to rate their health as poor. As the diverse immigrant population ages, the study of aging itself will need to change to reflect more critically on racial diversity and inequity in aging.

In addition, the intersections that disadvantage immigrant women in terms of health may position them as expected caregivers. As noted earlier, immigrant women are less likely to find employment outside the home, and tend to enter Canada while being more dependent on their family. Under the family reunification policy, families assume financial responsibility for their family members, and thus are not eligible for income security, hospi-talization, and home care – placing the responsibility of care on family car-egivers. Furthermore, language and cultural barriers may discourage some immigrants from using the formal health care system, or act as a barrier to effective communication with health care professionals, while others may favor non-Western approaches to medicine (Newbold, 2005; Stewart et al., 2006). Culturally-appropriate support may not be available outside the fam-ily, and immigrant women are positioned as the most available and seemingly appropriate source of support. Many of these assumptions about the role of, and support for, older women hinge on the structure of the family, which is also subject to diversity and change.

Marital Status

Marriage, family, and social support networks can help older women mediate experiences of disadvantage. Although not all married women accrue benefits from their intimate relationships (Abramsky et al., 2011), marriage is generally thought to have positive health effects for both men and women, such as improved mental health, and reduced smoking and alcohol consumption (Mair, 2010; Averett et al., 2013). Furthermore, marriage generally increases household income and resources. The greatest majority of low-income women in old age are those who identify as unattached (i.e. separated, divorced, widowed, and single), and the poorest of these women are separated and divorced (McDonald and Robb, 2004). Marital status intersects acutely with income and impacts decisions about labor force participation throughout women's lives, as some married women take on more family responsibilities in lieu of paid work. Married older women are likely to have been – and continue to be – caregivers in the family context, and to view caregiving in old age as a duty in their marriage, even as their own health declines (Herron and Skinner, 2011). In spite of their own care needs, women are more likely to be the primary caregivers or "committed amateurs" providing support to an older relative or spouse (LaPierre and Keating, 2013).

However, Canadian family structures are changing, with implications for older women's social support-giving and receiving. Families are smaller and more geographically dispersed, and increasing rates of divorce may weaken adult children's sense of duty and ability to care for two parents at separate times and in separate places (Williams and Crooks, 2008). An increasing number of couples without children may require more formal assistance, as they are less likely to find informal support for intimate care tasks when they experience poor health. We also have to wonder what the implications of emerging social networking technologies will be for older women in the future: will they enhance the emotional and psychosocial support that isolated older women receive from family and friends at a distance? Despite the availability of such technologies, the tangible support needs of older women will still be dependent on the physical presence of a spouse, family member, friend, or formal carer.

In addition to these changes, more older women will be married to, or have had, a lifelong partnership with another woman. Gendered constructions of caregiving in the home and institutional settings tend not to take into account the needs and experiences of lesbian and bisexual women, presenting barriers for these couples caring for one another outside of the home (Grigorovitch, 2013). Within the home, Reczek and Umberson (2012) indicate that health behaviors and caregiving in intimate lesbian relationships are more likely to be cooperative; thus, older lesbian women may face different expectations as caregivers and care recipients than their heterosexual counterparts. Certainly, how sexual orientation intersects with caregiving and receiving as well as other social identities requires further research.

As family structures change, so do the public health needs of older women. For example, more women are dating and having sex with more partners in their later years. Ross et al. (2013) found that older women in New Brunswick had moderately low sexual health knowledge, and that their knowledge of HIV/AIDS was very low. The increasing rates of HIV prevalence among older women indicates that there is a need for public health education that addresses older adults. Overall, the changing nature of social relationships have broad implications for the health and care needs of older women: they point to the need for public health interventions, income support, housing support, and social support for older women.

Living Arrangements

Marital status and living arrangements intersect to produce the most immediate and constant form of care for older women. Given women's longer life expectancy, higher rates of divorce, and distance to other family members, older Canadian women are more likely to find themselves living alone at some point in later life. This has many potential implications for older women as care recipients. For example, older women living alone may be challenged to provide high levels of self-care for longer periods of time, managing or coordinating their health needs such as medication, appointments, and problem recognition as well as other personal needs such as transportation, finances, cooking, and cleaning. In the absence of family support, they may rely more heavily on neighbors and friends who also may be older and in poorer health (Giesbrecht et al., 2012). Although some older women living alone may have social support networks around them (e.g. cultural or spiritual community), the changing geography of the family and changing labor structures have left many older women, particularly in small-town and rural Canada, with less social support (Ryser and Halseth, 2011). The support that older women living alone receive is contingent on where they live, and who is around them.

This view of older women's living arrangements takes for granted that women have a home in the first place. As Waldbrook (2013) explains, older Canadian women today have lived through a series of social, economic, and political transformations that have affected both their housing histories and their health. It may be the case that there are more single, separated, or divorced women who do not own a home, and thus find themselves unable to move into transitional housing, and are placed in long-term care before it is required. If public and private pensions continue to be cut, we may see more older women unable to afford housing.

In addition, older women living alone may be more at risk of experiencing affective inequality. That is, they may not have their needs for love and care met, while at the same time shouldering a great proportion of responsibility to provide love and care to others. For example, in a small qualitative study of older Irish women, Crawley and Lynch (2012) found that older women shared feelings of being devalued, an obligation to provide care, feeling excluded, and misrecognition. Although this study looks at older women as a relatively homogenous group, it identifies an often-overlooked area of inequality in old age. The intersections that produce and inhibit such affective inequalities should be given greater attention in research on aging.

Summarizing the Intersections of Older Women in Canada

We use data from the 2008–9 CCHS to summarize many of the intersections discussed above. Note that CCHS uses self-identified sex (i.e. male/female), and thus we can only use this information to make inferences about the role of gender (see Statistics Canada, 2013 for further details). Our focus is only on the results for women, and thus for ease of presentation we group the results with respect to four age cohorts: 45–64, 65–74, 75 and over, and for reference, 45 and older. In Table 11.1, the intersections of age and sex with marital status, family arrangements, household size, tenure of dwelling, education, personal income, household income deciles, immigration status, and time in Canada since immigration are highlighted. In Table 11.2, we highlight the intersections of age and sex with self-perceived health status, provided assistance, received formal care, received home care, and provided assistance and received home care.

Table 11.1 Demographic and socioeconomic characteristics of older women in Canada, 2008–9

	Age groups			
	45–64 *(%)*	*65–74* *(%)*	*75 and over* *(%)*	*45 and over* *(%)*
Marital status:				
Married/common law	77	62	35	67
Widowed	4	22	55	15
Divorced/separated	12	11	5	11
Single	7	5	4	6
Family arrangements:				
Unattached alone	14	30	49	22
Spouse/partner	40	53	30	41
Other	46	18	20	37
Household size:				
1 person in household	14	30	49	22
2 persons	46	58	39	47
3 persons	19	7	6	15
4 persons	13	2	3	10
5 persons	7	3	3	6
Tenure of dwelling:				
Not owned by respondent	17	23	36	21
Owned by respondent	83	77	64	79

continued

Table 11.1 (cont.)

	Age groups			
	45–64 (%)	65–74 (%)	75 and over (%)	45 and over (%)
Education:				
Less than than secondary	14	37	52	24
Secondary graduated	25	18	16	22
Other post-secondary	5	5	5	5
Post-secondary graduated	55	40	28	48
Personal income – all sources:				
Less than C$10,000	19	16	13	17
C$10,000–19,999	14	41	48	23
C$20,000–29,999	16	20	20	17
C$30,000–39,999	16	10	9	14
C$40,000–49,999	11	6	4	9
C$50,000 or more	25	8	6	20
Household income deciles:				
1 (lowest income group)	9	16	23	12
2	7	19	23	12
3	7	16	15	10
4	10	13	11	11
5	11	11	8	10
6	10	7	6	9
7	12	7	5	10
8	12	5	4	9
9	12	4	2	9
10 (highest income group)	11	4	2	8
Immigration status:				
Yes	23	27	25	24
No	77	73	75	17
Time in Canada since immigration:				
0–19 years	36	14	11	27
20–29 years	19	11	11	16
30–39 years	20	17	10	17
40–49 years	15	32	14	18
50 years or more	10	26	54	21

Source: Statistics Canada (2013).

What Table 11.1 emphasizes, first and foremost, are the differences among older Canadian women as they age. Women aged 75 and over are more likely to be:

- widowed;
- unattached and alone;
- living in a one-person household;
- more likely to own the home in which they live;

- have less than a secondary school education;
- have a personal income under C$20,000;
- live in a household which falls within the three lowest income deciles in Canada; and
- have immigrated to Canada more than 50 years ago than younger women.

What Table 11.1 also emphasizes is that women age 45–64 will have somewhat different profiles 20 years from now when they are between 65–84, than women who currently occupy this age range. Changes in divorce laws

Table 11.2 Health, caregiving and care receiving by older women in Canada, 2008–9

	Age groups			
	45–64 (%)	*65–74 (%)*	*75 and over (%)*	*45 and over %*
Self-perceived health status:				
Excellent	24	17	10	20
Very good	36	32	26	34
Good	29	31	36	30
Fair	11	14	21	13
Poor	4	5	7	4
Provided assistance:				
Did provide assistance	56	44	30	50
Did not provide assistance	44	56	70	50
Received formal home care:				
Received	3	7	22	7
Did not receive	97	93	78	93
Received home care:				
Did not receive home care	89	82	57	83
Received formal home care only	1	2	7	2
Received informal home care only	8	11	21	11
Received both formal and informal home care	2	4	15	4
Provided assistance and received home care:				
Did not receive home care and did provide assistance	50	36	19	42
Received formal home care only and did provide assistance	1	1	2	1
Received informal home care only and did provide assistance	5	5	6	5
Received informal and formal home care and did provide assistance	1	1	3	1
Did not provide assistance	44	56	70	50

Source: Statistics Canada (2013).

and same sex marriage are likely to mean that more women will be living alone or in same-sex marriages and households in the future. The next generation of older women is likely to be much better educated than the current generation of women aged 75 and older. While there certainly will be some improvements in income status and home ownership, whether this will offset the current trends in restructuring of health care services that place increasing responsibilities on families and friends to provide care is more difficult to say.

Table 11.2 highlights the intersections of older women as care receivers and caregivers. As much previous research has documented, the majority of older Canadian women live in good health but as they age, health status declines. More than half of women 45–64 and most women 65–74 provide assistance to others. Even among women aged 75 and over, 30 percent provide assistance to others. In contrast, only a small percentage of older women receive formal home care, and even if one sums up all women aged 75 and over who receive formal home care only, informal home care only, or both informal and formal care, it only amounts to fewer than half of all women in this age group. By looking at who provides assistance and also receives care, what stands out is that while the percentage of older women who only provide assistance declines with age as we might expect, the percentage of older women who provide assistance *and* receive care actually increases with age.

In essence, Tables 11.1 and 11.2 illustrate how demography, the socioeconomic characteristics of older women, and health status of older women converge to place them in "triple jeopardy" as their everyday lives intersect with care receiving and caregiving. Over the next 30 years, as women aged 45–64 become the women aged 75 and over, many of the characteristics of older women will change; but whether the positive gains that women are making will be offset by negative trends in other aspects of everyday life, and structurally with declines in public provision of services, remain open to speculation.

Future Research Directions

We have begun to explore some of the ways in which age, gender, sex, caregiving, and care receiving intersect with other social positions held by older Canadian women. Our investigation focused on women because of the gendered expectations that they face as caregivers, and their vulnerability as care recipients. In so doing, we have excluded the diversity of men's experiences and the impacts of masculinity on health from our chapter. We acknowledge that men are also a diverse group, and that some Canadian men are particularly vulnerable in later life. For example, single, never-married men are known to experience high levels of material and social deprivation (Arber, 2004). There are also an increasing number of studies demonstrating the involvement and challenges that older men caregivers face (Robinson et al., 2014). Nonetheless, our focus on the diversity of older women and their health and caregiving addresses a considerable gap in the literature.

Older Canadian women are not only different from younger women and different from men; they are also different from one another. Their identities are multiple, complex, and dynamic. This chapter addresses only a select few of these identities. Using the CCHS, we were unable to recognize the marginalized position of older racialized minority women in Canada, since the aggregated measures of "race" and ethnicity in CCHS are reduced to a small number of problematic categories, and on-reserve Aboriginal people are not included in the survey. Furthermore, the survey only includes community-dwelling older adults, and thus the multiple identities of the sickest and oldest women in Canada are not included in our secondary analyses. Future research needs to give voice to indigenous women's worldviews and lived realities, in order to look more comprehensively at the range of differences among older women in Canada and how they actually intersect to create either increased burdens or privileges (see also Chapter 3). Indeed, the views of marginalized and vulnerable women in general need to be taken into account to build larger-scale quantitative models that reflect the diverse experiences of older women.

Although there have been several innovative approaches in modeling intersectionality quantitatively, in this chapter we have illustrated the relationships among various social positions, in addition to age, sex, and caregiving and receiving, separately. Future research might model these axes as a composite whole, considering the weight of each variable in different contexts and at different times. Such an approach could reveal the contradictory and situated effects of different variables.

More qualitative research using an intersectional approach to older women's experiences would contribute greatly to our understanding of the lived experiences of the identities of older women, thereby providing the needed context for our CCHS-based analysis. For example, older Canadian women may identify as disabled or present as frail in a formal health care setting, while they may reject such identities in their home, or around their family members and friends (Crooks et al., 2008). As we have demonstrated, even the impacts of gender on health and care experiences will differ over the course of old age and in relation to place. In addition, qualitative approaches could be used to look more closely at the diverse meanings of sex and gender for older women, which we were unable to untangle using survey data. For example, scholars have only just begun to explore the experiences of older lesbian and bisexual women in later life (Grigorovich, 2013) (see also Chapter 4 for a discussion of the importance of considering diverse sexualities in health research). The experiences of transgendered and intersex peoples are required to build a more inclusive view of the diverse experiences of gender and aging in Canada.

Conclusion

The multiple social and physical positions that older women in Canada occupy are complex and changing. If we truly hope to make older women's health better, now and in the future, we need to be attentive to these changes and to look closely at the contexts in which people are left behind. Although more women in the future will have participated in the labor force, and will have higher incomes and higher levels of education than in the past, the shift towards more social and economic power for some women will not be felt by all older women. The absolute number of women experiencing the intersection of multiple forms of marginalization will still be large, and will require considerable investment in health and social support, if the simultaneous care receiver–care giver relationship, and the "triple jeopardy" of declining health, social supports and resources, are to be altered.

Acknowledgments

This research was undertaken in part thanks to funding from the Canada Research Chairs program and the Canadian Institutes of Health Research (CIHR).

References

Abramsky, T., Watts, C.H., Garcia-Moreno, C., Devries, K., Kiss, L., Ellsberg, M., Jansen, H. and Heise, L., 2011. What factors are associated with recent intimate partner violence? Findings from the WHO multi-country study on women's health and domestic violence. *BMC Public Health*, 11(1), pp. 109–26.

Angus, J.E., Lombardo, A.P., Lowndes, R.H., Cechetto, N., Ahmad, F. and Bierman, A.S., 2012. Beyond barriers in studying disparities in women's access to health services in Ontario, Canada: A qualitative metasynthesis. *Qualitative Health Research*, 23(4), pp. 476–94.

Arber, S., 2004. Gender, marital status and ageing: Linking material, health and social resources. *Journal of Aging Studies*, 18(1), pp. 91–108.

Armstrong, P. and Armstrong, H., 2004. Thinking it through: Women, work and caring in the new millennium. In: K.R. Grant, C. Amartunga, P. Armstrong, M. Boscoe, A. Pederson, and K. Wilson eds. *Caring for/caring about: Women, home and unpaid caregiving*. Aurora, ON: Garmond Press, pp. 5–44.

Armstrong, P., Armstrong, H. and Scott-Dixon, K., 2008. *Critical to care: The invisible women in health services*. Toronto: University of Toronto Press.

Aronson, J., 1991. Dutiful daughters and demanding mothers: Constraining images of giving and receiving care in middle and later life. In: C.T. Baines, P.M. Evans and S. Neysmith eds. *Women's caring: Feminist perspectives on social welfare*. Toronto: McClelland & Stewart. pp. 138–68.

Atkinson, S., Lawson, V. and Wiles, J., 2011. Care of the body: spaces of practice. *Social & Cultural Geography*, 12(6), pp. 563–72.

Atwood, M., 1985. *The handmaid's tale*. Toronto: McClelland & Stewart.

Averitt, S.L., Argys, L.M. and Sorkin, J., 2013. In sickness and in health: An examination of relationship status and health using data from the Canadian National Public Health Survey. *Review of Economics of the Household*, 11(4), pp. 599–633.

Bauer, G.R., 2014. Incorporating intersectionality theory into population health research methodology: Challenges and the potential to advance health equity. *Social Science & Medicine*, 110, pp. 10–17.

Bird, C.E. and Rieker, P.P., 2008. *Gender and health: The effects of constrained choices and social policies.* New York: Cambridge University Press.

Chow, H.P., 2010. Growing old in Canada: Physical and psychological well-being among elderly Chinese immigrants. *Ethnicity & Health*, 15(1), pp. 61–72.

Clarke, L.H. and Korotchenko, A., 2011. Aging and the body: A review. *Canadian Journal on Aging/Revue Canadienne du vieillissement*, 30, pp. 495–510.

Crawley, L. and Lynch, K., 2012. The emotional significance of affective inequalities and why they are important to women in old age. *Journal of Women & Aging*, 24(4), pp. 313–28.

Crenshaw, K., 1989. Demarginalizing the intersection of race and sex: A black feminist critique of antidiscrimination doctrine, feminist theory and antiracist politics. *University of Chicago Legal Forum*, 1, pp. 139–67. Available online at http://chicagounbound.uchicago.edu/cgi/viewcontent.cgi?article=1052&context=uclf (accessed February 12, 2016).

Crooks, V.A., Chouinard, V. and Wilton, R.D., 2008. Understanding, embracing, rejecting: Women's negotiations of disability constructions and categorizations after becoming chronically ill. *Social Science & Medicine*, 67(11), pp. 1837–46.

Dean, J.A. and Wilson, K., 2010. "My health has improved because I always have everything I need here...": A qualitative exploration of health improvement and decline among immigrants. *Social Science & Medicine*, 70(8), pp. 1219–28.

Do, E.K., Cohen, S.A. and Brown, M.J., 2014. Socioeconomic and demographic factors modify the association between informal caregiving and health in the Sandwich generation. *BMC Public Health*, 14(1), p. 362. Available online at http://bmcpublichealth.biomedcentral.com/articles/10.1186/1471-2458-14-362 (accessed February 12, 2016).

Dyck, I., Lewis, N.D. and McLafferty, S., 2001. *Geographies of women's health.* New York: Routledge.

Giesbrecht, M., Crooks, V.A., Williams, A. and Hankivsky, O., 2012. Critically examining diversity in end-of-life family caregiving: Implications for equitable caregiver support and Canada's Compassionate Care Benefit. *International Journal of Equity in Health*, 11, pp. 65–82.

Grigorovich, A., 2013. Long-term care for older lesbian and bisexual women: An analysis of current research and policy. *Social Work in Public Health*, 28(6), pp. 596–606.

Hankivsky, O., 2012. Women's health, men's health, and gender and health: Implications of intersectionality. *Social Science & Medicine*, 74(11), pp. 1712–20.

Herron, R.V. and Skinner, M.W., 2011. Farmwomen's emotional geographies of care: A view from rural Ontario. *Gender, Place & Culture*. 19(2), pp. 232–48.

Hinze, S.W., Lin, J. and Andersson, T.E., 2012. Can we capture the intersections? Older Black women, education, and health. *Women's Health Issues*, 22(1), pp. e91–8. Available online at http://www.whijournal.com/article/S1049-3867(11)00178-2/abstract (accessed January 30, 2016).

Joseph, G. and Joseph, A., 2014. Employment and eldercare: Engaging with embodied spaces of resistance. Paper presented at the International Medical Geography Symposium, Michigan State University, East Lancing, MI, July 8.

Kazanjian, A. and Hankivsky, O., 2008. Reflections on the future of women's health research in a comparative context: Why more than sex and gender matters. *Women's Health Issues*, 18(5), pp. 343–6.

Kobayashi, K.M. and Prus, S.G., 2012. Examining the gender, ethnicity, and age dimensions of the healthy immigrant effect: Factors in the development of equitable health policy. *International Journal of Equity in Health*, 11(1), pp. 8–10.

Koehn, S., Neysmith, S., Kobayashi, K. and Khamisa, H., 2013. Revealing the shape of knowledge using an intersectionality lens: Results of a scoping review on the health and health care of ethnocultural minority older adults. *Ageing and Society*, 33(3), pp. 437–64.

LaPierre, T.A. and Keating, N., 2013. Characteristics and contributions of non-kin carers of older people: A closer look at friends and neighbours. *Ageing and Society*, 33(8), pp. 1442–68.

Matheson, J. and McIntyre, L., 2004. Women respondents report higher household food security than do men in similar Canadian households. *Public Health Nutrition*, 17(1), pp. 40–8.

McDonald, J.T. and Kennedy, S., 2004. Insights into the "healthy immigrant effect": health status and health service use of immigrants to Canada. *Social Science & Medicine*, 59(8), pp. 1613–27.

McDonald, L. and Robb, A.L., 2004. The economic legacy of divorce and separation for women in old age. *Canadian Journal on aging/La Revue canadienne du viellissement*, 23(5), pp. S83–97.

Mair, C.A., 2010. Social ties and depression: An intersectional examination of black and white community-dwelling older adults. *Journal of Applied Gerontology*, 29(6), pp. 667–96.

Milligan, C. and Power, A., 2010. The changing geography of care. In: T. Brown, S. McLafferty and G. Moon, eds. *A companion to health and medical geography*. Malden, MA: Blackwell. pp. 567–86.

Newbold, K.B., 2005. Self-rated health within the Canadian immigrant population: Risk and the health immigrant effect. *Social Science & Medicine*, 60(6), pp. 1359–70.

Pillemer, K. and Suitor, J.J., 2013. Who provides care? A prospective study of caregiving among adult siblings. *The Gerontologist*, 54(4), pp. 589–98.

Reczek, C. and Umberson, D., 2012. Gender, health behavior, and intimate relationships: Lesbian, gay, and straight contexts. *Social Science & Medicine*, 74(11), pp. 1783–90.

Robinson, C.A., Bottorff, J.L., Pesut, B., Oliffe, J.L. and Tomlinson, J., 2014. The male face of caregiving: A scoping review of men caring for a person with dementia. *American Journal of Men's Health*, 8(5), pp. 409–26.

Ross, N.A., Garner, R., Bernier, J., Feeny, D.H., Kaplan, M.S., McFarland, B., Orpana, H.M. and Oderkirk, J., 2011. Trajectories of health-related quality of life by socio-economic status in a nationally representative Canadian cohort. *Journal of Epidemiology and Community Health*, 66, pp. 593–8.

Rooss, P., Humble, A.M. and Blum, I., 2013. Sexuality and HIV/AIDS: An exploration of older heterosexual women's knowledge levels. *Journal of Women and Aging*, 25(2), pp. 165–82.

Rozanova, J., Keating, N. and Eales, J., 2012. Unequal social engagement for older adults: Constraints on choice. *Canadian Journal on Aging/Revue Canadienne du viellissement*, 31(1), pp. 25–36.

Ryser, L. and Halseth, G., 2011. Informal support networks of low-income senior women living alone: Evidence from Fort St. John, BC. *Journal of Women & Aging*, 23(3), pp. 185–202.

Seaman, P.M., 2012. Time for my life now: Early boomer women's anticipation of volunteering in retirement. *The Gerontologist*, 52(2), pp. 245–54.

Seng, J.S., Lopez, W.D., Sperlich, M., Hamama, L. and Reed Meldrum, C.D., 2012. Marginalized identities, discrimination burden, and mental health: Empirical exploration of an interpersonal-level approach to modeling intersectionality. *Social Science & Medicine*, 75(12), pp. 2437–45.

Singh Setia, M., Lynch, J., Abrahamowicz, M., Tousignant, P. and Quesnel-Vallee, A., 2011. Self-rated health in Canadian immigrants: Analysis of the Longitudinal Survey of Immigrants to Canada. *Health & Place*, 17(2), pp. 658–70.

Sothern, M. and Dyck, I., 2010. "A penis is not needed in order to pee": Sex and gender in health geography. In: T. Brown, S. McLafferty and G. Moon, eds. *A companion to health and medical geography*. Malden, MA: Blackwell, pp. 258–77.

Springer, K.W., Hankivsky, O. and Bates, L.M., 2012. Gender and health: Relational, intersectional, and biosocial approaches. *Social Science & Medicine*, 74(11), pp. 1661–6.

Statistics Canada, 2013. *Canadian Community Health Survey (CCHS), 2008–2009: Health aging* (study documentation file). Ottawa: Health Statistics Division, Statistics Canada.

Stewart, M.J., Neufeld, A., Harrison, M.J., Spitzer, D., Hughes, K. and Makwarimba, E., 2006. Immigrant women family caregivers in Canada: Implications for policies and programmes in health and social sectors. *Health & Social Care in the Community*, 14, pp. 329–40.

Valentie, G., 2007. Theorizing and researching intersectionality: A challenge for feminist geography. *Professional Geographer*, 59(1), pp. 10–21.

Veenstra, G., 2013. Race, gender, class, sexuality (RGCS) and hypertension. *Social Science & Medicine*, 89, pp. 16–24.

Waldbrook, N., 2013. Formerly homeless, older women's experiences with health, housing, and aging. *Journal of Women & Aging*, 25(4), pp. 337–57.

Waldbrook, N., Rosenberg, M.W. and Brual, J., 2013. Challenging the myth of apocalyptic aging at the local level of governance in Ontario. *The Canadian Geographer/Le Géographe Canadien*, 57(4), pp. 413–30.

Warner, D.F. and Brown, T.H., 2011. Understanding how race/ethnicity and gender define age-trajectories of disability: An intersectionality approach. *Social Science & Medicine*, 72(8), pp. 1236–248.

Williams, A. and Crooks, V.A., 2008. Introduction: space, place and the geographies of women's caregiving work. *Gender, Place and Culture*, 15(3), pp. 243–7.

12 Does the Compassionate Care Benefit Adequately Support Vietnamese Canadian Family Caregivers?

A Diversity Analysis

Irene D. Lum and Allison M. Williams

Since the 1990s, Canada's health care system has been restructured to provide deinstitutionalized care (see Chapter 1 for a brief introduction to this system, and Chapter 10 for further discussion). As the Canadian population continues to age, the burden of caregiving has fallen largely on communities and families (Wilson et al., 2009; Klinger et al., 2014). As a result, more than 2 million informal family caregivers provide more than C$24 billion of unpaid labor each year in Canada (Hollander et al., 2009; Vuksan et al., 2011) (a reality echoed in the analysis presented in Chapter 11). As defined by Health Canada, an informal caregiver is "an individual who provides care and/or support to a family member, friend or neighbor who has a physical or mental disability, is chronically ill or is frail" (Health Canada, 2002, p. 6). To reduce the burden that caregivers face, which may be emotional, physical, mental, social, and/or financial in nature (Carretero et al., 2009; Kogan et al., 2013; Brazil et al., 2014), support is needed. Such support would be particularly meaningful for palliative and end-of-life (P/EOL) caregivers, as those who find themselves within this context often experience magnified emotional and psychosocial stress, and physical demands (Giesbrecht et al., 2012; Brazil et al., 2014). However, P/EOL care services remain accessible to less than one-third of the Canadian caregiving population (Carstairs, 2010).

While access to government support remains an issue for most caregivers, those from minority populations are especially disadvantaged due to cultural and language differences. Little research on family caregiving at the end of life has sought to understand how the caregiving experience is impacted by culture and ethnicity. Even fewer have explored the diversity that exists within particular cultural or ethnic groups. Given Canada's multicultural population, improving government support for minority family caregivers is essential for reducing caregiver burden and enhancing the caregiving experience. In order to accomplish this, it is necessary to understand both how the caregiving experience differs within a cultural or ethnic population, and how it differs between populations.

The purpose of the case study presented in this chapter is to explore how the caregiving experience differs within the Vietnamese Canadian family caregiver population in southern Ontario. By adopting a diversity framework, which recognizes that all individuals differ in, and are impacted by, their social location (Hankivsky and Christoffersen, 2008; Iyer et al., 2008; Sen et al., 2009; Springer et al., 2012) (see Chapter 2 for more details), our study aims to contribute to understanding the lived experiences of Vietnamese Canadian caregivers. Through employing a diversity approach, the complexity and nuances of the caregiving experience are revealed, demonstrating how caregiving is impacted by a number of intersecting factors (Milligan et al., 2007). In this chapter, we focus on the Vietnamese Canadian family caregiver population due to a lack of research concerning this group (Strumpf et al., 2001; Tran et al., 2006; Liu et al., 2008). Although some research has explored Vietnamese health care practices, these have been largely conducted in the USA, and have not addressed P/EOL care issues (Jenkins et al., 1996; Free et al., 1999; Purnell, 2008). Vietnamese Canadians are the thirty-first largest ethnic group in Canada, with an estimated population of approximately 180,000 (Statistics Canada, 2010). The majority of Vietnamese Canadians immigrated to Canada prior to 1991; the remainder arrived via three separate waves, two of which primarily consisted of political refugees (Richard and Dorais, 2003).

The Compassionate Care Benefit

This chapter considers the specific support needs of Vietnamese Canadian family caregivers living in Ontario, and the adequacy of Canada's Compassionate Care Benefit (CCB) in meeting some of these needs. We focus on the CCB because we want to offer an applied example of the ways in which support is being offered to Canadian family caregivers. The CCB is an employment insurance special program which was introduced by the federal government in 2004. Its purpose is to provide employed informal caregivers who are eligible for employment insurance programs with a paid leave of absence to provide informal care for a dying family member (broadly conceived), which can offer both financial support and job security as they balance their employee responsibilities with their caregiving roles. The CCB is funded directly by the federal government through employees' contributory payments to employment insurance: it is payable for a maximum of six weeks, and to a total of C$514 per week to eligible applicants (Service Canada, 2013).

Although the CCB was introduced just over a decade ago and has been recognized as a positive measure for supporting family caregivers (Klinger et al., 2014), it remains a greatly underused program (Osborne and Margo, 2005; Dykeman and Williams, 2013). For example, in the 2011/12 fiscal year, fewer than 6,000 successful claims for CCB were made, despite a significantly larger caregiver population (Employment and Social Development Canada, 2012). Uptake of the CCB is lower than initially anticipated for two primary reasons. First, there are several restrictions on who qualifies for this benefit, including having worked a minimum number of insurable hours in the 52-week period prior to application, and being able to prove that the care recipient is at risk of dying within 26 weeks (Giesbrecht et al., 2012). These restrictions limit both who is willing to apply, and who can qualify successfully for the benefit. Second, uptake of CCB is low due to a general lack of awareness about the program among eligible individuals and the wider Canadian population (Crooks et al., 2007; Giesbrecht et al., 2009; Dykeman and Williams, 2013). A survey conducted by Human Resources and Skills Development Canada (2011) found that 49 percent of Canadians are "somewhat or very aware of income benefits available to individuals who need to take time off work to care for a gravely ill or dying family member," while 39 percent are "not at all aware." Moreover, many front-line health care practitioners report poor knowledge of the CCB's eligibility requirements, and thus are unable to refer their patients to these available benefits (Williams et al., 2010).

Method

Participants and Data Collection

A total of seven Vietnamese family caregivers providing P/EOL care in southern Ontario were interviewed at multiple points over a span of 17 months from 2010–11. This 17-month window provided an opportunity to explore the changes experienced in the caregiving situation over time. In order to target both users and non-users of health care and government support services, participant recruitment occurred through various organizations (health, social service, and religious), as well as in community-at-large via brochures (both English and Vietnamese-language) posted in prominent locations and distributed by collaborating organizations. Vietnamese media sources also helped to advertise and promote the study.

Two female caregivers who were actively providing care, two female bereaved caregivers, and three male active caregivers participated in our interviews. All the participants provided home-based care and, at the time of this study, the care period ranged from three months to more than 25 years. In this chapter, all participants' names have been pseudonymised to protect their anonymity.

Procedure

One to five interviews were conducted with each participant ($n = 23$), lasting from one to three hours in duration. In addition to the formal interviews, a pre-assessment and information-gathering interview was conducted with each participant. The participants were asked specifically about the CCB in order to gauge their awareness of available, family caregiver support. A participant-driven strategy developed by Donovan et al. (2011) was used, whereby first the interview guide was examined by the participants to insure cultural appropriateness, and understanding of the context and meaning of ideas and terminology. In addition, the interview guide was pre-reviewed by cultural brokers or language interpreters, who insured that the research was conducted in a culturally sensitive way, and to better capture cultural norms and subtleties. These cultural brokers helped conduct the interviews and provided in situ translation in the presence of the primary researcher. The primary researcher also kept observational field notes.

Data Analysis

Data analysis took place concurrently with interviewing in order to direct ongoing data collection and identify gaps in the dataset. All the interviews were transcribed and translated, either verbatim or in situ. Transcripts were analysed thematically using a six-step process, with emergent themes being used as coding categories (Fereday and Muir-Cochrane, 2006). Then the coded transcripts were reviewed through the lens of each coding category, in order to explore the similarities and differences between the participants. Through this process, our axes of differences and their implications for the CCB were identified.

Following the style of a similar diversity analysis of the CCB conducted by Giesbrecht et al. (2012), in the next section we examine the key aspects of diversity that emerged from the interviews as being highly important in shaping the Vietnamese Canadian family caregiver experience. Following this, we consider the implications of these aspects of diversity for Vietnamese Canadian family caregivers' access to and use of the CCB, thereby considering the overall adequacy of the program for supporting this particular P/EOL caregiver group.

Findings

Key Aspects of Diversity among Vietnamese Canadian Family Caregivers

Despite sharing cultural beliefs and traditions, differences were observed in the participants' caregiving experiences, indicating that a diversity approach is appropriate for understanding the challenges that family caregivers may face in providing care. Our thematic analysis revealed four aspects of participants' identities to be particularly relevant to shaping these experiences:

1) gender – the constructed roles, values, beliefs, attitudes, and attributes assigned differently to men and women;
2) religion and spirituality – religion is defined here as any social institution which has accepted and shared beliefs and customs; whereas spirituality refers to a personal search for meaning and purpose in life;
3) socioeconomic status – level of income and educational attainment; and
4) length of residency and language – referring to the total time lived in Canada since arrival, and specifically English language acquisition.

Although we acknowledge the complex interrelationships between each of these aspects of participants' identities, for this analysis we examine in-depth each of these axes of difference separately.

Gender

Gendered expectations influenced a number of aspects of the caregiving experience, including why participants provided P/EOL care to their family members in the first place, as well as what sacrifices they made in order to do so. For example, the participants who were women seemed to place greater emphasis on gender expectations and/or gender socialization as a motivating factor for providing care. Several references were made by all four women about how caregiving is a job to be performed by women, and especially by daughters in the case of aging parents. The rationale behind this was the understanding that women were inherently better caregivers, and that by nature they are better suited to providing care, as this quote from Mai illustrates:

> It's not custom. Like English people, it's not just girls 'cause the boy is okay but the girl, in Vietnam, has to be like that. Because you know in Vietnamese, there is no way that a male could care for a female in that manner. The girl is more detailed and careful.

There was also discussion by women participants about how men could not handle certain aspects of caregiving, such as personal care. This seemed to be deeply rooted in cultural beliefs about modesty and norms specific to cross-gender interactions, where it is only acceptable and appropriate for women to perform these highly private and delicate tasks, as Ha states: "A boy couldn't provide care, because we have to wash and bathe and washroom and stuff, they just can't."

However, the participants who were men neither discussed whether or not they felt that caregiving was a role that only women should undertake, nor did they describe personal care situations as inappropriate for them to perform. In fact, for the men participants, gender expectations and/or gender socialization was absent as a motivator for care. Instead, all three expressed that they felt caregiving was part of their duty as a husband, exemplifying the ideal of a supportive, loving, and committed partner: "I have to bring her back home, I have to get her recovery, right? Not only my duty, but a human being – I have to do like that [sic] (Quan). As Duc states: "It's normal – it's my duty."

Among the men, reciprocity as a motivator for care was discussed, which was completely absent from the women participants' interviews. The men believed that if the situation was reversed and they were the ones that required care, their spouses would fulfill the caregiving role for them. Because of this, the men felt that they owed their spouses the same degree of self-sacrifice. Moreover, Duc described how his wife had spent their marriage taking care of him. He viewed caregiving as an opportunity to repay her for her previous devotion to him:

> When we were young and healthy, I asked her: cook this, treat me nice, she always did. ... So when she is sick now, I want to give back the same.

Ideas of reciprocity, love, and commitment were not apparent among the women interviewed. Instead, they seemed to be motivated primarily by perceptions of caregiving as a gendered role typically taken on by women, and by the belief that they alone in their families were capable of providing care. However, there was little discussion of whether or not the familial pressure on women to assume caregiving roles was present, or if the women caregivers simply took it upon themselves to assume the caregiving role.

Ha, who lived with her husband and father while providing care for her mother, also described how she was least essential as an income earner in her household. In order to provide at-home care, it was necessary for one member of her family to temporarily give up work in order to stay with her mother. Perhaps owing to gendered ideas of men being the breadwinners, or maybe because her job earned lower pay, it was decided that it was more important for Ha's husband and father to remain employed while she took on full-time caregiving:. As she states: "My father works and my husband has to work, right? And therefore because I am the daughter, I have to provide care. ... My father and husband work, so they don't have time to help."

For Quan, the need to learn new skills was highlighted as a challenge in providing care. This obstacle did not seem to be as strongly emphasized by the women interviewed, perhaps due to their socialization as carers and to their perception of caregiving as a role typically reserved for women. For Quan, the assistance of health care professionals in providing the necessary training was valuable:

> The hospital teach me a little bit. ... For example, change a diaper, and how to feed her, right? How to bath her, how to bring her in[to] the bathroom. ... Lifting like that, be careful. Legs, arms, how do you move, right? ... The first couple days, I didn't feel comfortable, right? Because I never do [that] before and I feel a little bit scared – but after one week, no problem.

Religion and Spirituality

Of the seven participants, one identified herself as Buddhist but a non-believer, two as Christian/Catholic, two as Buddhist, and one as non-religious but spiritual. Fluidity between religions was noted by another participant, who felt comfortable adopting practices from both Buddhism and Christianity: this was rationalized with the idea that religions share similar fundamental beliefs and can serve the same ends. This was echoed by one participant who described himself as Buddhist, but saw the value of all religions. Strong affiliation to a religion was lacking in most of the individuals, except for the two that identified themselves as Christian/Catholic. Rather, most of the participants appeared to have a moderate level of devotion to their specific faith and its teachings, but embraced personal understandings or interpretations of religion to serve their own needs.

For Linh, who identified herself as Christian/Catholic, religion was discussed as one of the motivators for providing P/EOL care to her husband:

> I will take care of everything, even if he was paralyzed and bedridden for years. I will take responsibility and care for him because I had made a promise in my religion that when he is bedridden, I will take care of him. That was my promise.

For other participants, religion or spirituality served as a facet of their lives, but not a motivator for providing care.

Religion as a coping mechanism was found to be extremely important to the participants, regardless of their level of devotedness to a specific religion. Prayer specifically was the most commonly referenced activity used for coping, as it seemed to provide comfort to caregivers through reassurance of a higher power that is omnipotent and benevolent. As Mai states: "I pray. I give it to God to look after because it's in part of His plan."

Prayer was also an active way for participants to resist pain or suffering, and allowed them to feel as though they were contributing to the recovery of the care recipient when nothing else could be done. Mai said: "[Religion] makes my caregiving experience less, less burden [sic]. ... When you have stress or you have challenge, you pray, and you feel peaceful."

Religious institutions were sources of much-needed social support for two participants who regularly attended church services. One participant joined a prayer group to pray for the health of her mother, and was supported by church friends who sometimes offered food or help. Church leaders also provided spiritual guidance to caregivers during times of emotional turmoil, such as at the death of Linh's husband. Religious institutions also offered a location for caregivers to access health-related information and services: churches and temples provided a place to connect with others who had used care-related services or had gone through similar experiences with family members, and was where Mai met the person she hired as a personal support worker.

When hiring both formal and informal support services, religious identity was not found to be a critical factor in the process. Instead, most of the participants stated that it was only important for support workers to be open-minded to their religious beliefs. Even so, it was beneficial if the worker did share the same religion as the caregiver and care recipient, and thus they could support one another religiously or spiritually, as Mai states: "It would help if [the homemaker is the same religion]. She is Christian – the homemaker, and sometimes she sings hymns and she's very uplifting."

Frequency of attendance at, and involvement with, religious institutions often decreased as the period of caregiving grew longer, because the

participants had less time for social activities. However, this did not necessarily mean that the frequency of religious and/or spiritual practices also
decreased. In fact, in many cases, religiosity and spirituality increased as
caregiving intensified. Caregiving often strengthened participants' faith,
even in cases where the care recipient experienced setbacks to their health.
Blaming a god or higher power was not observed by any participants, and
dissatisfaction with religion or spirituality as a result of the caregiving experience was absent, as Quan states: "I believe more [in my religion since my
wife became ill]. Because I pray every day. Before I sleep, I pray a little bit –
and wake up, I pray."

Spirituality and religion were important aspects of care for the religious participants. Providing medical care alone was not seen as sufficient in improving
the care recipient's health. Rather, engaging in religious or spiritual activities
also were seen as necessary. When care recipients made improvements, this
was attributed to religious or spiritual activity, in addition to medical interventions. As Hien states:

> You have to pray. Everything is related to a faithful heart. ... You pray,
> but you also have to give her medication, give her food, so that it con-
> verges together. If you only pray, and you don't give her the medication or
> food to eat, how can she be well? But in general, it's a faithful heart. You
> have to believe, and you have to do it with all of your heart and strength
> for your mom or your loved ones. You have to have a true spirit, and a
> true love.

Socioeconomic Status

Among the participants there were varying levels of educational attainment,
ranging from elementary school to a university graduate with a business
degree. Despite this variation, all the participants had relatively modest levels
of annual household income, with the highest being C\$40,000 to C\$60,000
per year. After migrating to Canada, all participants worked low-skilled jobs,
with the exception of a music teacher and a public servant.

Intersecting with gender, three of the four participants who were women
were forced to give up employment due to time constraints in order to provide
care. All three were members of the secondary labor market, with relatively
unskilled and low-paying jobs. For these women, their jobs did not provide
significant benefits that would permit them to balance their work responsibilities and their P/EOL care responsibilities. However, Mai was able to maintain
employment because of financial support from her brothers, as well as workplace flexibility that allowed her to work a compressed four-day work-week.
Unlike the other three women, she had a high-skill job:

> I work compressed hours. I work nine hours a day, and then every week
> I have a day off. ... On one day, I can do a few things. You know, some-
> times the weekend, you don't have time to do [anything].

Despite maintaining a career, P/EOL caregiving has impacted Mai's employment in other ways. For example, she described how caregiving limited her opportunities for moving up the career ladder:

> I like to ... with my job, I like to do something more. Let's say at one point, I want to work ... in Ottawa, and I cannot. You know, I'm limited to stay in Toronto. ... Even now, if I want to move, my mom doesn't want to move.

Of the three men participants, two were already retired and caring for their spouses, while the third continued working while providing P/EOL care for his wife. Thus, overall, only two participants were employed at the time of this study. These were also the only two participants who were aware of the CCB's existence, although both opted not to apply for the benefits. Quan opted not to apply due to its inadequate financial compensation; while Mai opted not to apply due to its requirement that the care recipient be at risk of dying within 26 weeks. The remaining five participants did not know about the CCB.

Length of Residency and Language

In general, it was found that of the study participants who had lived in Canada for more than 20 years, those who had arrived at a younger age had better language skills and were more familiar with Canadian culture than their older counterparts. When comparing the participants who had lived in Canada for fewer than 20 years to those who had lived in Canada longer, the latter, as would be expected, had assimilated better into Canadian society than the former. This provided these participants with better social networks and support to aid them in the P/EOL caregiving process. Moreover, they generally made better use of the health care system and its services, perhaps because they were more aware of what is available to them. For example, of the three participants who were men, Quan, who had immigrated to Canada at the youngest age, was able to access social work services, rehabilitative services, hospital care, and training (i.e. learning care skills), as well as personal home care for his wife. However, Duc, who had immigrated to Canada in late adulthood, did not make use of any of these same community services when providing P/EOL care.

English language acquisition was found to have the most significant impact on the caregiving experience, and the participants with low language skills were much more limited in terms of access to the health care system. The participants who had a poor grasp of English often needed to attend the P/EOL care recipient's medical appointments with a friend or relative who could provide informal translation. Alternatively, these participants also sought care exclusively from Vietnamese-speaking physicians, as Duc states: "We ask for the children ... if one is available, then that person will help. ... We ask for relatives, friends, or grandson, or ... we pick a Vietnamese doctor."

In general, caregivers with poorer English skills were more limited in how they could communicate and interact with health care professionals, as well as in what support and services they could access in the health care system.

Discussion

Revisiting the Compassionate Care Benefit

Analysis of these 23 interviews with Vietnamese Canadian family caregivers shows how acknowledging diversity within Canadian ethnic groups is essential for the identification of equitable and effective strategies for reducing caregiver burden. Our results indicate that four major axes of difference shape the experiences of Vietnamese Canadian family caregivers, and the types of support and services to which they have access. The results of this study are notable, both for reaffirming past research on caregiver support, and for bringing light to new challenges that may aggravate caregiver burden within this population.

The findings point to four particularly vulnerable groups *within* the Vietnamese Canadian family caregiver population:

1) non-English speakers who are limited in communication with health care professionals, leading to a poorer grasp of medical information and available services and support;
2) employed caregivers who are women with low-skilled jobs, many of whom give up these jobs with few benefits to provide P/EOL care;
3) caregivers who are men and who must navigate what has been previously viewed as a women-dominated role; and
4) newcomers who lack familiarity with the health care system in Canada.

It is critical that diversity within the caregiver experience be considered, such that caregiver support, programs, and policies such as the CCB can be more responsive to the needs of these vulnerable populations.

Implications for the Compassionate Care Benefit

In the first axis of difference we examined, gender, we found that Vietnamese participants who were men differed from those who were women in terms of what motivated them to assume the caregiving role. Expectations for women to take on this position were vocalized by all four participants who were women, and this gendered reality is a phenomenon observed within the larger caregiver population in Canada (Williams and Crooks, 2008; Carstairs, 2010), where an estimated two-thirds of all of Canada's family caregivers are women (Vuksan et al., 2011). In contrasted with the men participants, who expressed a greater sense of personal choice in deciding to provide care, the women seemed to feel comparatively more pressured into the caregiving role.

Thus, one way to increase support for women caregivers may be to appreciate them better for their care work, and consequently reduce their sense of solitude in their caregiving role. This assistance may be well received if provided by health care professionals – particularly when family support is absent. As previous research has recognized, health care professionals can play a crucial role not only in treating the patient, but also in offering social support for both the patient and the family, the latter of which often includes the caregiver (Williams et al., 2011; Guerriere et al., 2013). This support could extend to such professionals actively discussing the CCB with women caregivers whom they believe are eligible for the benefit, and ensuring that they have the skills and resources necessary to complete the paperwork.

In the second axis we examined, religion and/or spirituality, the findings show that despite mixed levels of devotedness and differences in beliefs, religion and spirituality were important coping mechanisms for all seven participants. This trend is echoed in the larger literature examining the relationship between religion or spirituality and health, which finds that, in general, religion and/or spirituality can help individuals maintain hope, happiness, and self-esteem when providing P/EOL care (Dew et al., 2010; Harvey and Cook, 2010; Visser et al., 2010; Chen et al., 2011; Marini and Glover-Graf, 2011). For caregivers specifically, religion and/or spirituality may be important in helping one focus on the rewards of the caregiving experience (Parveen et al., 2011; Delgado-Guay et al., 2012). Our study also found that the participants relied on religious institutions as sources of social support, which again is seen elsewhere in the research literature (Dew et al., 2010; Peterson, 2011; Delgado-Guay et al., 2012; Svalina and Webb, 2012). However, beyond social support, the research also identified that participants sought information regarding community health services within these institutions. This is an important finding, as it suggests that these organizations should be targeted in the outreach process about the CCB, given that the benefit is reported to have low uptake, and that there is a general lack of awareness about its existence.

In the third axis of difference examined, socioeconomic status, we found that three of the four participants who were women were forced to give up their jobs to fulfill the P/EOL caregiving role. Contrasted with the one employed man in our study who continued to work while caring for his wife, our study reflects larger trends in the literature which suggest that women in particular often sacrifice their employment in order to provide care (Clemmer et al., 2008; Reid et al., 2010; Vuksan et al., 2011). Women working in the unskilled labor market (such as those who gave up their jobs in our study) are most vulnerable to this job loss, as such part-time and low-paying positions typically have few benefits and high turnover rates (Vuksan et al., 2012). Moreover, with the CCB eligibility requirement of working a minimum of 600 insurable hours in the last 52 weeks prior to applying, this population of workers is excluded from eligibility for these benefits; consequently, these caregivers also lack government financial support which may have helped to protect their jobs (Williams et al., 2010). Thus, one way that government support can be improved is by extending CCB coverage, such that all employed caregivers can qualify – which would require it to be removed from the employment insurance program and housed elsewhere.

For Mai, who was able to keep her job after she began providing care for her mother, she did not apply for the CCB but instead relied on flexibility from her workplace, which offered her a compressed work schedule. Quan, the one employed man in our study, also did not apply for the CCB, due to the requirement that the care recipient must be at risk of dying within 26 weeks. These findings are significant, because they highlight how the CCB is inadequate in meeting the needs of the Vietnamese Canadian family caregivers with whom we spoke. For these two participants, the decision not to apply stemmed from the benefit not providing adequate financial support, as well as from its strict restrictions on who can qualify. Past research on the CCB has cited both these reasons as deterrents for potential applicants, and thus are major criticisms of the program (Williams et al., 2010, 2011; Giesbrecht et al., 2012). In situations where the CCB is inadequate or inaccessible to family caregivers, workplace flexibility and support for employed P/EOL caregivers through this flexibility are vital. The remaining five participants were unaware of the CCB's existence, which echoes larger literature findings that lack of awareness of the CCB contributes to its low uptake (Giesbrecht et al., 2009, 2010; Dykeman and Williams, 2013).

In the fourth and final axis of difference, length of residency and language, we found that language barriers were a major problem for some participants in providing P/EOL care. These participants were typically new immigrants to Canada, or had settled in Canada at an older age; consequently, they had to rely on friends or relatives to provide informal translation, or had to seek Vietnamese-speaking health care professionals. Past research on immigrant health has found that language is often the most significant barrier to immigrants' use of the health care system (Reitmanova and Gustafson, 2007; Asanin and Wilson, 2008; Wang et al., 2008; Sun et al., 2010; Klassen et al., 2012). Our study agrees with the existing literature in respect of having more interpreters on site, a culturally and linguistically-diverse health care workforce, and multilingual documentation for forms, applications, and informational leaflets (Asanin and Wilson, 2008; Giesbrecht et al., 2012; Klassen et al., 2012). In regard to the CCB, the need to complete the necessary paperwork and application process is complicated by issues of language competency as well as literacy among Vietnamese Canadian P/EOL caregivers, thus acting as obstacles to accessing financial support through the program (Klassen et al., 2012).

Future Research Directions

While caregiving has been generally understood as a role filled by women, studies have found that caregivers in Canada come from all ethnic, linguistic, gender, religious, and socioeconomic backgrounds (Donovan et al., 2011;

Giesbrecht et al., 2012). As such, it is important to explore how diversity among differing population groups, including Vietnamese Canadians, could shape caregiving experiences. For example, despite a growing number of men providing care, their experiences have not been well documented, and thus our study is unique in that it has explored this perspective in addition to those of women among Vietnamese Canadians. Previous research has shown that lack of expertise in providing care can greatly aggravate caregiver burden (van Ryn et al., 2011; Stajduhar et al., 2013; Kanter et al., 2014). Thus, the relative newness of men in the caregiver role, in addition to other variables such as lack of English language proficiency, suggests that they may be especially vulnerable and requiring greater attention and support from health care professionals.

The research also explored how length of time in Canada impacted the caregiving experience. We found that participants who had lived in Canada for a longer period of time typically had better access to available services; this was the result of having increased familiarity with the Canadian health care system, stronger social networks in the location of settlement, and a better grasp of the English language. Thus, in addition to improving health care system access for minorities, special attention must be paid to better outreach to newcomers. This issue needs to be further examined through first-hand research prior to identifying strategies for such outreach, in order to insure cultural relevancy among Vietnamese Canadians.

Conclusion

Such findings point to the need to understand better the nuances of the caregiving experience, and to tease out the highly intricate relationships between social dimensions – both within a specific group such as the Vietnamese Canadians, and between groups in the larger Canadian population. This process of identifying how social dimensions shape the caregiving experience has the potential to capture a more accurate picture of social inequity and power relations in Canadian society, and thus better equip researchers, policymakers, and other stakeholders with more equitable ways to reform health and social care programs, such as the CCB, to reduce systemic disparities (Hankivsky and Christoffersen, 2008; Iyer et al., 2008; Hankivsky et al., 2010; Hankisvky and Cormier, 2011). Thus, this research confirms the need for more researchers to apply diversity frameworks to family caregiver research in order to understand better how complex social locations can impact the caregiving experience. Moreover, it follows a growing trend in health literature that recognizes the importance of conducting diversity-based health research for generating policy-relevant findings (Hankivsky and Cormier, 2011; Springer et al., 2012).

Given the four axes of difference examined in this analysis, we put forth several recommendations for improving government support for family caregivers. To support women better who may have felt pressured to take on the caregiving role, health care professionals should help these individuals feel more appreciated for their work, and less isolated in providing care and accessing the support they need, including the CCB.

For caregivers who are men, health care professionals may play an important role in helping them navigate and learn what has been previously viewed as a role fulfilled only by women. In addition, training health care professionals in cross-religious and cross-cultural situations may be beneficial, as religion and/or spirituality was found to be powerful coping mechanisms. Furthermore, targeting religious institutions in disseminating information related to health care services and government support may help with increasing family caregiver awareness of available programs, including the underutilized CCB.

Our study also indicates that support for family caregivers must be improved to meet the needs of a diverse family caregiver population better. This includes lowering eligibility requirements for the CCB, such that more family caregivers can qualify; increasing the amount of the benefits, such that more family caregivers will apply; providing language services for family caregivers not speaking English or French in order to enable them to apply; and targeting informational outreach to newcomers, so they know that they can apply.

Acknowledgments

This work was supported by a Canadian Institutes of Health Research grant titled "Cultural Influences on Caregiving at End-of-Life" (201724). We would like to thank Rhonda Donovan, who tirelessly played a key role in data collection.

References

Asanin, J. and Wilson, K., 2008. "I spent nine years looking for a doctor": Exploring access to health care among immigrants in Missisauga, Ontario, Canada. *Social Science & Medicine*, 66(6), pp. 1271–83.

Brazil, K., Kaasalainen, S., Williams, A. and Dumont, S., 2014. A comparison of support needs between rural and urban family caregivers providing palliative care. *American Journal of Hospice and Palliative Medicine*, 31(1), pp. 13–19.

Carretero, S., Garcés, J., Ródenas, F. and Sanjose, V., 2009. The informal caregiver's burden of dependent people: Theory and empirical review. *Archives of Gerontology and Geriatrics*, 49(1), pp. 74–9.

Carstairs, S., 2010. *Raising the bar: A Roadmap for the future of palliative care in Canada* Available online at www.chpca.net/media/7859/Raising_the_Bar_June_2010.pdf (accessed February 4, 2016).

Chen, R.K., Glover-Graf, N.M. and Marini, I., 2011. Religion and spirituality in the lives of people with multiple sclerosis. *Journal of Religion, Disability & Health*, 15(3), pp. 254–71.

Clemmer, S.J., Ward-Griffin, C. and Forbes, D., 2008. Family members providing home-based palliative care to older adults: The enactment of multiple roles. *Canadian Journal on Aging*, 27(3), pp. 267–83.

Crooks, V.A., Williams, A., Stajduhar, K.I., Allan, D.E. and Cohen, R., 2007. The information transfer and knowledge acquisition geographies of family caregivers: An analysis of Canada's Compassionate Care Benefit. *Canadian Journal of Nursing Research*, 39(3), pp. 36–54.

Delgado-Guay, M.O., Parsons, H.A., Hui, D., De la Cruz, M.G., Thorney, S. and Bruera, E., 2012. Spirituality, religiosity, and spiritual pain among caregivers of patients with advanced cancer. *American Journal of Hospice and Palliative Medicine*, 30(5), pp. 455–61.

Dew, R.E., Daniel, S.S., Goldston, D.B., McCall, W.V., Kuchibhatla, M., Schleifer, C., Triplett, M.F. and Koenig, H.G., 2010. A prospective study of religion/spirituality and depressive symptoms among adolescent psychiatric patients. *Journal of Affective Disorders*, 120(1–3), pp. 149–57.

Donovan, R., Williams, A., Stajduhar, K., Brazil, K. and Marshall, D., 2011. The influence of culture on home-based family caregiving at end-of-life: A case study of Dutch reformed family care givers in Ontario, Canada. *Social Science & Medicine*, 72(3), pp. 338–46.

Dykeman, S. and Williams, A., 2013. The importance of place and time in translating knowledge about Canada's Compassionate Care Benefit to informal caregivers. *Journal of Social Work in End-of-Life & Palliative Care*, 9(4), pp. 289–307.

Employment and Social Development Canada, 2012. *EI special benefits*. Available online at www.esdc.gc.ca/eng/jobs/ei/reports/mar2012/chapter2_4.shtml (accessed September 28, 2014).

Fereday, J. and Muir-Cochrane, E., 2006. Demonstrating rigor using thematic analysis: A hybrid approach of inductive and deductive coding and theme development. *International Journal of Qualitative Methodology*, 5(1), pp. 1–11.

Free, C., White, P., Shipman, C. and Dale, J., 1999. Access to and use of out-of-hours services by members of Vietnamese community groups in South London: A focus group study. *Family Practice*, 16(4), pp. 369–74.

Giesbrecht, M., Crooks, V.A. and Williams, A. 2010. Scale as an explanatory concept: Evaluating Canada's Compassionate Care Benefit. *Area*, 42(4), pp. 457–67.

Giesbrecht, M., Crooks, V.A., Schuurman, N. and Williams, A., 2009. Spatially informed knowledge translation: Informing potential users of Canada's Compassionate Care Benefit. *Social Science & Medicine*, 69(3), pp. 411–19.

Giesbrecht, M., Crooks, V.A., Williams, A. and Hankivsky, O., 2012. Critically examining diversity in end-of-life family caregiving: Implications for equitable caregiver support and Canada's Compassionate Care Benefit. *International Journal for Equity in Health*, 11(65), pp. 1–13.

Guerriere, D.N., Zagorski, B. and Coyte, P.C., 2013. Family caregiver satisfaction with home-based nursing and physician care over the palliative care trajectory: Results from a longitudinal survey questionnaire. *Palliative Medicine*, 27(7), pp. 632–8.

Hankivsky, O. and Christoffersen, A., 2008. Intersectionality and the determinants of health: A Canadian perspective. *Critical Public Health*, 18(3), pp. 271–83.

Hankivsky, O. and Cormier, R., 2011. Intersectionality and public policy: Some lessons from existing models. *Political Research Quarterly*, 64(1), pp. 217–29.

Hankivsky, O., Reid, C., Cormier, R., Varcoe, C., Clark, N., Benoit, C. and Brotman, S., 2010. Exploring the promises of intersectionality for advancing women's health research. *International Journal for Equity in Health*, 9(5), pp. 1–15.

Harvey, I.S. and Cook, L., 2010. Exploring the role of spirituality in self-management practices among older African-American and non-Hispanic White women with chronic conditions. *Chronic Illness*, 6(2), pp. 111–24.

Health Canada, 2002. *National profile of family caregivers in Canada – 2002: Final Report.* Ottawa: Health Canada.

Hollander, M.J., Liu, G. and Chappell, N.L., 2009. Who cares and how much? The imputed economic contribution to the Canadian health care system of middle aged and older unpaid caregivers providing care to the elderly. *Healthcare Quarterly*, 12(2), pp. 42–59.

Human Resources and Skills Development Canada, 2011. *Employment Insurance (EI) Tracking Survey 2011.* Available online at http://epe.lac-bac.gc.ca/100/200/301/pwgsc-tpsgc/por-ef/human_resources_development/2011/086-10-e/EItracking Study11-eng.html#cc (accessed October 23, 2014).

Iyer, A., Sen, G. and Ostlin, P., 2008. The intersections of gender and class in health status and health care. *Global Public Health*, 3(Supp. 1), pp. 13–24.

Jenkins, C.N., Le, T., McPhee, S.J., Stewart, S. and Ha, N.T., 1996. Health care access and preventive care among Vietnamese immigrants: Do traditional beliefs and practices pose barriers? *Social Science and Medicine*, 43(7), pp. 1049–56.

Kanter, C., D'Agostino, N.M., Daniels, M., Stone, A. and Edelstein, K., 2014. Together and apart: Providing psychosocial support for patients and families living with brain tumours. *Support Care Cancer*, 22(1), pp. 43–52.

Klassen, A.F., Gulati, S., Watt, L., Banerjee, A.T., Sung, L., Klassen, R.J., Dix, D., Poureslami, I.M. and Shaw, N., 2012. Immigrant to Canada, newcomer to childhood cancer: A qualitative study of challenges faced by immigrant parents. *Psycho-oncology*, 21(5), pp. 558–62.

Klinger, C.A., Howell, D., Zakus, D. and Deber, R.B., 2014. Barriers and facilitators to care for the terminally ill: A cross-country case comparison study of Canada, England, Germany and the United States. *Palliative Medicine*, 28(2), pp. 111–20.

Kogan, N.R., Dumas, M. and Cohen, S.R., 2013. The extra burdens patients in denial impose on their family caregivers. *Palliative and Supportive Care*, 11(2), pp. 91–9.

Liu, D., Hinton, L., Tran, C., Hinton, D. and Barker, J.C., 2008. Reexamining the relationships among dementia, stigma, and aging in immigrant Chinese and Vietnamese family caregivers. *Journal of Cross Cultural Gerontology*, 23(3), pp. 283–99.

Marini, I. and Glover-Graf, N.M., 2011. Religiosity and spirituality among persons with spinal cord injury: Attitudes, beliefs, and practices. *Rehabilitation Counseling Bulletin*, 54(2), pp. 82–92.

Milligan, C., Atkinson, S., Skinner, M. and Wiles, J., 2007. Geographies of care: A commentary. *New Zealand Geographer*, 63(2), pp. 135–40.

Osborne, K. and Margo, N., 2005. *Analysis and evaluation of Canada's Compassionate Care Benefit.* Ottawa: Health Council of Canada.

Parveen, S., Morrison, V. and Robinson, C.A., 2011. Ethnic variations in the caregiver role: A qualitative study. *Journal of Health Psychology*,16(6), pp. 862–72.

Peterson, J.L., 2011. The case for connection: Spirituality and social support for women living with HIV/AIDS. *Journal of Applied Communication Research*, 39(4), pp. 352–69.

Purnell, L.D., 2008. Traditional Vietnamese health and healing. *Urologic Nursing*, 28(1), pp. 63–7.

Reid, C., Stajduhar, K.I. and Chappell, N., 2010. Impact of work interference on family caregiver outcomes. *Journal of Applied Gerontology*, 29(3), pp. 267–89.

Reitmanova, S. and Gustafson, D.L., 2007. "They can't understand it": Maternity health and care needs of immigrant Muslim women in St. John's, Newfoundland. *Maternal Child Health Journal*, 12(1), pp. 101–11.

Richard, E. and Dorais, L.J., 2003. Statistical profile of immigrants of Vietnamese origin in Quebec and in Canada: Comparison of 1991, 1996 and 2001 data. *Review of Vietnamese Studies*, 3(1), pp. 1–9.

Service Canada, 2013. *Employment Insurance Compassionate Care Benefits*. Available online at www.servicecanada.gc.ca/eng/ei/types/compassionate_care.shtml (accessed October 1, 2014).

Sen, G., Iyer, A. and Mukherjee, C., 2009. A methodology to analyze the intersections of social inequalities in health. *Journal of Human Development and Capabilities*, 10(3), pp. 397–415.

Springer, K.W., Hankivsky, O. and Bates, L.M., 2012. Gender and health: Relational, intersectional, and biosocial approaches. *Social Science & Medicine*, 74(11), pp. 1661–6.

Stajduhar, K.I., Funk, L. and Outcalt, L., 2013. Family caregiver learning – how family caregivers learn to provide care at the end of life: A qualitative secondary analysis of four datasets. *Palliative Medicine*, 27(7), pp. 657–64.

Statistics Canada, 2010. *Visual census, ethnic origin and visible minorities, Ontario: 2006 census*. Available online at www12.statcan.gc.ca/census-recensement/2006/dp-pd/fs-fi/index.cfm?Lang=ENG&TOPIC_ID=11&PRCODE=35 (accessed September 28, 2014).

Strumpf, N., Glicksman, A., Goldberg-Glen, R., Fox, R. and Logue, E., 2001. Caregiver and older adult experiences of Cambodian, Vietnamese, Soviet Jewish, and Ukranian refugees. *International Journal of Aging and Human Development*, 53(3), 233–52.

Sun, Z., Xiong, H., Kearney, A., Zhang, J., Liu, W., Huang, G. and Wang, P.P., 2010. Breast cancer screening among Asian immigrant women in Canada. *Cancer Epidemiology*, 34(1), pp. 73–8.

Svalina, S.S. and Webb, J.R., 2012. Forgiveness and health among people in outpatient physical therapy. *Disability and Rehabilitation*, 34(5), pp. 383–92.

Tran, J.N., Tran, C.G. and Hinton, L., 2006. Working with Vietnamese American families. In: G. Yeo and D. Gallager-Thompson, eds. *Ethnicity and the dementias*. New York: Routledge, pp. 263–83.

van Ryn, M., Sanders, S., Kahn, K., van Houtven, C., Griffin, J.M., Martin, M., Atienza, A.A., Phelan, S., Finstad, D. and Rowland, J., 2011. Objective burden, resources, and other stressors among informal cancer caregivers: A hidden quality issue? *Psycho-oncology*, 20(1), pp. 44–52.

Visser, A., Garssen, B. and Vingerhoets, A., 2010. Spirituality and well-being in cancer patients: A review. *Psycho-oncology*, 19(6), pp. 565–72.

Vuksan, M., Williams, A.M. and Crooks, V., 2011. The workplace perspective on supporting family caregivers at end of life: Evaluating a new Canadian social program. *Community, Work & Family*, 15(3), pp. 317–33.

Vuksan, M., Williams, A. and Crooks, V., 2012. Family friendly policies: Accommodating end-of-life caregivers in workplaces. *International Journal of Workplace Health Management*, 5(1), pp. 4–14.

Wang, L., Rosenberg, M. and Lo, L., 2008. Ethnicity and utilization of family physicians: A case study of mainland Chinese immigrants in Toronto, Ontario. *Social Science & Medicine*, 67(9), pp. 1410–22.

Williams, A. and Crooks, V., 2008. Space, place, and the geographies of women's caregiving work. *Gender, Place & Culture*, 15(3), pp. 243–47.

Williams, A., Crooks, V., Giesbrecht, M. and Dykeman, S., 2010. *Evaluating Canada's Compassionate Care Benefit from the perspective of family caregivers*. Hamilton: McMaster University.

Williams, A., Eby, J., Crooks, V.A., Stajduhar, K., Giesbrecht, M., Vuksan, M., Cohen, R., Brazil, K. and Allan, D., 2011. Canada's Compassionate Care Benefit: Is it an adequate public health response to addressing the issue of caregiver burden in end-of-life care? *BMC Public Health*, 11, pp. 335–49.

Wilson, D.M., Truman, C.D., Thomas, R., Fainsinger, R., Kovacs-Burns, K., Froggatt, K. and Justice, C., 2009. The rapidly changing location of death in Canada, 1994–2004. *Social Science & Medicine*, 68(10), pp. 1752–8.

13 Conclusion

Ways Ahead in Diversity-based Health Geography Research

Valorie A. Crooks and Melissa D. Giesbrecht

As mentioned in Chapter 1, across sectors of Canadian society (e.g. government, policy and planning initiatives, social conventions), diversity is defined often in terms of cultural and ethnic variations among and between people (Citizenship and Immigration Canada, 2010; Clow et al., 2015). Recognizing this kind of diversity is critical in health research, as culture and ethnicity affect our values, beliefs, and behaviors, which in turn shape our understandings and experiences of health. However, it is important to keep in mind that while cultural and ethnic variations are important, if we focus only on this kind of "visible" diversity, we overlook all those other forms of difference that simultaneously shape our health and well-being (Hankivsky and Christoffersen, 2008; Clow et al., 2009, 2015). For example, we are likely to ignore those other important variables that are not always as obvious, such as sexual orientation, education, and religious beliefs. Together, the chapters in this book have moved beyond this common understanding of "cultural" diversity to reflect on what diversity means across a variety of peoples and places, and what it can mean within the context of health geography. The result is this unique collection, which we hope has given multiple examples of how diversity can be understood and applied in differing research specializations, thus providing readers with model studies from which they can draw in their own health geography scholarship.

Thematic Reflection

As noted in Chapters 1 and 2, the most common approach to diversity-focused analyses are in-depth examinations of the diversity that exists *within* particular populations which, in general, tend to be viewed largely as homogenous groups by society, researchers, and policy alike. Chapters 3, 4, 10, 11, and 12 in particular all disrupt this common assumption and contribute valuable knowledge regarding the different health experiences, needs, and outcomes that exist among or within some of Canada's minority and/or more marginalized populations.

In Chapter 3, Castleden, Martin and Lewis acknowledged the common experiences that Aboriginal people in Canada collectively share: in particular, a history of colonization and a generally higher risk of having poorer health, compared to non-Aboriginal Canadians. Much contemporary health research on this topic tends to stop here – comparing Aboriginal with non-Aboriginal health status, and assuming that all Aboriginal peoples are the same. However, the authors looked deeper to demonstrate the vast diversity that exists *within* this population group: specifically, how culture, geographic place of residence, gender, sexuality, and socioeconomic status all complexly intersect to create diverse understandings and experiences of health, and ultimately health outcomes, among Canada's various Aboriginal populations. Similarly, in Chapter 12, Lum and Williams moved beyond culture and ethnicity alone to emphasize that differences in gender, religion, culture, and socioeconomic status exist within Canada's Vietnamese population, which ultimately shapes their unique family caregiver experiences and their needs for support. Both of these chapters disrupted the common notion of diversity as being simply based on culture and ethnicity, and importantly draw attention to those other variables of difference that often tend to go unseen within health research focused on minority ethnic, racial and cultural groups.

Chapters 10 and 11 explored diversity within particular groups of women who share common experiences either of aging or illness diagnosis. Both chapters highlighted how differing lived positions can shape experiences of health and health care, as well as opportunities to access the support and services needed. In Chapter 10, Crooks explored the complex relationship between macro and micro health care experiences in the lives of women living with the chronic illness, fibromyalgia syndrome. She found that their experiences as recipients of formal health care are shaped by their unique social location, access to care, and bodily experiences as well as the larger organization and workings of Canada's health care system. In Chapter 11, Herron and Rosenberg explored diverse experiences of health among Canada's aged women. More specifically, they examined how social and physical roles intersected in older women's lives, and shaped their opportunities over time and across space. They contended that while today many older women face a "triple jeopardy" of declining health, declining social support, and declining resources while simultaneously being expected to be caregivers in the home, some will find the opportunity to position themselves outside of caregiving.

In Chapter 4, Holmes explored diversity within gender and sexuality: categories of difference that continue to be seen by many health researchers as simply binary – man/woman, male/female, homosexual/heterosexual, and/or gay/straight. Here, Holmes shed light on the complexity that exists within gender and sexuality by exploring the links between trans and gender nonconforming people, violence, and mental health in particular places. Importantly, she demonstrated that the concept of diversity also includes sex and gender, as well as other factors such as "race" and place of residence – all of which together influence how we see ourselves and how others see us, how we behave, and how easy it is to achieve and maintain a sense of health and well-being.

Some particularly unique and novel approaches illustrated in this collection included exploring diversity in services and within the health care system. For example, in Chapter 9, Temenos and Johnston not only investigated the differences, but also the similarities, in the use of language and ideological concepts between private service care providers which have emerged in light of the limitations inherent within Canada's public health care system. Here, medical tourist and harm reduction service providers were found to position themselves similarly as providing "personal choice" in care, but in fact were providing a very "radical" sense of choice in similar consumerist ways to two very different patient groups. Building from here, diversity in practices was explored in Chapter 5, where Evans and Wilton highlighted the diversity that exists in Canadian workplaces, emphasizing how social enterprises are designed explicitly to be inclusive, while conventional workplaces still pose many barriers to meaningful employment for many Canadians.

In Chapters 7 and 8, the authors focused their attention on deprivation mapping: a contemporary area of health geographic research in Canada and beyond which examines the social determinants of health among populations in order to identify who are most "vulnerable," and where they reside. Here, both chapters demonstrated the harm that can be done by such mapping, and the knowledge that can be missed when deprivation mapping researchers take a top-down approach, fail to engage with populations, and thus undermine their equity-based goals. For example, in Chapter 7, Masuda and Skinner present an alternative "relational" deprivation index, which is based on input by those residents living in so-called "deprived" neighborhoods. In Chapter 8, also engaging with those residing in "deprived" or "Code Red" neighborhoods, Cahuas, Malik, and Wakefield examined the inherent power dynamics that exist in deprivation mapping research, and provided an example of how underlying, often unconscious narratives of dominance are reproduced in and through the media on health inequities. In both chapters, the authors presented perspectives and concerns of residents that challenge and transform dominant narratives.

The general approach taken by all the authors in their chapters was critical, with many of the chapters drawing links to those diverse, broader structures that complexly intersect to shape lived experiences, which in turn create the health inequities experienced by Canadians today. For example, racism, colonialism, sexism, classism, agism, ableism, and cisnormativity were raised in various chapters throughout this collection as social structures that hold significant implications for the health of individual Canadians. The analytic techniques and methods used by the contributing authors also varied and include literature reviews, content analyses, interviews, observational field notes, descriptive statistical analyses, spatial analyses, intersectionality, participatory action, as well as mixed and multi-method approaches. Cinnamon and Sui, in Chapter 6, made a call for more researchers to engage with mixed-methods research in particular in order to gain more nuanced understandings in diversity-based research. For example, they demonstrated the valuable role that mixed-methods approaches play in merging the spatial-analytical with contextual qualitative data, in order to identify specific locations and population groups that are disproportionately at risk of pedestrian injury. This call for more mixed-method research was echoed by Masuda and Skinner in Chapter 7.

Together, this collection provides multiple examples of diversity-based health geography research in various Canadian contexts. These various applications of diversity frameworks – to populations, systems, services, practices, and structures that shape sociospatial life – help us to gain a more nuanced understanding of how people who share many commonalities ultimately have radically different health and life outcomes.

Ways Ahead in Diversity-based Health Geography Research

We believe that each chapter in this volume offers specific directions for future health geography research, while the collection as a whole also offers insights into how and where health geographers should depart from, in terms of conducting their own diversity-focused research. While this collection is anchored by a consistent focus on Canada and the Canadian experience, by no means are these research directions bound only to health geographers studying Canada. One useful way to conceptualize these directions is through considering six main messages emerging from this collection.

First, diversity can mean different things in different health geography research contexts. Second, an array of methods and research approaches can be used to explore diversity in health geography research. Third, it is essential that health geographers acknowledge diversity within populations that are commonly conceptualized as homogeneous. Fourth, it is similarly important for health geographers to recognize the value held in uncovering experiential perspectives. Fifth, diversity frameworks need not only be applied to populations, but also systems (e.g. health care systems), services (e.g. access to social support), practices (e.g. inclusive workplaces), and other structures (e.g. social structures such as racism, sexism, and colonialism) that shape sociospatial life. Such applications by health geographers can help us to understand how people who share many commonalities ultimately can have radically different health and life outcomes. Finally, health geographers are particularly well positioned to uncover the ways in which care practices happen in diverse spaces; health and well-being are achieved through exposure to healthful spaces; and health-promoting activities account for space in their place-focused diversity analyses. These messages are woven throughout the discussion in the previous section.

To embrace both the potential and the challenge of taking up diversity-based approaches in health geography, health geographers need to ask themselves questions during the inception, data collection, and analysis phases of their research which can assist them in seeing health-related problems in completely new ways. While there is neither a "master list" of such questions, nor a set order in which they should be asked, we believe the following offer some meaningful direction.

- Which voices or perspectives are not currently reflected in my research questions? What does their absence mean for my ability to speak to the full scope of factors that shape participants' lives and experiences?

- Do my questions and/or analytic approaches favor a dominant positioning, population group, or perspective? If they do, how will this limit my ability to engage with truly understanding the root causes of the results generated by my analyses?
- What is the relationship between the methods I use and my ability to use diversity, intersectionality, and/or a related issue as a central explanatory concept?
- Why does the existing research on this topic privilege particular axes of difference or perspectives, and is it my responsibility to unsettle them through identifying new ways of answering these questions?
- Where are the spaces and places within which diversity is mute, silent, or invisible? How has such lack of voice or visibility shaped existing approaches to similar research?
- How do I go about posing questions and identifying approaches to research that truly uncover the full spectrum of differences (and similarities) in people, places, structures, and systems that support a diversity approach to my research?

We encourage health geographers seeking to undertake diversity-focused research to ask themselves these and other critical questions throughout the course of their research, in order to insure that they never lose sight of the criticality needed to engage with such complex concepts. Further to this, we recommend that students and trainees at the undergraduate and graduate levels be exposed to the types of diversity approaches introduced in Chapter 2, the six main messages of this collection summarized above, and the critical thinking questions synthesized here in order to prepare the next generation of health geographers to undertake research that introduces complex aspects of diversity yet even to be considered.

References

Citizenship and Immigration Canada, 2010. *Mulitculturalism.* Available online at www.cic.gc.ca/english/multiculturalism/index.asp (accessed November 29, 2010).

Clow, B., Pederson, A., Haworth-Brockman, M. and Bernier, J., 2009. *Rising to the challenge: Sex- and gender-based analysis for health planning, policy and research in Canada.* Halifax: Atlantic Centre of Excellence for Women's Health.

Clow, B., Hanson, Y. and Bernier, J., 2015. *Diversity.* Center of Excellence for Women's Health. Available online at http://sgba-resource.ca/en/concepts/diversity/ (accessed March 21, 2015).

Hankivsky, O. and Christoffersen, A., 2008. Intersectionality and the determinants of health: A Canadian perspective. *Critical Public Health*, 18(3), pp. 271–83.

Index

Note: page numbers in *italic* type refer to Figures; those in **bold** refer to Tables.

ableism 23, 70, 240
Aboriginal people, Canada: and health
    inequities 6–7, 9, 238–9; and HIV/
    AIDS 6; and injury rates 97 *see
    also* First Nations people, Canada;
    Indigenous people; Inuit people,
    Canada; Métis people, Canada
Aboriginal rights 41–2 *see also* Treaty
    rights, of Indigenous people
Aboriginal Two-Spirit and LGBTQ
    Migration, Mobility, and Health
    Research Project 61, 63–4, 70
abuse, in residential schools 35
access to health care services 3, 8–9;
    HRSPs (harm reduction service
    providers) 163, 166–7, 168, 169,
    170, 171, 172, 173–4, 174–5, 176–80,
    240; Indigenous peoples 36; MTFs
    (medical tourism facilitators) 19, 163,
    164–6, 169, 170, 171, 172, 173, 174,
    175–80, 240; T/GNC (transgender and
    gender nonconforming) people 53, 57,
    66–7, 239; women with fibromyalgia
    syndrome (FMS) study 183–4,
    187–97, 239
Act to Amend the Indian Act, An,
    1985 44
acupuncture 184, 192
age: ageing population 3, 44, 97, 202;
    older women as providers and
    recipients of care study 10, 200–2,
    205–16, **211–12**, **213**, 239
ageism 202, 205, 240
Ahmed, S. 144
Albany Treaty, 1701 146
allopathic medicine, and chronic
    illness 184

alternative medicine 33, 192–3; costs of
    184, 189–91, 195 *see also* traditional
    knowledge
American Psychiatric Association 56
Anderson, Jordan River 41
Anderson, K. 143
Anishinaabe people 37
anti-colonial theory 68
anti-smoking campaigns: GSBA+
    approaches to 18
"arenas of recovery" 91
Assembly of First Nations 46
Atwood, Margaret 200
Australia: and the UN Declaration on
    the Rights of Indigenous
    Peoples 43
autonomy of Indigenous people 41–4
Axworthy, Lloyd 122, 123

Baltimore Food and Farm Map 112
Bauer, G. R. 57, 65
benefit trap 88, 91
Benoit, C. 21–2
Berger Inquiry 46
bigender people 54 *see also* T/
    GNC (transgender and gender
    nonconforming) people
bisexual people 54; women caregivers
    and care recipients 209, 215 *see also*
    T/GNC (transgender and gender
    nonconforming) people
black Canadians 145, 146
black feminism 23
black women, multiple
    marginalizations of 203
Boleg, L. 24
Borg, M. 80

British Columbia: federal responsibility for health care services 3 *see also* Vancouver, British Columbia
British Columbia Trauma Registry 102
Brown, Nicola 61
Brown, T. H. 204
Browne, Kath 62
Buddhism 225–6
Buffalo, New York 107
Buist, Steve 152, 154–5
Butchart, A. 100

Cahuas, Madelaine C. 10, 141–62, 240
CAI (Core Area Initiative), Winnipeg 122–3
Cairns, K. 24
Cajete, Gregory 34
Canada: as an innocent nation 142–3; context of 2–4; injury rates 96–7; physical geography 2; social demographics of T/GNC (transgender and gender nonconforming) people 55–6; and social determinants of health 4–5; and the UN Declaration on the Rights of Indigenous Peoples 43; urbanization 2
Canada Health Act, 1984 3
Canada Pension Plan disability benefits 190
Canadian Community Health Survey 10, 24–5; older women study 200, 211–12, 211–14, **213**, 215
Canadian Constitution Act, 1982 42
Canadian Institutes of Health Research (CIHR) 17, 33, 44, 45, 46
Canadian Multiculturalism Act, 1988 1
Cape Town, South Africa: pedestrian injury research 98, 108–9, *109*, **110**, 111, *111*
cardiovascular disease: GSBA+ approaches to 18–19
care-giving: older women as providers and recipients of care study 200–2, 205–16, **211–12**, **213**, 239; Vietnamese Canadians family caregiving study 10, 220–1, 222–33, 239
care-receiving: older women as providers and recipients of care study 200–2, 205–16, **211–12**, **213**, 239
Caspi, O. 186
Castleden, Heather 9, 29–52, 238–9
CCB (Compassionate Care Benefit) 204, 221–2, 229–31, 232

Centennial neighborhood, Winnipeg 130, 131–2, 133, 135
Central Park, Winnipeg 133
Chamberlain, Mark *153*
Cherokee people 112
children, denial of spaces for 13, 20, 134
chiropractic treatment 184, 189, 190, 192
Chouinard, V. 196, 197
Chow, H. P. 208
Christianity 225–6
chronic illness: health care system challenges 184–5; women with fibromyalgia syndrome (FMS) study 183–4, 187–97, 239
CIHR (Canadian Institutes of Health Research) 17, 33, 44, 45, 46
Cinnamon, Jonathan 10, 96–118, 240
Circle of Life Thunderbird House 134
cisgender 55
cisnormativity 55, 69, 240
class: classism 23, 70, 240; and intersectionality 204 *see also* socioeconomic status
climate change, impact on Indigenous people 34
Clow, B. 18
"Code Red" health inequities study, Hamilton, Ontario 22, 141–2, 141–52, *153*, 154–9, 240
Collins, K. M. 99, 101, 106
colonialism 58, 70, 123, 240; and Indigenous people 29, 30–2, 34–6, 39–40
colonization, reversal of 6
Columbus, Ohio, pedestrian injury research 98, 112–13, *113*
Commission on Social Determinants of Health 5
common spaces, denial of 131–2
Compassionate Care Benefit (CCB) 204, 221–2, 229–31, 232
comprehensive land claims 42 *see also* Treaty rights, of Indigenous people
"contested chronic illnesses" 183
Cope, M. 107
Core Area Initiative (CAI), Winnipeg 122–3
Core Area, Winnipeg 122–3, 124, 128
counternarratives/counter story-telling 144, 155–7, 159
Craddock, S. 143
Crawley, L. 210–11
Cree people 37

Crenshaw, Kimberlé 203
Crescentwood, Winnipeg 132
critical GIS 106
critical trans politics 68–9
Crooks, Valorie A. 1–13, 14–28, 183–99, 238–42, 239
cross-dressers 54 *see also* T/ GNC (transgender and gender nonconforming) people
cultural safety 46–7
cultural spaces, denial of 134–5

D/deaf people 24
Daley, Andrea 56
Daniel McIntyre neighborhood, Winnipeg 132
De Silva, Karen 151–2
Declaration of Alma-Ata (WHO) 5, 20
decolonial theory 58
degenerate space, cities as 142
Dene people 37
Denyes, M. J. 168
depression, and T/GNC (transgender and gender nonconforming) people 53, 65
deprivation mapping 10, 119–20, 136–8, 240; limitations of 123–5; Winnipeg 119, 120–3, 124, 126–36, *128*, **129**, 139, 240
Diagnostic and Statistical Manual of Mental Disorders (DSM), American Psychiatric Association 56
Ding, G. X. 107
disabilities, people with, human rights of 196
disability benefits 190; benefit trap 88, 91; and mental health 78, 79, **79**, 80, 85–7, 88
disability, language of 82
diversity: as a concept 1–2; and health 4–9; and intersectionality and health 203–5; and place 7–9
diversity-based analyses 14–15
diversity-based research 14–16; future directions 25, 241–2; gender and sex-based research (GSBA) 16–19, 21, 23, 25; health impact assessments (HIA) and health equity impact assessments (HEIA) 21–2, 23, 25; intersectionality 22–5; social determinants of health (SDOH) approach 19–22, 23, 25
Doan, Petra 62–3

domestic violence 59, 61 *see also* intimate partner violence; violence
dominance 141–2, 144
Downtown Eastside, Vancouver, British Columbia 102–4, *103*, 105, 114
drug users, HRSPs (harm reduction service providers) 163, 166–7, 168, 169, 170, 171, 172, 173–4, 174–5, 176–80, 240
DSM (Diagnostic and Statistical Manual of Mental Disorders), American Psychiatric Association 56
Dunn, J. R. 7, 22
Dyck, I. 197

education, level of, older women as providers and recipients of care study 205–6, 211, **211**, 213
Eisenberger, Fred *153*
Elwood, S. 107
employment: and mental health 9–10, 79–81; older women as providers and recipients of care study 205, 206, 209
"ensoulment" 34
environmental pollution, impact on Indigenous people 34
environmental protests 46, 146
Environmental Systems Research Institute (ESRI) 112
erasure, of T/GNC (transgender and gender nonconforming) people 57–8, 69
ethical research 44–5, 144
ethnicity: and injury rates 97; T/ GNC (transgender and gender nonconforming) people 55, 56
European Union, violence against T/ GNC people 59
Evans, Joshua 9–10, 76–95, 240
experts, as saviors 142, 143, 152, *153*, 154–5, 157–8

Faludi, E. G. 146
family doctors: change of 194–5, 196; and chronic illness 185, 191–2, 193, 195; continuity of care 185, 195
federal government: responsibility for health care system 3; responsibility to Indigenous people 42, 43
Fellows, M. L. 142
feminism: anti-violence movement 61–2; feminist analysis of care 201–2
feminist geography 23, 144

feminist GIS 106
fibromyalgia syndrome (FMS) study 10,
    183–4, 187–97, 239
First Nations people, Canada 2,
    37–8; child poverty 40; culturally
    appropriate food 135; denial of
    cultural space in Winnipeg 134;
    federal responsibility for health care
    services to 3; and gender diversity
    39–40; Hamilton, Ontario 146; Treaty
    rights 42
food: ethnic-cultural diets 135; growing
    spaces in urban areas 132

gay people 54 *see also* T/GNC
    (transgender and gender
    nonconforming) people
Geiger, S. 144
gender: as a concept 17, 18, 54,
    202–3; and injury rates 96; and
    intersectionality 204; and Vietnamese
    family care-giving 223, 224–5, 229–30,
    233, 239; and women 202–3
gender and sex-based research (GSBA)
    16–19; GSBA + 18–19, 21, 23, 25
gender diversity 9; and Indigenous
    people 39–40 *see also* T/
    GNC (transgender and gender
    nonconforming) people
Gender Dysphoria 56
gender fluid people 54 *see also* T/
    GNC (transgender and gender
    nonconforming) people
Gender Identity Disorder 56
gender nonconforming people *see* T/
    GNC (transgender and gender
    nonconforming) people
gender variant people 54 *see also* T/
    GNC (transgender and gender
    nonconforming) people
genderqueer people 54 *see also* T/
    GNC (transgender and gender
    nonconforming) people
geographic information systems (GIS)
    see GIS (geographic information
    systems)
GeoWeb mapping 108
Gesler, W. M. 183
Giesbrecht, Melissa D. 1–13, 14–28,
    204–5, 223, 238–42
GIS (geographic information systems)
    99, 100, 102, 106 *see also* qualitative
    GIS (geographic information systems)
Global Burden of Disease 96, 97

Goldberg, Joshua 61–2
Google Earth/Google Maps 108
Greaves, L. 20–1
grocers, as supporters of ethnic-cultural
    diets 135
GSBA: see gender and sex-based
    research (GSBA)

*Hamilton Health Sciences Corp. v.
    D. H.* 46
Hamilton Spectator 141, 145, 147,
    148, 156
Hamilton, Ontario: "Code Red" health
    inequities study 22, 141–2, 141–5,
    147–52, *153*, 154–9, 240; context
    145–7; women with fibromyalgia
    syndrome (FMS) study 187, 190, 191
Hankivsky, O. 204
harm reduction service providers *see*
    HRSPs (harm reduction service
    providers)
Harper, Stephen 35
hate-based violence 58, 59–60 *see also*
    violence
Haudenosaunee people 145, 146
health: and diversity 4–9, 203–5;
    individuals' responsibility for 143–4;
    and intersectionality 203–5; and
    place 7–9 *see also* social determinants
    of health
Health Canada 220
health care services: access to (*see*
    access to health care services);
    responsibilities for 3–4; structural and
    organizational challenges in 184–5;
    women with fibromyalgia syndrome
    (FMS) study 183–4, 187–97, 239
health equity impact assessments
    (HEIA) 21–2, 23, 25
health geography 7, 183; diversity-based
    research 14–25; future directions
    241–2; and mixed-methods
    research 99
health impact assessments (HIA)
    21–2, 25
health inequities: "Code Red" study,
    Hamilton, Ontario 22, 141–2, 141–52,
    153, 154–9, 240; geographic disparities
    (Chapter 8 - review) 10; Indigenous
    people 30–2, 44–7, 238–9; relational
    nature of 125; and socioeconomic
    status 6 *see also* deprivation mapping
health information, online sources of 186
health storymaps 112

HEIA (health equity impact assessments) 21–2, 23, 25
Herman, Jody 63
Herron, Rachel V. 10, 200–19, 239
heterosexism 23
HIA (health impact assessments) 21–2, 25
Híjar, M. 100–1
Hinze, S. W. 204
HIV/AIDS: and health inequities in Canada 6; and Indigenous people 38; and older women 210
Holmes-Rover, M. 186–7
Holmes, Cindy 9, 53–75, 239
homoeopathy 184, 192
hospital closures, Saskatchewan 196–7
HRSPs (harm reduction service providers) 10, 163, 166–7, 168, 169, 170, 171, 172, 173–4, 174–5, 179–80, 240; agency-as-choice 177–8; and expertise 176–7; and risk management 178–9
Human Development Index 40
human rights, of people with disabilities 196
Hunt, Sarah 58

IAPH (Institute of Aboriginal Peoples' Health) 45
"Idle No More" movement 46
immigration 3; countries of origin 207; healthy immigrant effect 19, 208; older women as providers and recipients of care study 205, 207–8, 211, **212**, 213
income: of older women as providers and recipients of care study 205, 206–7, 209, 211, **212**, 213 *see also* socioeconomic status
Indian Act, 1876 31, 43
Indigenous feminism 23
Indigenous healing practices 30, 31
Indigenous knowledge 33, 44
Indigenous people 2, 29–30; autonomy and self-determination 41–4; denial of cultural space in Winnipeg 134–5; diversity amongst 37–41; embeddedness in place 32–4; federal responsibility for health care services to 3; as a growing population 44; health issues 30–2, 44–7, 238–9; land dispossession 29, 34–5; marginalization of 6, 34–7; multigenerational trauma of 35–6; origin stories 30, 32; political action

by 45–6; racism towards 36–7, 46; relationship to land 32–7; and unethical research 44–5 *see also* Aboriginal people, Canada; First Nations people, Canada; Inuit people, Canada; Métis people, Canada
Indigenous women, violence against 46
infectious diseases, and colonial settlers 30–1
informal care-giving, Vietnamese Canadians family caregiving study 10, 220–1, 222–33, 239
injury 96–7
inner cities 120; as degenerate spaces 149–50, 157; as racialized spaces 143, 150 *see also* deprivation mapping
Institut National de Santé Publique du Québec (INSPQ) 120–1, *121*
Institute of Aboriginal Peoples' Health (IAPH) 45
Insurance Corporation of British Columbia 102
intersectionality 10; and diversity-based research 22–5; and hate-based violence 60; and health and diversity 203–5; older women as providers and recipients of care study 200–2, 205–16, **211–12**, **213**, 239; and T/GNC (transgender and gender nonconforming) people 54, 60–1, 68–9, 69–70, 239; Vietnamese Canadians family caregiving study 10, 220–1, 222–33, 239 *see also* "Code Red" health inequities study, Hamilton, Ontario
intimate partner violence 58–9, 60–1 *see also* domestic violence; violence
Inuit people, Canada 2, 37–8; and gender diversity 39–40; Treaty rights 42 *see also* Aboriginal people, Canada; Indigenous people, Canada

James, A. 196–7
Johannesburgh, South Africa 100
Johnston, Rory 10, 163–82, 239–40
Jordan's Principle 41
Joseph, A. 206
Joseph, G. 206
Jung, J.-K. 107

Kearns, R. A. 7, 25, 183
Kirk, D. L. 112
Knigge, L. 107

knowledge production, erasure of T/
GNC (transgender and gender
nonconforming) people from 57–8
Kobayashi, K. M. 208
Kristiansen, K. 80
Kwakwaka'wakw people 58
Kwan, M. P. 107

labor force participation, older women
as providers and recipients of care
study 205, 206, 209
Lalonde, M. 4
land: dispossession of Indigenous people
29, 34–5, 42; Indigenous people's
relationship to 32–7
language proficiency, and Vietnamese
family care-giving 223, 228–9, 231,
232, 239
Larner, W. 168
LaScala, E. A. 100
lesbian women 54; caregivers and
care recipients 209, 215 *see also* T/
GNC (transgender and gender
nonconforming) people
Lewis, Diana 9, 29–52, 238–9
LGBTQ2S people 54 *see also* T/
GNC (transgender and gender
nonconforming) people
liberalism, in Canadian healthcare
system 168, 180
living arrangements, older women as
providers and recipients of care study
205, 210–11, **211**, 212
Los Angeles, California 101
Loukaitou-Sideris, A. 101
Lum, Irene D. 10, 220–37, 239
Lynch, K. 210–11

MacDonald, John 31
MacFarlane, Devon 68
Mackenzie Valley Pipeline 46
Mair, C. A. 204
Malik, Mannat 10, 141–62, 240
Manhattan, New York 111
marital status, older women as providers
and recipients of care study 205,
209–10, 211, **211**, 212
Martin, Debbie 9, 29–52, 238–9
massage therapy 190, 192
Masuda, Jeffrey R. 10, 119–40, 240
McIntyre, J. 65
McMaster University 147
medical geography 7, 99

medical tourism *see* MTFs (medical
tourism facilitators)
Medicine Wheel 33
men: as care-givers 224–5, 233; older
men 214
mental health: and employment
9–10, 79–81; and injury rates
96; and poverty 78–9, **79**; and T/
GNC (transgender and gender
nonconforming) people 9, 53, 64–8,
70; terminology 83 *see also* mental
health recovery
mental health recovery 76; and
supportive workplaces 9–10,
77–8, 81–90
Métis people, Canada 2, 37–8; denial
of cultural space in Winnipeg 134;
and gender diversity 39–40 *see
also* Aboriginal people, Canada;
Indigenous people, Canada
Mexico 100
Mi'kmaq people 37, 40
military personnel, federal responsibility
for health care services to 3
"minority stress" 65, 70
mixed-methods research 16, 113–15, 240;
pedestrian injury research 98–101 *see
also* deprivation mapping
mobility, denial of 135–6
Monette, L. E. 6
Mooney, James 112
Morgan, Jeffrey 1–13, 14–28
MTFs (medical tourism facilitators)
10, 19, 163, 164–6, 169, 170, 171,
172, 173, 174, 175, 179–80, 240;
agency-as-choice 177–8; and expertise
176, 177; risk management 178–9
Mulé, Nick 56
multigeneraltional trauma of Indigenous
people 35–6

Nagar, R. 144
Namaste, Viviane K. 57, 58, 62, 69
Nash, Catherine 62–3
National Aboriginal Health
Organization 45
National Collaborating Center for
Aboriginal Health 6, 21
National Indian Brotherhood 46
National Sciences and Engineering
Research Council of Canada 44
National Transgender Discrimination
Survey 60, 66

Native Friendship Centers 39
naturopathy 189, 190, 192
Neighbourhood Action Strategy, Hamilton, Ontario 148, 157
Nelson, J. 143
Neo Eamas, Tien 68
Network Environments for Aboriginal Health Research (NEAHRs) 45
New York Times 111
New Zealand: gender, and health care reform 19; and the UN Declaration on the Rights of Indigenous Peoples 43
Newbold, K. B. 208
North Bay, Ontario 187, 190, 191, 193
North End, Winnipeg 128, 132, 133, 136
nutritionists 192
Nuu-chah-nulth people 34, 37

OCAP™ (Ownership, Control, Access, and Possession of Data involving Indigenous People in Canada) 45
Odoi, A. 128
ODSP (Ontario Disability Support Program) 85–7, 88
Ohio State University, pedestrian injury research 112–13, *113*
Oka Crisis, 1990 46
Ontario: human rights, of people with disabilities 196; mental health recovery, and supportive workplaces 9–10, 77–8, 81–90; T/GNC (transgender and gender nonconforming) people 55; Vietnamese Canadians family caregiving study 10, 220–1, 222–33, 239; women with fibromyalgia syndrome (FMS) study 183–4, 187–97, 239
Ontario Disability Support Program (ODSP) 85–7, 88
Orem, D. E. 168
origin stories of indigenous people 30, 32
Ownership, Control, Access, and Possession of Data involving Indigenous People in Canada (OCAP™) 45

P/EOL (palliative and end of life) care, Vietnamese Canadians family caregiving study 10, 220–1, 222–33, 239
Pampalon, R. 126

participatory GIS 106
patients, agency of 186–7
Paul, Ken 33
pedestrian injury research 10, 97–8, 113–15; Cape Town, South Africa 98, 108–9, *109*, **110**, 111, *111*; Columbus, Ohio 112–13, *113*; mixed-methods approach 98–101; storymapping 111–13; Vancouver, British Columbia 98, 101–6, *103*
penitentiary inmates, federal responsibility for health care services to 3
personal recovery *see* mental health recovery
photography, Winnipeg neighbourhood deprivation assessment research 126–36, *128*, **129**
physiotherapy 192
place: and diversity 7–9; and health 7–9; and health geography 25; and T/GNC (transgender and gender nonconforming) people 62–4, 70
Point Douglas, Winnipeg 130, 131–2, 133, 134, 136
postcolonial theory 23
poverty: and the "Code Red" narratives 156–7; impact on health 40–1
prayer 226
private health providers *see* HRSPs (harm reduction service providers); MTFs (medical tourism facilitators)
provincial governments, responsibility for health care system 3–4
Prus, S. G. 208
psychiatric disabilities, people with: and employment 9–10, 79–81; and poverty 78–9, **79**; recovery, and supportive workplaces 9–10, 77–8, 81–90 *see also* mental health; mental health recovery
"psychiatric ghettoes" 76
Public Health Agency of Canada 5, 6, 20
public spaces 125–6; denial of 131–2

qualitative GIS (geographic information systems) 98, 106–8, 114; Cape Town, South Africa research 98, 108–9, *109*, **110**, 111, *111*; storymapping 111–13
qualitative research 15–16; and intersectionality 24, 203, 204–5, 215; and mixed-methods research 98, 99

quantitative research 16; and
intersectionality 24, 203–4, 205; and
mixed-methods research 98, 99–100
queer people 54 *see also* genderqueer
people; T/GNC (transgender and
gender nonconforming) people
queer theory 23

"race": critical "race" theory 144; and
intersectionality 204
racialized space 143
racism 70, 124, 240; and black
Canadians 146; and Indigenous
people 36–7, 46
Rainbow Health Network 56
rape 61 *see also* sexual assault
"rational agency" 186–7
Razack, S. 142–3
reciprocity, in care-giving 224–5
Reczek, C. 209
Red Hill Valley expressway, Hamilton,
Ontario 146
refugee protection claimants, federal
responsibility for health care
services to 3
religion and spirituality, and Vietnamese
family care-giving 223, 225–7,
230, 239
research ethics 144; and Indigenous
people 44–5; and T/GNC (transgender
and gender nonconforming)
people 58, 60
research methods: mixed-methods
research 10, 16, 98–101, 113–15, 240
see also diversity-based research;
qualitative research; quantitative
research
researchers, epistemological
stances of 15
reserves, and Indigenous people 31,
38, 39, 42
residency, length of, and Vietnamese
family care-giving 223, 228–9, 231,
232, 239
residential schools, treatment of
Indigenous people in 31, 35–6, 46–7
Richmond, C. A. 6, 22
risk management 178–9
Ristock, Kanice 61
road traffic injuries 96, 97 *see also*
pedestrian injuries
Rose, G. 144
Rosenberg, Mark W. 10, 200–19, 239

Ross, N. A. 6, 22, 206, 210
Royal Commission on Aboriginal
Peoples 46
rural areas, and Indigenous people
38–9, 42

Saskatchewan, hospital closures 196–7
Scott, Duncan Campbell 31–2
self-care deficit nursing theory 164,
167–8; self-care agency domain 169,
170, 172; self-care domain 169, **170**,
171–2; self-care practices and systems
169, **170**, 174–5; self-care requisites
domain 169, **170**, 173; therapeutic
self-care demand domain 169, **170**,
173–4
self-determination of Indigenous people
6–7, 41–4
Sells, D. 91
Senese, L. 42
Seng, J S. 203
Setia, M. S. 19, 208
Seven Oaks, Winnipeg 132, 133
sex, as a concept 17, 18, 54, 202
sexism 23, 202, 205, 240
sexual abuse, in residential schools 35
sexual assault 59, 60 *see also* rape;
violence
sexual health, of older women 210
SFU Medical Tourism Group 169
Shumka, L. 21–2
Sinclair, Brian 46
Skinner, Emily 10, 119–40, 240
social determinants of health 4–7; social
determinants of health (SDOH)
research approach 19–22, 23, 25
social enterprises 81; mental health
recovery and supportive workplaces
study 82–90
social exclusion, T/GNC (transgender
and gender nonconforming) people 57
social inclusion, and mental health
84–5, 89
Social Sciences and Humanities
Research Council of Canada 44
socioeconomic status: impact on
health 6, 22; and Indigenous people
40–1; older women as providers and
recipients of care study 205, 206–7,
209, 211, **212**, 213; and Vietnamese
family care-giving 223, 227–8,
230–1, 239
solastalgia 34–5

Spade, Dean 68–9
St Boniface, Winnipeg 134
Status of Women Canada 17
stereotypes: and Indigenous people 36,
    38; and T/GNC (transgender and
    gender nonconforming) people 67
stigmatization: and deprivation mapping
    124, 137; of inner cities 143, 148, 158
storymapping 111–13
Stotzer, R. L. 59
stress 36
Sudbury, Ontario 187, 191
Sui, Daniel Z. 10, 96–118, 240
suicide 66, 97; and T/GNC (transgender
    and gender nonconforming) people
    53, 65, 67
Sundberg, J. 144
Survivor Project, The 60–1

T/GNC (transgender and gender
    nonconforming) people 9, 53–4,
    215, 239; context of study 56–8; and
    critical trans politics 68–9; health
    geography research directions 69–71;
    and intersectionality 54, 68–9, 69–70;
    mental health and well-being 53, 64–8,
    70; and place 62–4, 70; resilience of
    71; social demographics of in Canada
    55–6; terminology 54–5; violence
    against 53, 58–62, 63, 68–9, 70
Tashakkori, A. 98
Taylor, Catherine 61
Teddlie, C. 98
Temenos, Cristina 10, 163–82, 239–40
territorial governments, responsibility
    for health care system 3
"Third World" discourses 149, 150
Third World feminism 23
Tjepkema, M. 38
traditional knowledge 33
traditional medicines 46
Trans PULSE Project 55, 57, 63,
    65, 66, 69
trans* people 54 *see also* T/
    GNC (transgender and gender
    nonconforming) people; transgender/
    trans people
Transgender Sexual Violence Project 60
transgender/trans people 9, 54 *see also*
    T/GNC (transgender and gender
    nonconforming) people
transitioning (gender) 55, 63
transphobia 55, 57

Treaty rights, of Indigenous people 42–3
Tri-Council Policy Statement on
    Research Ethics involving Human
    Subjects 44
"triple jeopardy", of older women 200,
    214, 216, 239
Truth and Reconciliation Commission,
    Canada 35
Tuxedo, Winnipeg 132, 133
Two-Spirit people 9, 39–40, 54, 58, 70
    see also T/GNC (transgender and
    gender nonconforming) people

Umberson, P. 209
unethical research: and Indigenous
    people 44–5; and T/GNC (transgender
    and gender nonconforming)
    people 58, 60
United Nations Declaration on the
    Rights of Indigenous Peoples
    29, 43–4
urban areas, and Indigenous people 38–9
urban planning 146
USA: hate-based violence 59, 60, 66;
    relationship between education
    levels and health 205–6; and the
    UN Declaration on the Rights of
    Indigenous Peoples 43

Valentine, G. 24
Vancouver Island Trans* Needs
    Assessment 66–7
Vancouver Island, British Columbia:
    T/GNC (transgender and gender
    nonconforming) people 56
Vancouver, British Columbia:
    Aboriginal Two-Spirit and LGBTQ
    Migration, Mobility, and Health
    Research Project 61, 63–4; pedestrian
    injury research 98, 101–6, *103*, 114
Veenstra, G. 24–5, 204
Vietnamese Canadians family caregiving
    study 10, 220–1, 222–33, 239
violence: against Indigenous women
    46; and mental illness 66; against
    T/GNC (transgender and gender
    nonconforming) people 53, 58–62,
    68–9, 70

Wakefield, Sarah 10, 141–62, 240
Waldbrook, N. 210
"War in the Woods" 46
Warner, D. F. 204

welfare benefits 190; benefit trap 88, 91; CCB (Compassionate Care Benefit) 204, 221–2, 229–31, 232; and mental health 78, 79, **79**, 80, 85–7, 88

West Broadway, Winnipeg 130, 131–2, 133, 134, 135

White, Caroline 61–2

WHO (World Health Organisation) 33; Commission on Social Determinants of Health 5; Declaration of Alma-Ata 5, 20; and HEIA/HIAs 21; mental health definition 64; and social determinants of health 4, 5–6, 19–20

wholistic health, and Indigenous people 33

Wiles, J. 19

Wilkinson, L. 14, 24

Willcox, Cunsolo 34–5

Williams, Allison M. 10, 220–37, 239

Wilson, K. 22, 42

Wilson, M. W. 106

Wilton, Robert 9–10, 76–95, 240

Winnipeg: Aboriginal Two-Spirit and LGBTQ Migration, Mobility, and Health Research Project 61, 63–4; deprivation mapping 119, 120–3, 124, 126–36, *128*, **129**, 139, 240; marginalization of Indigenous people 39

Winnipeg Area Characterization Study 122

women: and gender 202–3; and hate-based violence 60; and injury rates 96–7; as irresponsible victims ("Code Red" narratives) 142, 150–2, 157; life expectancy 202; older women as providers and recipients of care study 10, 200–2, 205–16, **211–12**, **213**, 239; violence against Indigenous women 46; women with fibromyalgia syndrome (FMS) study 10, 183–4, 187–97, 239 *see also* gender and sex-based research (GSBA)

World Health Organisation *see* WHO (World Health Organisation)

Yates, I. 92

Yokoyama, Gary 152

young people: denial of spaces for 132–4; road traffic injuries 96